HAND ECZEMA

EDITED BY

Torkil Menné, M.D.
Professor and Chairman
Department of Dermatology
Gentofte Hospital
University of Copenhagen
Hellerup, Denmark

and

Howard I. Maibach, M.D.
Professor
Department of Dermatology
School of Medicine
University of California
San Francisco, California

CRC Press
Boca Raton   Ann Arbor   London   Tokyo

Library of Congress Cataloging-in-Publication Data

Hand eczema/edited by Torkil Menné, Howard I. Maibach.
   p. cm. — (CRC series in dermatology)
   Includes bibliographical references and index.
   ISBN 0-8493-7355-7 (alk. paper)
   1. Eczema. 2. Hand—Diseases. I. Menné, Torkil. II. Maibach,
Howard I. III. Series.
   [DNLM: 1. Eczema. 2. Hand Dermatoses. 3. Occupational Diseases.
WR 190 H236 1993]
RL251.H35 1993
616.5'21—dc20
DNLM/DLC
for Library of Congress   93-19124
                      CIP

No claim to original U.S. Government works
International Standard Book Number 0-8493-7355-7
Library of Congress Card Number 93-19124
Printed in the United States of America   3 4 5 6 7 8 9 0
Printed on acid-free paper

CRC Series in
DERMATOLOGY: CLINICAL AND BASIC SCIENCE
Edited by Dr. Howard I. Maibach

The CRC Dermatology Series combines scholarship, basic science, and clinical relevance. These comprehensive references focus on dermal absorption, dermabiology, dermatopharmacology, dermatotoxicology, and occupational and clinical dermatology.

The intellectual theme emphasizes in-depth, easy to comprehend surveys that blend advances in basic science and clinical research with practical aspects of clinical medicine.

Published Titles:

**Health Risk Assessment: Dermal and Inhalation Exposure
and Absorption of Toxicants**
Rhoda G. M. Wang, James B. Knaak, and Howard I. Maibach

Pigmentation and Pigmentary Disorders
Norman Levine

Forthcoming Titles:

Bioengineering of the Skin: Water and the Stratum Corneum
Peter Elsner, Enzo Berardesca, and Howard I. Maibach

Bioengineering of the Skin: Cutaneous Blood Flow and Erythema
Enzo Berardesca, Peter Elsner, and Howard I. Maibach

Handbook of Contact Dermatitis
Christopher J. Dannaker, Daniel J. Hogan, and Howard I. Maibach

Human Papillomavirus Infections in Dermatovenereology
Gerd Gross and Geo von Krogh

**Mouse Mutations with Skin and Hair Abnormalities:
Animal Models and Biomedical Tools**
John P. Sundburg

Protective Gloves for Occupational Use
Gunh Mellstrom, J.E. Walhberg, and Howard I. Maibach

Skin Cancer: Mechanisms and Relevance
Hasan Mukhtar

The Contact Urticaria Syndrome
Arto Lahti and Howard I. Maibach

The Irritant Contact Dermatitis Syndrome
Pieter Van der Valk, Pieter Coenrads, and Howard I. Maibach

PREFACE

Hand eczema is one of the most common clinical conditions treated and evaluated both among general dermatologists and in dermatological departments. Depending on country and referral habits, 5 to 10% of all patients seen by dermatologists have hand eczema.

Hand eczema is the most common occupational skin disease and one of the most frequent occupational disorders over all. Hand eczema can be long-standing and incapacitating. Research within the last decade has evaluated the epidemiology and risk factors concerning hand eczema. Much of this knowledge has not yet entered dermatologic textbooks.

This book discusses the common varieties of hand eczema. Further, indications for patch testing in this condition are clarified. As hand eczema is often an occupational disorder, several chapters are devoted to specific occupational exposures.

EDITORS

Torkil Menné, M.D., is Professor and Chairman, Department of Dermatology, Gentofte Hospital, University of Copenhagen, Denmark. Dr. Menné obtained his M.D. from the University of Copenhagen in 1971 and received a Ph.D. in 1983 at the same university for investigations on genetic and epidemiologic aspects of nickel dermatitis.

Dr. Menné is Chairman of the European Environmental Contact Dermatitis Research Group and a member of the Danish Contact Dermatitis Research Group. He is author of 180 articles and co-author and editor of 5 books.

Howard I. Maibach, M.D., is Professor of Dermatology, School of Medicine, University of California, San Francisco. Dr. Maibach graduated from Tulane University, New Orleans, Louisiana (A.B. and M.D.) and received his research and clinical training at the University of Pennsylvania, Philadelphia. He received an honorary doctorate from the University of Paris Sud in 1988.

Dr. Maibach is a member of the International Contact Dermatitis Research Group, the North American Contact Dermatitis Group, and the European Environmental Contact Dermatitis Group. He has published more than 1100 papers and 40 volumes.

CONTRIBUTORS

Tove Agner, M.D., Ph.D.
Department of Dermatology
Gentofte Hospital
University of Copenhagen
Hellerup, Denmark

C.F. Allenby, M.D.
Lister Hospital
Herts, United Kingdom

Klaus E. Andersen, M.D., Ph.D.
Department of Dermatology
Odense University Hospital
Odense, Denmark

David A. Basketter, B.Sc.
Environmental Safety Lab
Unilever Research
Sharnbrook, United Kingdom

Derk P. Bruynzeel, M.D.
Department of Dermatology
Free University Academic Hospital
Amsterdam, The Netherlands

Magnus Bruze, M.D., Ph.D.
Department of Occupational Dermatology
Lund University
Malmö General Hospital
Malmö, Sweden

Ole B. Christensen, M.D., Ph.D.
Department of Dermatology
Lund University
Malmö General Hospital
Malmö, Sweden

Edith M. De Boer, M.D.
Department of Dermatology
Free University Academic Hospital
Amsterdam, The Netherlands

Thomas L. Diepgen, M.D.
Department of Dermatology
Friedrich-Alexander-University Erlangen-
  Nuremberg
Erlangen, Germany

Björn Edman, M.Sc., D.M.Sc.
Department of Dermatology
Lund University
Malmö General Hospital
Malmö, Sweden

Tuula Estlander, M.D., Ph.D.
Section of Dermatology
Institute of Occupational Health
Helsinki, Finland

Manigé Fartasch, M.D.
Department of Dermatology
Friedrich-Alexander-University Erlangen-
  Nuremberg
Erlangen, Germany

Sigfrid Fregert, M.D., Ph.D.
Department of Occupational Dermatology
Lund University
Malmö General Hospital
Malmö, Sweden

Peter J. Frosch, M.D.
Department of Dermatology
Städt Kliniken
University of Witten/Herdecke
Dortmund, Germany

**Chee-Leok Goh, M.B.B.S., M.Med.,
  M.R.C.P.**
National Skin Centre
Singapore

Lars Halkier-Sørensen, M.D.
Department of Dermatology
Marselisborg Hospital
Aarhus, Denmark

Daniel J. Hogan, M.D.
Dermatology and Cutaneous Surgery
School of Medicine
University of South Florida
Tampa, Florida

Riitta Jolanki, D.Tech.
Section of Dermatology
Institute of Occupational Health
Helsinki, Finland

Lasse Kanerva, M.D., Ph.D.
Section of Dermatology
Institute of Occupational Health
Helsinki, Finland

Kaija Lammintausta, M.D., Ph.D.
Department of Dermatology
Turku University Central Hospital
Turku, Finland

Antti I. Lauerma, M.D., Ph.D.
Department of Dermatology
School of Medicine
University of California, San Francisco
San Francisco, California

Bernt Lindelöf, M.D., Ph.D.
Department of Dermatology
Danderyd Hospital
Stockholm, Sweden

Howard I. Maibach, M.D.
Department of Dermatology
School of Medicine
University of California
San Francisco, California

Birgitta Meding, M.D., Ph.D.
Department of Occupational Dermatology
National Institute of Occupational Health
Solna, Sweden

Torkil Menné, M.D., Ph.D.
Department of Dermatology
Gentofte Hospital
University of Copenhagen
Hellerup, Denmark

Halvor Möller, M.D., Ph.D.
Department of Dermatology
Lund University
Malmö General Hospital
Malmö, Sweden

Eskil Nilsson, M.D.
Department of Dermatology
Sundsvall Hospital
Sundsvall, Sweden

Beate Pilz, M.D.
Department of Dermatology
Städt Kliniken
University of Witten/Herdecke
Dortmund, Germany

Jytte Roed-Petersen, M.D.
Department of Dermatology
Gentofte Hospital
Hellerup, Denmark

Ingela Rystedt, M.D., Ph.D.
Department of Dermatology
Karolinska Hospital
Stockholm, Sweden

Hans J. Schwanitz, M.D., Ph.D.
Department of Dermatology and Theory of
 Health
University of Osnabrück
Osnabrück, Germany

Kyllikki Tarvainen, M.D.
Section of Dermatology
Institute of Occupational Health
Helsinki, Finland

Kristian Thestrup-Pedersen, M.D.
Department of Dermatology
University of Aarhus
Marselisborg Hospital
Aarhus, Denmark

Kristiina Turjanmaa, M.D., Ph.D.
Department of Dermatology
Tampere University Hospital
Tampere, Finland

Henk B. van der Walle, M.D., Ph.D.
Center of Occupational Dermatology
Ziekenhuis Rijnstate GZ
Arnhem, The Netherlands

Niels K. Veien, M.D.
The Dermatology Clinic
Aalborg, Denmark

D. S. Wilkinson, M.D., F.R.C.P.
Whitecroft
Amersham, Bucks,
United Kingdom

ACKNOWLEDGMENT

The editors are grateful for the sponsoring of the color slides in this book by Brocades Pharma A/S, Yamanouchi Group.

In honor of
Etain Cronin
a special friend of dermatology, her patients,
and her many admiring colleagues

CONTENTS

HAND
ECZEMA

1

Introduction, Definition, and Classification

D. S. Wilkinson

CONTENTS

I. INTRODUCTION

The eczematous group of skin disorders embraces a number of entities in which endogenous, exogenous, environmental, and cultural factors are often interwoven. This is particularly true of eczema affecting the hands, a condition that is frequently multifactorial, usually disabling or distressing to the sufferer, and often difficult to treat. This difficulty is partly due to the intrinsic nature of eczema itself and the special anatomical features of the palmar skin but also because of the role of the hands in everyday social life and work and the inability of the patient to comply fully with avoidance techniques.

This chapter is designed to present a general overview of the subject. All the aspects touched on here are dealt with more fully in subsequent chapters. The views expressed are personal and in no way invalidate the more detailed analyses and conclusions reached by those working in particular fields of the subject. Indeed, some may be considered to be idiosyncratic.

A. Historical Background

It may be considered curious to single out eczema of the hands as being worthy of special study. The dermatologists of the 19th century, although well aware of variations due to site, were more concerned with morphological forms of the disease (eczema solare, rubrum, or impetiginodes and, later, squamosum, papulosum, and marginatum). In his long treatise on eczema, Hebra[1] devoted less than a page to eczema of the hands and feet, and this in morphological terms. Fox[2] stated that eczema in these sites is "chiefly remarkable for the peculiar tenacity and persistence of the vesicles" and mentioned grocers' and bakers' itch but little else. Radcliffe-Crocker[3] emphasizes the role of external irritants. It is noteworthy, however, that all these outstanding clinicians devoted far more space to a detailed discussion of treatment than is usually the case today.

The recognition of the hands as a region of particular interest has come about gradually during this century and increasingly so in the last 50 years. There are several reasons for this. The most important was the rapid growth of industrialization of Western Europe and the U.S., accelerated by two world wars, and especially the enormous development in the dye and chemical industries. This led to an increasing realization of the importance of both irritant and allergic dermatitis and to legislation to prevent this or to indemnify workers suffering from it. Industrial dermatology finally came into its own,[4] 215 years after Ramazzini's seminal treatise.[5]

In the increasingly complex environment of the 20th century the housewife, too, encountered new causes of hand dermatitis. The "soda rash" of the past gave rise to more subtle and sophisticated forms of irritant and allergic dermatitis in the house[6] and the garden.[7]

Finally, with increasing affluence and media role-making, personal adornment flourished and the social, professional, and psychological effect of disfigurement on a visible area, such as the hands, undoubtedly prompted the increased use of potentially sensitizing hand creams and a greater desire for medical attention.

B. Allergic Contact Dermatitis and the Patch Test

The ability of certain specific substances to cause dermatitis by external contact had, of course, long been recognized. The early writers spoke of sulfur, mercury, croton oil, and other such agents. As early as 1609 Captain John Smith had recognized the effect of poison ivy, and Lady Mary Wortley Montague, in 1718, wrote a dramatic description of the disastrous result of applying "balm of Mecca" to her own face.[8] Although irritant dermatitis from physical and chemical agents was well known, anomalous reactions were regarded as examples of constitutional idiosyncrasy. It was not until the experimental work of Bloch and Steiner-Woerlich in 1926[9] and 1930[10] that the concept of allergic sensitization was established; Jadassohn[11] had devised the epicutaneous patch test 30 years earlier. The importance of this diagnostic tool was quickly recognized and established on a firm basis by Sulzberger and Wise.[12] In the subsequent 60 years the technique of patch testing has continually been extended and improved; innumerable publications have attested to its value. As an investigative procedure that is applied to human beings, it has its limitations and requires careful interpretation, but it remains at present the best means of determining the presence of cutaneous delayed-type allergy, if not always its relevance.

The introduction of the concept of "atopy" by Cocä and Cooke[13] at about the same time provided a further stimulus to the investigation of hand eczema and gave a new dimension to the concept of the "constitutional diathesis" of the older authors.

II. DEFINITION

A. Definition of Eczema

This has had a checkered career in dermatology. The older writers referred to eczema as a non-contagious "catarrhal inflammation" of the skin and recognized the importance of the vesicle and the accompanying pruritus or burning sensations (although Hebra[1] considered that vesicles were not essential for the diagnosis). However, not everyone would accept all cases of dermatitis under this title, and Norman Walker,[14] an influential writer and teacher, would not have it at all — a "chaotic conglomeration" and a "name which is a cloak for ignorance." This dichotomy has bedevilled the literature ever since.

We owe to the histopathologists a more precise approach to a definition. Spongiosis and a dermal lymphohistiocytic infiltrate are always present at some stage and the spongiotic vesicle is the hallmark of the disease, although spongiosis is seen in other conditions. Yet these histopathological features are the result of a dynamic sequence of events, influenced by intensity, site and time, and modified by trauma, infection or treatment.

A current and acceptable definition of eczema is that it is "a pattern of inflammatory response of the skin which can be defined histologically by the presence of a predominantly lymphohistiocytic infiltrate around the upper dermal blood vessels, associated with spongiosis and varying degrees of acanthosis. The clinical features of eczema may include itching, redness, scaling and clustered papulovesicles. The condition may be induced by a wide range of external and internal factors acting singly or in combination."[15]

Calnan[16] regarded eczema as having an analogy with conditions such as iritis and colitis, in which a diverse etiology and a variable and unpredictable course are also features. He also stressed the infinite variety of the quality and quantity of the limited number of signs that make up the disease. It is the "lack of orderly or homogenous arrangement of [these] in the area which is most characteristic of eczema."[16] He further commented that "writing an account of eczema does not necessarily denote a fixed position."[16] Nowhere is this more true than in discussing some of the aspects of eczema affecting the hands.

B. Definition of Eczema and Dermatitis

The word "eczema has an obscure origin. It was first used by Aëtius Amidenus, physician to the Byzantine Court in the sixth century, in referring to a phlyctenular condition the Greeks commonly (vulgo) called "eczemata", but it is uncertain whether he was describing eczema, boils, or something else. "Dermatitis" means nothing more than inflammation of the skin (derma).

There is no universal agreement on the use of these two terms and they are the cause for some confusion. Most dermatologists now regard them as synonymous for all practical purposes, although some will continue to use one or other term preferentially. Dermatitis has a broader application in that it embraces all forms of inflammation of the skin, including eczema, but not all forms of dermatitis are eczematous.[15]

In common usage, at least in Great Britain and parts of Europe, "eczema" is too entrenched a term to be abandoned,[16] although many efforts have been made to dislodge it. Both terms are in general use in the context of hand eczema. We speak of "soluble oil dermatitis" and (usually) of "housewives' dermatitis" rather than eczema, but of palmar or discoid forms of the condition. Another nuance is apparent in many published reports; those authors who are dealing with exogenous or occupational causes of the disease tend to prefer the term "dermatitis" and those concerned with endogenous or constitutional causes prefer eczema.[17] There are, of course, good historical reasons for this.

A final twist is given by the legal and psychological implications, in Great Britain at least, of the use of the term "dermatitis" in dealing with patients with occupational disease. In an effort to avoid prejudging the issue, many dermatologists will avoid using this word when manual workers present with an eczema of the hands, at least until the connection with their work is firmly established.

In this book both terms are used, and in this chapter the terms are to be regarded as synonymous unless otherwise stated. After nearly 1450 years, the word "eczema" remains, then, one that is in common use, as it was in Byzantium when "Graeci vulgo appellant".

C. Definition of Eczema of the Hands

For the purpose of this chapter, and indeed of the book as a whole, the term "hand eczema" is taken to refer to eczema wholly or largely confined to the hands, although it is accepted that pompholyx and hyperkeratotic eczema may affect the feet concurrently and subsequently. It does not exclude the presence of a mycotic infection of the feet or of noneczematous lesions elsewhere, but the patients studied have presented with a complaint of hand eczema and not of lesions elsewhere.

It is not always possible to be absolutely precise on what constitutes the borders and boundaries of the hands, which, properly defined, is the "terminal part of the arm beyond the wrist, consisting of the palm and five digits" (O.E.D). Some involvement of the wrists or distal forearms may occur as an extension of hand eczema, for instance, as part of a contact dermatitis due to rubber gloves, and some latitude must be allowed. In practice, this does not usually cause any great difficulty to most observers and is really a matter of common sense.

Of more importance are the boundaries in time. The dermatologist impinges on the patient's life at one, or perhaps a few consecutive, periods in the course of his illness. He classifies the disease as he sees it at that time, but in the course of a few weeks or months it may have taken on a different appearance or distribution or changed its characteristics, just as etiological factors may change or may not have been recognized at the earlier stage. This is especially true of eczema. A long history of dry skin of the legs gives place to xerotic eczema; dry or chapped skin on the hands grades imperceptibly into irritant dermatitis. The line dividing noneczema from eczema may be hard to define. Some dermatologists would insist on the presence of vesicles, but these may not always be present at any one time.

Finally, eczema has a natural tendency to spread. With continuing exposure to irritants the forearm may become involved, with allergens the face or other sites of contact and in constitutional forms the feet or other areas. It is important to distinguish between primary and secondary diagnoses in such cases. If such a spread has already occurred when the patient is first seen, he is not likely to be included in the material studied, but if it occurs during the course of such a study, he is unlikely to be excluded. To this extent the concept of hand eczema may appear flawed. Nevertheless, it remains a valid and practical method of grouping together similar cases and of studying the various factors involved.

III. PREVALENCE AND SIGNIFICANCE

Hand eczema is a common condition and one that has a particular social and occupational significance for many of the patients affected.[18]

A. Prevalence

It is difficult to obtain even an approximate estimate of the prevalence of hand eczema because there have been few relevant population studies, even with regard to eczema itself. A lack of conformity in classification makes tenuous any comparison between those that do exist. Agrup,[19] who examined 1659 of 2499 persons with hand lesions in a survey of 107,206 of the population in southern Sweden, estimated the prevalence at 1.2 to 2.4%, with a female-to-male ratio of 2:1. The large HANES study in the U.S.[20] gave lower totals, but a different classification was used. Menné et al.[21] calculated a prevalence in women of 2.3 to 6.2%, with a cumulative prevalence of 22%. Other authors have given higher figures over various prevalence periods. Meding and Swanbeck,[22] for instance, found that 10.6% of 20,000 persons in an industrial city in southern Sweden considered themselves to have had hand eczema during the preceding 12 months, with a point prevalence of 5.4%. Studies from heavily industrialized areas do not necessarily reflect the prevalence in the population at large, but the 2:1 female predominance found here is a similar ratio to that found by Agrup[19] in a mixed rural and urban population.

Data for hospital attendance are more easily available, but methods of classification differ and the material is selected by severity, persistence, the interests of the dermatologist, and other factors.[23] Many patients with minor degrees of hand eczema will not have seen any doctor[19,24] let alone have been referred to a hospital center.

All forms of eczema and contact dermatitis accounted for 10 to 24% of 137,565 patients seen in eight hospital centers in Great Britain between 1978 and 1981.[23] It is likely that at least 20 to 25% of these had eczema confined to the hands. A personal analysis of material over a 30-year period from one of these areas[25] (and one with little heavy industry) is in this range. Thus, it accounts for 3 to 5% of all cases seen, a percentage not far different from that for psoriasis or acne, conditions that have received far more attention. In larger industrial centers or occupational dermatitis units the percentage is higher. The hands alone were affected in 36% of 424 patients seen in a small industrial clinic,[26] and even higher figures were found in a larger occupational unit in Lund.[27] In an analysis of 4825 patients patch tested in 8 European centers the International Contact Dermatitis Research Group found that the hands along were involved in 36% of males and 30% of females.[28]

These are merely indicators of the size of the problem. The epidemiology is discussed in more detail in Chapter 17.

B. Significance

Although minor degrees of hand dermatitis are often accepted as a normal hazard of life, a major breakdown in the integrity of the skin of the hands may cause, at least, social embarrassment and, at most, a devastating change in the working capacity of a patient and thus his livelihood itself. The significance and consequences of hand eczema can be considered under the following headings: occupational, domestic, social, and psychological.

1. Occupational

The worker affected with a severe or persistent hand eczema, whether it is occupational in origin or endogenous, risks having to change or even lose his job in a competitive market. It is not overstating the case to say that this affliction may be of more consequence and importance to him than the loss of a leg. For this he would get adequate compensation, considerable rehabilitation, and a great deal of sympathy. In due course he would, in most cases, be able to return to his work, but with hand eczema his condition is different. The condition itself and the factors involved are often complex and may be poorly assessed. The doctors who look after him may be poorly trained in occupational dermatology. Rehabilitation procedures are often lacking or inadequate. Advice for him to change his job is easier for the doctor to pronounce than for the worker to carry out, and there is no certainty that he will be better off in new employment.[29] He may come to regard himself as being unemployable and in any case is likely to suffer loss of income and self-esteem in being unable to continue in the trade in which he was trained.[30] The importance of an expert assessment of his condition is obvious, but it is too often dealt with cursorily and without adequate explanation and investigation of all the parameters involved. The problem is dealt with more fully in later chapters of this book and in other publications.[31,32]

2. Domestic

Although women in western Europe are increasingly engaged in work outside the home (and men within it), it is still the woman and mother who has to bear the burden of work in the house and who is in repeated contact with the numerous irritants and allergens associated with this. To the housewife the home is a minifactory,[6] with all the hazards of such but without any statutory regulations or guidelines, except those of common sense and upbringing. The combination of soaps, detergents, cleansers and solvents provides the background risk. To these, if she is also a mother, are added the effects of extra washing, bathing and shampooing of her children. The onset of hand eczema is more frequently after the arrival of the first or second child than after marriage and the start of housework itself. The care of infants and young children is the equivalent of her taking up a job — and one associated with all the risks of wet work[33] and of cumulative irritant dermatitis.[34]

In a study of 1000 women patch tested in a 5-center European survey,[35] 281 had contact dermatitis of the hands. Half of these gave positive patch tests, notably to balsams (there was no perfume mix then), nickel, cobalt, chromate, and paraphenylenediamine. Reactions to rubber chemicals and medicaments were also frequent, reflecting the wearing of gloves and the use of hand creams to protect or treat a skin already damaged. This may account for the finding that allergic dermatitis was as common as irritant dermatitis.

The housewife is also more at risk from houseplants and, usually, from gardening hazards.[7] And, finally, the young atopic, with a lowered threshold to irritants, may suffer a relapse of an earlier hand eczema when faced with the extra burden of housework and young children.

Although minor degrees of hand chapping and dryness are probably common in housewives, these are not usually presented to the dermatologist until painful fissuring occurs or a cumulative dermatitis develops, or perhaps until topical treatment induces a secondary allergic eczema.

The onset of hand eczema in a housewife does not imperil her job or threaten her livelihood. Paradoxically, it is expected that she will somehow continue to carry out her everyday duties; there is no compensation and no redress, but the presence of exudative lesions or painful fissures may greatly limit her working capacity, curtail her normal activities, and restrict the enjoyment of those pastimes in which she may have found a necessary relaxation from her work. As a housewife, mother, and individual she loses her pride and becomes dejected. This sense of failure, although often well disguised, may lead to a feeling of depression and to tension within the household. Indeed, her affliction may provoke resentment rather than sympathy on the part of those who have grown accustomed to the well-ordering of their daily existence.

The activities of the man in the house should not be forgotten. Contact with petrol, solvents, paints and glues in servicing cars and motorcycles, repairing and decorating, compounded by friction, abrasions and general wear and tear may themselves be the cause of both irritant and allergic dermatitis. If this is already present, such activities are often an unsuspected cause of perpetuation.[36]

3. Social

The social implications of hand eczema may be considerable. The hands are a highly visible area of the body. They are used for greeting and grooming and are organs of communication and expression in everyday life. Any eczematous eruption will excite attention and may cause difficulties in social intercourse. These may be the declared reason for the patient seeking advice. The sales manager, representative, shop assistant, or professional man or woman, perhaps already insecure in their jobs, may feel unable to meet clients on equal terms. The wife whose husband is embarking on a year's official duties in his field may be anxious about having to shake hands with so many. The young may feel embarrassed in their pursuit and grooming of each other. Even the schoolboy may feel ostracized in playing with his friends. These limitations (perhaps partly self-imposed by an undue exaggeration of concern about it) may even lead to a partial withdrawal from social or professional life and further increase an anxiety that is not always openly expressed by the patient.

A more restricted effect is on hobbies and sports. Some of these are purely domestic and have been dealt with, but others, such as golf, tennis, or squash, are carried out in a social context. The retired man who passes his time with his friends on the golf course may be incapacitated by a fissured hyperkeratotic palmar eczema, the younger tennis or squash enthusiast by the pressure and friction of holding a racket. Similarly, the amateur musician is impeded by a fingertip eczema. In all such activities the patient's social life is thereby diminished.

4. Psychological

The belief of many patients that stress initiates or, more commonly, causes relapses or exacerbations of hand eczema is widely held. This vexed problem is outside the scope of this chapter. We are concerned here with the effect of a severe, recurrent, or protracted hand eczema on the individual who suffers from it. Some of these have already been touched on earlier in this section.

The affected worker may feel both aggrieved and anxious about his future prospects. The eczematous skin takes some time to return to normality, and even when a definitive allergen has been found it may be several weeks before he can return to work. In chronic eczema with a less well-defined cause, the anxiety it arouses may itself lead to a perpetuation of the condition.[36] Scratching or rubbing may lead to lichenification and perpetuate the itch-scratch cycle; at the worst, self-manipulation and artifactual lesions may fulfill a conscious or unconscious need to let the lesion remain visible during the long period of legal dispute. But this is rarer than the post-insult constitutional hand eczema, which may follow an occupational dermatitis and is so often the cause of medicolegal problems.[29]

An overconscious preoccupation with the condition may, in other cases, lead to excessive hand-washing, rubbing or fiddling, habits that are often evident during consultation and which should be regarded as a sign of heightened anxiety. These obsessional traits of hand-washers and hand-watchers are bad omens in prognosis.

The problem of young atopics with hand eczema brought about or rekindled by starting work in an unsuitable occupation can also be distressing. They may not have the experience or find the support to guide them through a period in which entry to a worthwhile life and occupation seems to them to be blocked and their standing with the opposite sex disadvantaged.

In all such cases the hands become magnified in the patient's body imaging; his mirror distorts reality. The hands are an important organ of communication between the person and the environment. As symbols of power, prayer, and hope, their significance is often better expressed in folklore and appreciated by artists than by doctors in the consulting room.

IV. CLASSIFICATION

There are several ways in which hand eczema can be classified. The simplest is into acute, subacute and chronic forms. This is certainly useful as a guide to treatment but of little value in assessing the factors responsible. Classification by the type of elemental eczematous lesion present, much used by the earliest dermatologists, is also unproductive, although remnants persist in descriptions of vesicular and hyperkeratotic forms.

An anatomical approach is more interesting and has a logical basis. The skin of the hands is not homogeneous. The thick skin of the palmar surfaces adapted for gripping and holding, abundant in eccrine sweat glands but lacking hairs and sebaceous glands, differs markedly from the dorsal surfaces. Vascular reactivity is also more marked. Functional differences determine variations in anatomical susceptibility. The wearing of rings provides entrapment sites for irritants, as do the finger-webs; laterality is of great importance in all exogenous etiological factors; endogenous hand eczema tends to be symmetrical. Cronin,[37] in an analysis of 263 women, divided the cases into four groups: palms and fingers involved, dorsa and fingers, fingers only, and the entire hand. Cronin found that allergic sensitization and atopy were equally common in all groups. The only distribution characteristic of an endogenous cause was the central-to-proximal palmar and, to some extent, the "apron" pattern of the distal palm. The rather high percentages of positive patch tests in all four patterns may be because the patients were seen in a contact dermatitis clinic. This detailed study, which should be read in its entirety, demonstrated that it is impossible to differentiate between endogenous and exogenous or between irritant and allergic contact dermatitis and that the latter can commonly cause eczema of the palmar surfaces of the hands and fingers as well as the dorsa.

This study suggests that an etiological classification as such is not feasible. All the factors that may be responsible must be considered in all cases, although some are more applicable to one site than to another.

For everyday clinical purposes it is useful to have a starting point and a reference frame within which the relevant factors and behavior of similar patterns can be studied. A morphological classification is best suited to this, but it must be regarded as both pragmatic and tentative: pragmatic in the sense that it consists of ill-defined groupings of cases of a similar nature and tentative in that the placing of a patient in one group or another depends on the view of the dermatologist concerned and his beliefs and teaching. It is also subject to the varying nature of hand eczema itself. All clinicians who deal with these patients realize that in a process as dynamic as that of eczema they are seeing (at any one consultation) only one phase of the eruption. What starts in one pattern may change to another, through interaction of irritants and allergens on damaged skin, the intervention of treatment, changes in the environment, situations of stress, or the natural tendency of eczema to spread. The classification that follows is therefore a tentative one. It is based on a retrospective study of routine unselected patients, many of whom were seen on several occasions.[25] In a minority of patients in each group a change from one pattern to another was evident. A well-designed prospective analysis of such cases would certainly produce a more logical arrangement. But in our limited knowledge, at the present time, of the mechanisms involved, it offers a practical working system.[15]

The morphological classification of hand eczema that follows is suggested as a guide. The categories are not absolute but are capable of being merged or redefined in light of advances in knowledge or further studies.

A.   Diffuse or Patchy, Dorsal, and Palmar

Most cases of hand eczema are of a patchy nature and without any special morphological characteristics. They can be considered together in one category, although some may prefer to separate those that are predominantly dorsal in distribution from those that affect any part of the hands and fingers in various patterns. There is, however, some merit in considering separately those cases in which the palmar surfaces are solely or predominantly affected because they embrace a number of conditions that deserve special attention, such as pompholyx, dry palmar, and hyperkeratotic types. Cronin[37] did not find any material difference between dorsal and palmar types in the frequency of atopic or nickel sensitivity. Although allergic and irritant contact dermatitis have traditionally been associated with dorsal hand eczema, this has not been borne out by closer inquiry and patch testing. Purely constitutional cases, "id" reactions and the effect of ingested allergens, tend to affect the palmar surfaces, whereas involvement of the finger-webs is often an indication of irritant dermatitis. In an atopic, irritant dermatitis may present in any one of several patterns.

With the exception of the special types mentioned previously, most cases of palmar hand eczema are of a nonspecific vesiculosquamous nature and without special characteristics. It would be imprudent to attempt to define these too closely. Only about a third of all cases of hand eczema present with a morphological pattern that deserves special recognition, and even these are, in the present state of our knowledge, qualified distinctions.

B.   Particular Patterns

1.   Ring Eczema

This characteristic form of hand eczema starts under a ring but frequently spreads to the adjacent side of the third finger or of the palms. It is far more common in women, often starting after marriage or the arrival of a child, but it may affect men under a signet (or wedding) ring. The onset is usually in the third decade but may be earlier, especially in girls wearing cheap metal rings. Patch tests show a low yield, except for nickel, but this is common in women of this age and it is usually irrelevant unless associated with cheap jewelry or white gold rings. This form of hand eczema is considered to be an irritant reaction to the concentration of soap and detergent residues under the ring, but certain anomalies remain unexplained. Ring eczema is usually a primary manifestation of hand eczema, but a spread to other patterns is common.

2.   Discoid Hand Eczema

The pattern of lesions in this form of hand eczema is similar to that of discoid eczema elsewhere but is localized to the hands and fingers, usually the backs. One or more round, nummular lesions develop and remain fixed in place. They may be exudative or scaly in type. The intervening skin remains normal in appearance. The patches are resistant to treatment, and when they recur they do so in the same site. These characteristics distinguished the condition from the more common patchy form of hand eczema.

Discoid hand eczema affects both sexes, and young atopics entering unsuitable occupations are particularly susceptible. In a personal series[38] the onset usually occurred between 15 and 25 years, although some cases continued to appear into the 60s, particularly in men. Sometimes the first lesions appear at the site of burns, injury, or irritant reactions, and the condition is likely to be irritant in type. The relevance of the positive patch tests that may be found is usually difficult to establish.

3. Hyperkeratotic Hand Eczema

Although clinically characteristic, this form of hand eczema, which is more common in males and which has a later age of onset, is the most contentious form. Many dermatologists would regard all cases as being psoriatic. It is certainly not always easy to distinguish between the two conditions, but there are some features that lead us to regard it as different: the age bias, the selective age of onset, the absence of any close family or personal history of psoriasis, and any signs of this disease on the skin, scalp, or nails. The condition is pruritic and there is often an initial vesicular stage. Indeed, it is one form of progression of chronic vesicular eczema of the palms.

Because neither palmar hand eczema nor a psoriatic constitution is a rare condition, it is reasonable to suggest that the former could take on a psoriatic character and behave as such. An attractive alternative view was put forward by Hersle and Möbacken,[38] who regarded it as an entity. This certainly commands some respect. The subject is dealt with in Chapter 11.

4. Fingertip Eczema

This is known as "pulpite" in France, a term that accurately localizes it to the pulps rather than the backs of the fingers. These become dry and glazed parchment pulps, then cracked and even fissured and extremely painful. Many patients do not present to the dermatologist until this stage is reached and they are unable to carry out their normal activities. Women are affected about three times as often as men.

Two patterns can be recognized. The first involves most or all of the fingers, although preferentially the thumb and forefinger of the master hand. It may gradually extend down the palmar surface of the fingers, merging into the dry palmar pattern. Patch tests are usually negative or relevant. It is best considered as a form of irritant dermatitis from cumulative degreasing and trauma. The second affects the thumb and first two fingers of either the master or serving hand, occasionally others but in an asymmetric pattern. It may be traumatic, as in repetitive handling of newspapers, or allergic, as from colophony, formaldehyde, tulip bulbs, or certain foods held in the fingers of the serving hand during preparation. In some cases the affected finger pulps become more acutely eczematous. Patch tests and 20-min contact tests are indicated.

5. Palmar Eczema

Most cases are vesiculosquamous and a component of the common patchy form of hand eczema in which endogenous and exogenous factors vie for supremacy in the etiology. Ingested allergens may play a role, but this remains undecided and is always difficult to evaluate. There may be etiological differences, also at present unclear between those cases involving chiefly the center of the palms and those affecting the thenar or hypothenar eminences. Three minor and less common forms of eczema involving the palms do, however, show characteristic features that justify separate mention.

a. Dry palmar

Also termed "wear and tear" or "housewives" dermatitis, dermatitis palmaris sicca and asteatotic hand eczema, this form is characterized by a dry fractured horny layer with a pattern of superficial criss-crossing of superficial cracks but without deeper fissuring. Usually, although not always bilateral, it affects the palms and palmar surfaces of the fingers. It may occur as an extension of fingertip eczema or be preceded by ring eczema. It is more common in women and is regarded as a response to the repeated effect of soaps, detergents, and washing.

b.   "Apron" pattern

This rather unusual pattern accounted for 18 of 115 cases of palmar eczema.[16] The term, given by Calnan,[16] describes a localized eczema extending from the proximal part of two or more adjacent fingers and the metacarpophalangeal joints to the contiguous part of the palm in a semicircular fashion. More common in women, it is regarded by Cronin[37] as endogenous.

c.   Subacute recurrent vesicular type

This variety of palmar eczema is often referred to as "pompholyx" in the literature, but it differs in the longer duration of the recurrent attacks and the rupture of the vesicles, features alien to pompholyx as originally described. After a variable time, the condition fails to heal between attacks and the condition becomes chronic. It may not be valid to separate this group from the majority of cases of palmar eczema. Indeed, in some endogenous cases an allergen or irritant may be discovered that explains the episodic behavior of the cases, but in others (perhaps the majority) this is not so and in our present state of ignorance of the endogenous mechanisms involved, it is perhaps as well to leave the door open.

6.   Pompholyx

This term has been and still is the cause of much confusion in the literature and in practice. Tilbury Fox, in 1873, first described the condition as a disturbance of sweat gland function and separate from eczema.[39] Hutchinson, 3 years later, gave it the name "pompholyx" without any etiological connotation.[40] The first term is now known to be inaccurate and the second merely descriptive of severe forms. Both are in use, but the more evocative "pompholyx" is preferred by most British and many other European writers.

These early authors noted certain characteristics that seemed to them to set it apart from other forms of eczema of the hands. "Nothing could be more different than the origin and course." "They (the vesicles) never by any chance result in eczema."[40] Attacks occur suddenly and sometimes explosively, in an episodic or cyclical manner. The sides of the fingers and the palms, or both, are affected. The eruption is monomorphic, with deeply set vesicles resembling "boiled sago-grains",[39] which resorb without rupturing, often leaving a light scaling in their wake. Each attack lasts 10 to 30 days, and the hands are normal between these. In severe cases the palmar vesicles merge to form large bullae, justifying the name.

In the course of time these criteria have expanded considerably, sometimes to the point of extinction of the original description. Although histological studies have been sparse, the changes are consistent with those of eczema.[15] This has encouraged those who would include cases that are asymmetric or more chronic cases of a vesiculosquamous nature. This tendency to merge pompholyx with the more common chronic or recurrent vesicular eczema of the palms has considerably broadened the etiological possibilities but perhaps at the expense of those relating specifically to the short-lived cyclical disease. There is some merit in retaining it as a separate entity because the responsible factors may differ.

Fox[39] and Hutchinson[40] regarded the condition as a vasomotor neurosis and were impressed by the depressed or "neurotic" nature of their patients, although the latter did mention the possibility of food or drugs as causes. With the development of the concepts of atopy and of allergic contact dermatitis, the field of inquiry has been extended to include reactions to both topical ingested allergens,[41,42] bacterial and fungal infections, and atopy.[43] Further studies are required, but for the present it is perhaps best to regard pompholyx as a nonspecific reaction pattern of the skin,[44] the "réaction cutaneé" of the French writers.

Variations include the recurrent digital vesiculation already referred to, a form in which vesicles are sparse or absent but shows as a recurrent palmar peeling, "dyshidrotic lamellosa sicca"[43] and ridging of the nails alone in the absence of recognized attacks.[44]

7.   Rare Forms

a.   Gut (slaughterhouse) eczema

A transient vesicular eczema affects the webs and sides of the fingers of those engaged in eviscerating pigs' carcasses.[45] The cause is uncertain.

b. Chronic acral dermatitis

Winkelmann and Gleich[46] described a pruritic hyperkeratotic papulovesicular eczema of the palms and soles in middle-aged subjects. Immunoglobulin E levels are considerably elevated, but there is no personal or family history of atopy. It is probably underdiagnosed.

c. Other patterns

Other forms of hand eczema may become recognized and accepted, although it is more likely that existing categories will be better defined and rearranged as the responsible factors are more accurately established by newer techniques of investigation.

REFERENCES

1. Hebra, F., *On Diseases of the Skin,* New Sydenham Society, London, 1868, chap. 19.
2. Fox, T., *Skin Diseases,* 3rd ed., Henry Renshaw, London, 1873, chap. 10.
3. Radcliffe-Crocker, H., *Diseases of the Skin,* 3rd ed., H. K. Lewis, London, 1903, 147.
4. Prosser-White, R., *The Dermatergoses or Occupational Affections of the Skin,* 4th ed., H. K. Lewis, London, 1934.
5. Ramazzini, B., *Treatise on the Diseases of Tradesmen,* London, 1746.
6. Wilkinson, D. S., Contact dermatitis in the home: the house, in *Current Concepts in Contact Dermatitis,* Verbov, J., Ed., MTP Press, Lancaster, England, 1987, chap. 1.
7. Shaw, S. and Wilkinson, J. D., Contact dermatitis in the home: the garden, in *Current Concepts in Contact Dermatitis,* Verbov, J., Ed., MTP Press, Lancaster, England, 1987, chap. 2.
8. Montague, W., *Letters,* Vol. 3, Dodd and Riley, London, 1776, 3, 21.
9. Bloch, B. and Steiner-Woerlich, A., Die Willkurliche Erzengung der Primeluberengfindlichkeit bein Menschen und ihre Bedeutung für das Idiosyncrasieproblem, *Arch. Dermatol. Syphilol.,* 152, 283, 1926.
10. Block, B. and Steiner-Woerlich, A., Die Sensibilirierung des Meerschweinchens gegein Primeln, *Arch. Dermatol. Syphilol.,* 162, 349, 1930.
11. Jadassohn, J., Zur Kenntniss der Arzneiexantheme, *Arch. Dermatol. Syphilol.,* 34, 103, 1896.
12. Sulzberger, M. B. and Wise, F., The contact or patch test in dermatology: its uses, advantages and limitations, *Arch. Dermatol.,* 23, 519, 1931.
13. Coca, A. F. and Cooke, R. A., On the classification of the phenomenon of hypersensitiveness, *J. Immunol.,* 8, 163, 1923.
14. Walker, N., *An Introduction to Dermatology,* 6th ed., Green, W., Ed., Edinburgh, London, 1913, 94.
15. Burton, J. L., Eczema, lichenification, prurigo and erythroderma, in *Textbook of Dermatology,* 5th ed., Champion, R. H., Burton, J. L., and Ebling, F. J. G., Eds., Blackwell Scientific, Oxford, 1992, chap. 14.
16. Calnan, C. D., Eczema for me, *Trans. St. John's Hosp., Dermatol. Soc.,* 54, 54, 1968.
17. Wilkinson, D. S. and Wilkinson, J. D., Nickel allergy and hand eczema, in *Nickel and the Skin: Immunology and Toxicology,* Maibach, H. I. and Menné, T., Eds., CRC Press, Boca Raton, FL, 1989, chap. 13.
18. Wilkinson, D. S., Contact dermatitis of the hands, *Trans. St. John's Hosp. Dermatol. Soc.,* 58, 163, 1972.
19. Agrup, G., Hand eczema and other hand dermatoses in South Sweden, *Acta Derm. Venereol. Suppl.,* 49, 61, 1969.
20. Johnson, M. L. T. and Roberts, J., *Skin Conditions and Related Needs of Medical Care among Persons 1-74 Years,* DHEW Publication No. (PHS) 79-1668, Hyattsville, U.S. Dept. Health, Education and Welfare, National Center for Health Statistics, 1978.
21. Menné, T., Borgan, Ö., and Green, A., Nickel allergy and hand dermatitis in a stratified sample of the Danish female population: an epidemiological study including a statistic appendix, *Acta Derm. Venereol.,* 62, 35, 1982.

22. Meding, B. and Swanbeck, G., Prevalence of hand eczema in an industrial city, *Br. J. Dermatol.,* 116, 627, 1987.

23. Burton, J. L., Savin, J. A., and Champion, R. H., Introduction, epidemiology, and historical biography, in *Textbook of Dermatology,* 5th ed., Champion, R. H., Burton, J. L., and Ebling, F. J. G., Eds., Blackwell Scientific, Oxford, 1992, chap. 1.

24. Rea, J. N., Newhouse, M. L., and Halil, T., Skin disease in Lambeth: a community study of prevalence and use of medical care, *Br. J. Prev. Soc. Med.,* 30, 107, 1976.

25. Wilkinson, D. S., Unpublished data, 1992.

26. Wilkinson, D. S., Budden, M. G., and Hambly, E. M., A 10-year review of an industrial dermatitis clinic, *Contact Dermatitis,* 6, 11, 1980.

27. Fregert, S., Occupational dermatitis in a 10-year material, *Contact Dermatitis,* 1, 96, 1975.

28. Fregert, S., Hjorth, N., Magnusson, B., Bandmann, H.-J., Calnan, C. D., Cronin, E., Malten, K., Meneghini, C. L., Pirilä, V., and Wilkinson, D. S., Epidemiology of contact dermatitis, *Trans. St. John's Hosp. Dermatol. Soc.,* 55, 17, 1969.

29. Wall, L. M. and Gebauer, K. A., A follow-up study of occupational skin disease in Western Australia, *Contact Dermatitis,* 24, 241, 1991.

30. Burrows, D., Industrial dermatitis today and its prevention, in *Essentials of Industrial Dermatology,* Griffiths, W. A. D. and Wilkinson, D. S., Eds., Blackwell Scientific, Oxford, 1985, chap. 2.

31. Maibach, H. I., Ed., *Occupational and Industrial Dermatology,* 2nd ed., Year Book, Chicago, 1986.

32. Griffiths, W. A. D. and Wilkinson, D. S., Eds., *Essentials of Industrial Dermatology,* Blackwell Scientific, Oxford, 1985.

33. Lammintausta, K., Kalimo, K., and Havu, V. K., Occurrence of contact allergy and hand eczema in hospital wet work, *Contact Dermatitis,* 8, 84, 1982.

34. Malten, K. E., Thoughts on irritant contact dermatitis, *Contact Dermatitis,* 7, 238, 1981.

35. Calnan, C. D., Bandmann, H.-J., Cronin, E., Fregert, S., Hjorth, N., Magnusson, B., Malten, K., Meneghini, C. L., Pirilä, V., and Wilkinson, D. S., Hand dermatitis in housewives, *Br. J. Dermatol.,* 82, 543, 1970.

36. Wilkinson, D. S., Causes of unexpected persistence of an occupational dermatitis, in *Essentials of Industrial Dermatitis,* Griffiths, W. A. D. and Wilkinson, D. S., Eds., Blackwell Scientific, Oxford, 1985.

37. Cronin, E., Clinical patterns of hand eczema in women, *Contact Dermatitis,* 13, 153, 1985.

38. Hersle, K. and Möbacken, H., Hyperkeratotic dermatitis of the palms, *Br. J. Dermatol.,* 107, 195, 1982.

39. Fox, T., Clinical lectures on dyshidrosis (an undescribed eruption), *Br. Med. J.,* 1, 365, 1873.

40. Hutchinson, J., Cheiropompholyx: notes of a clinical lecture, *Lancet,* 1, 630, 1876.

41. Meneghini, C. L. and Angelini, G., Contact and microbial allergy in pompholyx, *Contact Dermatitis,* 5, 46, 1979.

42. Menné, T. and Hjorth, N., Pompholyx: dyshidrotic eczema, *Semin. Dermatol.,* 2, 75, 1983.

43. Schwanitz, H. J., *Atopic Palmoplantar Eczema,* Springer-Verlag, Berlin, 1988.

44. Strempel, R., Zur Ätiologie und Pathogenese der Dyshidrosis, *Hautartzt,* 7, 241, 1956.

45. Hjorth, N., Gut eczema in slaughterhouse workers, *Contact Dermatitis,* 9, 49, 1978.

46. Winkelmann, R. K. and Gleich, G. J., Chronic acral dermatitis: association with extreme elevations of IgE, *J. Am. Med. Assoc.,* 225, 378, 1973.

2

Biology of Skin Inflammation Related to Dermatosis of the Hands

Kristian Thestrup-Pedersen

CONTENTS

I. INTRODUCTION

Eczema is a prolonged lymphocyte-mediated inflammation of skin, in which activated T lymphocytes attack the epidermis. This leads to formation of microvesicles and breakage of the normal epidermal structure with scaling and dryness. Increased vascular flow is reflected in erythema, and itching is the prominent sign of mediators related to the T cell activation.

Although hand eczema is clinically restricted to less than 5% of the skin area, every dermatologist knows how the entire skin of the patient is in a hyperirritative state, indicating that eczema affects the immune system in a more generalized manner.

The well-known clinical features are contrasted by our lack of knowledge concerning the inflammatory events, although recent years have brought much detailed information.[1-3] We are still faced with the basic question of why some persons under similar exposures develop eczema and others do not. We tend to understand the concept of allergic contact dermatitis but lack an answer as to why eczema develops as a response to irritants, which are clearly not of an allergic nature.

The most central question in our understanding of eczema is still not answered: are the T lymphocytes in eczema always activated via antigen-specific T cell receptors and, if so, what is the nature of the antigen in irritant contact dermatitis?

The accumulation of CD4+ T lymphocytes in eczematous skin must be the end-result of a well-controlled series of events. It includes expression of adhesion molecules on endothelial cells, attachment of the CD4+ T lymphocytes, and an ensuing response to an existing chemotactic gradient, enabling the cells to migrate into the surrounding tissue and later toward epidermis. Finally, a cytolytic event from activated T cells probably explains the structural changes.

This chapter will summarize new knowledge of inflammation related to contact eczema.

II. ADHESION MOLECULES

Adhesion molecules are important not only for cell adhesion and migration, but for T lymphocyte stimulation.[4-8] Blocking of adhesion molecules during antigen presentation and T cell stimulation will under experimental conditions lead to a lack of T cell proliferation, indicating development of anergy toward the antigen in question.

The presently known adhesion molecules are divided into four families: the immunoglobulin family (CAMs); integrins, which are the complementary molecules for the CAMs; selectins, which are only found on leukocytes but not on solid tissue; and cadherins.

Migration includes several steps, such as rolling, adhesion, chemotaxis, and an ensuing activation of the cells. When cells are not expressing adhesion molecules, the existence of a chemotactic gradient will not induce chemotaxis. Expression of adhesion molecules on circulating cells and endothelial cells will allow cell adhesion and migration if a chemotactic gradient exists and provided the adhesion forces are not too strong. Very strong adhesion will keep cells immobilized despite the existence of a chemotactic gradient.

Some adhesion molecules carry a similar function as membrane-bound cytokines and act via secondary messengers. Thus, integrins can activate cells via protein-tyrosine kinases. Not all adhesion molecules have a transmembranous sequence. The selectin family and certain members of the immunoglobulin superfamily do not. The membrane-bound adhesion molecules may also be shed via proteolytic activity and thus function as soluble products with biological activity. Soluble ICAM-1 has been found to show T cell chemotactic activity.[9]

The selectin family consists of E-selectin (ELAM-1), G-selectin (GMP 140), and P-selectin (Mel-14), which are found on a variety of cells, including T lymphocytes. The molecules are glycoproteins. Their binding affinity is calcium-dependent and often low. Selectins function as "rolling-inducers", i.e., cells in the bloodstream are slowed down for a brief moment, thereby allowing binding between integrins and their counterparts on the endothelial cells, provided these are expressed.

Integrin molecules consist of two chains, an α chain in which 17 different chains are recognized, and a β-chain, in which 9 are known. So far, 24 combinations of these chains are known. The integrins bind to members of the CAM family; these bindings are the most important for T lymphocyte adhesion. The integrin binding is a much stronger binding than the selectin binding. Examples are LFA-1 binding to ICAM-1 or -2 and VLA-4 binding to VCAM-1.

The T lymphocyte LFA-1 binding can be influenced by cross-linking of CD3 epitopes with anti-CD3 antibody, which will within 20 min increase the affinity of the binding of T lymphocytes via LFA-1 by a factor 5 to 6. The integrin family is dependent upon calcium and manganese ions, and a change in the calcium ion concentration seems to be able to switch the integrin molecule into either an "ON" or "OFF" position. This switch may be related to or caused by the presence or absence of calcium in the extramembraneous part of the molecule.

The molecules in the CAM family are similar to immunoglobulin in structure. The complementary molecules to the CAM family are the integrins. Expression of CAM molecules can be influenced by certain cytokines, such as interferons, which can up-regulate ICAM-1.[10] ICAM-1 and -2 are important for binding to LFA-1 and other adhesion molecules on T lymphocytes. ELAM-1 is expressed on endothelial cells and seems to be of particular importance for T lymphocytes in their homing to skin.[11-13]

So far, cadherins have not been shown on solid tissue cells, and their role in eczema has not been studied.

A. Lymphocyte Traffic and Homing

Naive T lymphocytes carry adhesion molecules (L-selectins), which preferentially bind to the high endothelial cells in the lymph nodes.[11] It has been observed in animal experiments that naive T cells will leave the bloodstream and go into the lymph node and return to the blood via the afferent lymph vessels. In contrast, memory or activated T lymphocytes express other receptors, including cutaneous lymphocyte antigen (CLA) and/or VLA-4α, and they can leave the blood in an area where signals for an inflammation exist.[6,12] Such signals include up-regulation of selectin receptors and CAM receptors on endothelial cells, presence of cytokines, presence of chemotactic gradients, and presence of activation factors, such as augmenting pro-inflammatory cytokines, antigens, possibly superantigens, or mitogens.

B. Adhesion Molecules and Dermatology

Boehncke et al.[14] recently reviewed and demonstrated that a variety of integrins and immunoglobulin superfamily adhesion molecules are up-regulated in various dermatological disorders, in which T-lymphocytes are often a prominent cell type in the inflammatory process. Vejlsgaard et al.[15] studied adhesion molecules in particular in allergic and irritant patch tests and observed that ICAM-1 is up-regulated and present as early as 4 h after initiation of a positive patch test. Only 1 of 14 irritant tests demonstrated ICAM-1 expression in epidermis. The HLA-DR staining was significantly less than that of ICAM-1. Cleavage of ICAM-1 from keratinocytes could be as biologically relevant as chemotactic factors for T lymphocytes.[9]

Adhesion molecules are most likely to be of primary importance for the development of a lymphocyte-mediated skin inflammation. It must be studied whether patients with eczema have an increased or prolonged expression of integrins and CAMs on their endothelial cell surfaces and T lymphocytes, thereby increasing their risk for eczema development.

III. MAJOR HISTOCOMPATIBILITY ANTIGENS

The human lymphocyte antigen (HLA) system is necessary for antigen stimulation of T lymphocytes. In normal skin Langerhans cells and interdigitating dermal cells express HLA class II antigens. There seems to be no difference between irritant and allergic contact dermatitis when studying class II expression.[16]

Keratinocytes are able to express class II molecules during eczema, but the consequences for the immune inflammation are uncertain. First, they appear to occur several days after the initiation of a positive patch test,[16] and their *in vitro* capacity to function as antigen-presenting cells is much less than that of Langerhans' cells.[17] Certain experimental observations could indicate that keratinocyte class II antigen expression could function as down-regulators of lymphocyte activation. Thus, injection of interferon-γ (IFN-γ) into rats with allergic contact dermatitis strongly up-regulates keratinocyte class II antigens but at the same time inhibits allergic contact dermatitis.[18]

TABLE 1   Pro-inflammatory Cytokines and T Lymphocyte
Cytokines

Pro-inflammatory cytokines
TNF-α
IL-1
IL-6
IL-8-family
GRO/MGSA
PF 4
PBP/NAPII
IP10
MCAF
LD78
Act-2
RANTES
I-309
T lymphocyte cytokines
T_{h1}
IL-2
IFN-γ
T_{h2}
IL-4
IL-5
IL-10

The role of major histocompatibility complex (MHC) class II expression is thus of importance for the immune competent cells in the skin, but maybe not on nonimmune cells. Again, it is puzzling that irritant eczema is similar to allergic contact eczema and no difference seems obvious. This could be due to the fact that MHC class II expression is determined by the release of IFN-γ from activated T lymphocytes.[19]

IV.   CYTOKINES

The observations of epidermal T lymphocyte activating factor (ETAF) more than 10 years ago brought a new important aspect into our concept of contact dermatitis.[20] The overwhelming field of cytokines is growing exponentially, but so far no skin disease has been shown to be a consequence of either an overproduction or deficiency of a cytokine(s), including eczema.

The cytokine cascade could be an important part in the development of eczema. Many cytokines are expressed and secreted during inflammation. The sustained lymphocyte inflammation of eczema could be caused of an up-regulation of pro-inflammatory cytokines, an increased secretion of cytokines from activated T lymphocytes, or the lack of cytokine synthesis inhibitors.

The cytokines can be simplified as pro-inflammatory cytokines and T lymphocyte-derived cytokines (Table 1). This oversimplification may help in our understanding of their role in eczema. Pro-inflammatory cytokines can be produced by almost any nucleated cell when stimulated. Some cytokines are inducted by other cytokines, and some may need induction from supraphysiological concentrations of cytokines or stimuli, such as tumor-promoting factors. All nucleated cells in the skin can up-regulate their production of pro-inflammatory cytokines, but they do so in a different time sequence and amount. This has been documented in detail for IL-8 and MCAF.[21,22]

The T lymphocyte-derived cytokines are only released by T cells after activation. The cytokine profile of activated T lymphocytes probably depends upon the activation signals. Thus, human T cells can at least *in vitro* be brought to express both a T_{h1} and T_{h2} cytokine profile.[23] Nickel-specific T cell clones mostly secrete the T_{h1} cytokine profile (IL-2 and IFN-γ), but little IL-4 and IL-5.[24]

A.   Experimental Studies

Several *in vitro* and *in vivo* experiments have tried to elucidate the role of cytokines in contact eczema. Recent and preliminary *in vitro* studies have shown that nickel added to human endothelial cells can up-regulate the expression of IL-8 mRNA[25] and ICAM-1.[26] Monocytes can up-regulate their mRNA for IL-8 followed by secretion of IL-8, when exposed to metal ions, of which manganese and mercury were the most potent inducers.[27]

Recent studies in mice have shown that breakage of the lipid barrier will induce the up-regulation of TNF-α, IL-1α, IL-1β and colony-stimulating factor–granulocyte macrophage (GM-CSF), whereas IL-6 and IFN-γ were not detected.[28] These experiments document that a pro-inflammatory cytokine cascade is initiated after irritant trauma to the epidermis. Similar studies in humans are needed.

In vivo studies have shown that injection of anti-TNF antibodies into mice will prevent the ensuing development of both allergic and irritant contact dermatitis.[29] This finding contrasts the observation that TNF injection into skin of mice will reduce an ensuing contact eczema reactivity and that TNF seems to exert its effect via *cis*-urocanic acid.[30] Injection of TGF-β into mice can also inhibit the elicitation of both the early and late phase of delayed-type hypersensitivity reactions.[31] Injection of anti-IL-8 antibodies into rabbits can prevent the development of arthritis induced by intraarticular (LPS) injection.[32]

Studies of contact dermatitis in humans have shown the occurrence of both ETAF/IL-1 and epidermal lymphocyte chemotactic factor(s) (ELCF) in allergic patch test reactions.[33] ELCF, but not ETAF/IL-1, was increased in irritant patch tests using 3% (SLS).[34] These studies were performed by studying suction blister homogenates and using biological activity assays.

Immunohistological studies of cytokines have given somewhat contrasting results among various investigators and when compared with other techniques. Several groups have found an up-regulation of TNF-α in epidermis during the development of an allergic reaction, and recent time-course studies of the urushiol reaction demonstrated an up-regulation of TNF-α, IL-8, and ECAM-1 in keratinocytes and ELAM-1, VCAM-1, and ICAM-1 on endothelial cells.[35] Kristensen et al.[36] performed similar studies using antibodies toward IL-1α, TNF-α, IL-1, and TNF receptors, IRAP, and IL-8. All cytokines and receptors were expressed in normal skin except the TNF R-75 receptor. IL-1α was increased in a positive patch test, but not the remaining cytokines. There was an increased expression of the TNF R-55 and TNF R-75 and IL-1R corresponding to the perivascular and interstitial cellular infiltrate seen in the allergic patch test reaction.

The immunohistological techniques depend upon the reactivity of the antibodies used. The use of a quantitative polymerase chain reaction technique allows for the measurement of mRNA for various cytokines,[37] and we have recently observed that IL-8 seems to be the most strongly up-regulated pro-inflammatory cytokine in the skin during the development of both allergic and irritant reactions. The concomitant occurrence of T lymphocyte cytokines needs to be studied in time-sequence experiments.[38]

The many cytokines demonstrated in skin cells have the potential to create chemotactic gradients especially for T lymphocytes, establish a setting for augmentation of T lymphocyte activity, and augment adhesion molecule expression. The up-regulation of IL-8 and other pro-inflammatory cytokines is sufficient to create a lymphocyte chemotactic gradient. Experiments in rats support that small amounts of IL-8 will preferentially attract T lymphocytes, whereas larger amounts will attract neutrophil granulocytes.[39] Therefore, an initial release of IL-8 would create a T cell gradient. IL-8 will at the same time be able to up-regulate CAMs on endothelial cells, and endothelial cells are themselves strong IL-8 producers.[40] Even nonactivated human T lymphocytes will show adhesion in such an area and then go into the tissue.[41] We have found that human T lymphocytes up-regulate their CD45RO after chemotaxis toward IL-8.[42]

We have recently demonstrated that IL-10 is able to specifically attract CD8 + human T lymphocytes and at the same time block the response of CD4 + T cells in their ensuing reaction toward IL-8.[43] IL-10 is known to be mostly up-regulated between 24 and 48 h after stimulation.[44] The ensuing release of IL-10 in the area will then lead to a chemotactic gradient for CD8 + T lymphocytes and at the same time inhibit the ability of CD4 + T lymphocytes to respond to a still existing gradient of IL-8. Thus, cytotoxic and suppressor functioning cells would then be brought into the area. The CD4/CD8 ratio in skin is two to three times above the ratio in blood. It will be interesting to determine whether IL-10 is lacking in epidermis and dermis in patients with eczema.

The diversified capacities of cytokines will allow for the speculative possibility that patients with eczema are those who have a defect in their cytokine cascade regulation by up-regulation ''too-much'' pro-inflammatory cytokines for ''too long time'', or by a lack of ability to produce cytokine synthesis inhibitory factors thus being unable to bring suppressor lymphocytes into the area and end the reaction.

These possibilities are still speculative and require further work. The coming years will show whether new molecular biology techniques will lead us to discoveries that will help our patients with eczema.

REFERENCES

1. Thestrup-Pedersen, K., Larsen, C. G., and Rønnevig, J. R., The immunology of contact dermatitis: a review, *Contact Dermatitis,* 20, 81, 1989.
2. Nickoloff, B. J., Griffiths, C. E. M., and Barker, J. N. W. N., The role of adhesion molecules, chemotactic factors and cytokines in inflammatory and neoplastic skin disease: 1990 update, *J. Invest. Dermatol.,* 94 (Suppl.), 151, 1990.
3. Barker, J. N. W. N., Role of keratinocytes in allergic contact dermatitis, *Contact Dermatitis,* 26, 145, 1992.
4. Picker, L. J., Mechanisms of lymphocyte homing, *Curr. Opin. Immunol.,* 4, 277, 1992.
5. Issekutz, T. B., Lymphocyte homing to sites of inflammation, *Curr. Opin. Immunol.,* 4, 287, 1992.
6. Issekutz, T. B., Inhibition of *in vivo* lymphocyte migration to inflammation and homing to lymphoid tissues by the TA-2 monoclonal antibody: a likely role for VLA-4 *in vivo, J. Immunol.,* 147, 4178, 1991.
7. Mackay, C. R., T-cell memory: the connection between function, phenotype and migration pathways, *Immunol. Today,* 12, 189, 1991.
8. Deckert, M., Kubar, J., and Bernard, A., CD58 and CD59 molecules exhibit potentializing effects in T cell adhesion and activation, *J. Immunol.,* 148, 672, 1992.
9. Takagawa, M., personal communication.
10. Picker, L. J., Kishimoto, T. K., Smith, C. W., Warnock, R. A., and Butcher, E. C., ELAM-1 is an adhesion molecule for skin-homing T cells, *Nature,* 349, 796, 1991.
11. Berg, E. L., Yoshino, T., Rott, L. S., Robinson, M. K., Warnock, A., Kishimoto, T. K., Picker, L. J., and Butcher, E. C., The cutaneous lymphocyte antigen is a skin lymphocyte homing receptor for the vascular lectin endothelial cell-leukocyte adhesion molecule 1, *J. Exp. Med.,* 174, 1461, 1991.
12. Shimizu, Y., Shaw, S., Graber, N., Vopal, T. V., Horgan, K. J., Van Seventer, G. A., and Newman, W., Activation-independent binding of human memory T cells to adhesion molecule ELAM-1, *Nature,* 349, 799, 1991.
13. Bruynzeel, I., Nickoloff, B. J., van der Raaij, E. M. H., Boorsma, D. M., Stoof, T. J., and Willemze, R., Induction of ICAM-1 expression by epidermal keratinocytes via a paracrine pathway possibly involving dermal dendritic cells, *Arch. Dermatol. Res.,* 284, 250, 1992.
14. Boehncke, W.-H., Kellner, I., Konter, U., and Sterry, W., Differential expression of adhesion molecules on infiltrating cells in inflammatory dermatoses, *J. Am. Acad. Dermatol.,* 26, 907, 1992.
15. Vejlsgaard, G., Ralfkiær, E., Avnstorp, C., Czajkowski, M., Marlin, S. D., and Rothlein, R., Kinetics and characterization of intercellular adhesion molecule-1 (ICAM-1) expression on keratinocytes in various inflammatory skin lesions and malignant cutaneous lymphomas, *J. Am. Acad. Dermatol.,* 20, 782, 1989.
16. Gawkrodger, D. J., Carr, M. M., McVittie, E., Guy, K., and Hunter, J. A. A., Keratinocyte expression of MHC class II antigens in allergic sensitization and challenge reactions and in irritant contact dermatitis, *J. Invest. Dermatol.,* 88, 11, 1987.
17. Gaspari, A. A. and Katz, S. I., Induction and functional characterization of class II MCH (Ia) antigens on murine keratinocytes, *J. Immunol.,* 140, 2956, 1988.
18. Scheynius, A. and Skoglund, C., Interferon-gamma and the contact allergic reaction, *Contact Dermatitis,* 23, 230, 1990.

19. Basham, T. Y., Nickoloff, B. J., Merigan, T. C., and Morhenn, V. B., Recombinant gamma-interferon induces HLA-DR on cultured human keratinocytes, *J. Invest. Dermatol.,* 83, 88, 1984.

20. Luger, T. A., Stadler, B. M., and Katz, S. I., Epidermal cell derived thymocyte activating factor, *J. Immunol.,* 127, 1493, 1981.

21. Kristensen, M., Paludan, K., Larsen, C. G., Zachariae, C., Deleuran, B., Jensen, P. K. A., Jørgensen, P., and Thestrup-Pedersen, K., Quantitative determination of IL-1 alfa-induced IL-8 mRNA levels in cultured human keratinocytes, dermal fibroblasts, endothelial cells, and monocytes, *J. Invest. Dermatol.,* 97, 506, 1991.

22. Kristensen, M. S., Deleuran, B. W., Larsen, C. G., Thestrup-Pedersen, K., and Paludan, K., Expression of monocyte chemotactic and activating factor (MCAF) in skin related cells: a comparative study, *Cytokine,* in press.

23. Yssel, H., Johnson, K. E., Schneider, P. V., Wideman, J., Terr, A., Kastelein, R., and De Vries, J. E., T cell activation-inducing epitopes of the house dust mite allergen Der p I: proliferation and lymphokine production patterns by Der p I-specific CD4+ T cell clones, *J. Immunol.,* 148, 738, 1992.

24. Kapsenberg, M. L., Wierenga, E. A., Stieckema, F. E., Tiggelman, A. M., and Bos, J. D., Th 1 lymphokine production profiles of nickel specific CD4+ T lymphocyte clones from nickel contact allergic and nonallergic individuals, *J. Invest. Dermatol.,* 98, 59, 1992.

25. Kristensen, M., Deleuran, B. W., Larsen, C. G., and Thestrup-Pedersen, K., Nickel induces upregulation of IL-8 mRNA in endothelial cell cultures, submitted.

26. ICAM-1 upregulation on endothelial cells: Abstract from ESDR, Copenhagen.

27. Matsushima, K., personal communication.

28. Wood, L. C., Jackson, W. M., Elias, P. M., Grunfeld, C., and Feingold, K. R., Cutaneous barrier perturbation stimulates cytokine production in the epidermis of mice, *J. Clin. Invest.,* 90, 482, 1992.

29. Piquet, F. P., Grau, G. E., Hauser, C., and Vassalli, P., Tumor necrosis factor is a critical mediator in hapten-induced irritant and contact hypersensitivity reactions, *J. Exp. Med.,* 173, 673, 1991.

30. Kurimoto, I. and Streilein, J. W., *cis*-Urocanic acid suppression of contact hypersensitivity induction is mediated via tumor necrosis factor-alfa, *J. Immunol.,* 148, 3072, 1992.

31. Meade, R., Askenase, P. W., Geba, G. P., Neddermann, K., Jacoby, R. O., and Pasternak, R. D., Transforming growth factor-beta 1 inhibits murine immediate and delayed type hypersensitivity, *J. Immunol.,* 149, 521, 1992.

32. Matsushima, K., personal communication.

33. Larsen, C. G., Ternowitz, T., Larsen, F. G., and Thestrup-Pedersen, K., Epidermis and lymphocyte interactions during an allergic patch test reaction: increased activity of ETAF-IL-1, epidermal derived lymphocyte chemotactic factor and mixed skin lymphocyte reactivity in persons with type IV allergy, *J. Invest. Dermatol.,* 90, 230, 1988.

34. Larsen, C. G., Ternowitz, T., Larsen, F. G., and Thestrup-Pedersen, K., ETAF/interleukin 1 and epidermal lymphocyte chemotactic factor in epidermis overlying an irritant patch test, *Contact Dermatitis,* 20, 335, 1989.

35. Griffiths, C. E. M., Barker, J. N. W. N., Kunkel, S., and Nickoloff, B. J., Modulation of leucocyte adhesion molecules, a T-cell chemotaxin (IL-8) and a regulatory cytokine (TNF-alfa) in allergic contact dermatitis (rhus dermatitis), *Br. J. Dermatol.,* 124, 519, 1991.

36. Kristensen, M., Brennan, F. M., Feldmann, M., and Thestrup-Pedersen, K., Detection of interleukin 1 receptor antagonist protein (IRAP), IL-lafla, TNFalfa, their receptors and IL-8 in allergic patch test reactions, submitted for publication.

37. Paludan, K. and Thestrup-Pedersen, K. Quantification of interleukin 8 mRNA in minute epidermal samples of the polymerase chain reaction, *J. Invest. Dermatol.,* 99, 340, 1992.

38. Paludan, K., Lund, M., Larsen, C. G., and Thestrup-Pedersen, K., Time-course studies of the cytokine cascade during allergic and irritant skin reactions in man, in preparation.

39. Larsen, C. G., Anderson, A. O., Appella, E., Oppenheim, J. J., and Matsushima, K., The neutrophil-activating peptide (NAP-1) is also chemotactic for T lymphocytes, *Science,* 243, 1464, 1989.

40. Huber, A. R., Kunkel, S. L., Todd, R. F., and Weiss, S. J., Regulation of transendothelial neutrophil migration by endogenous interleukin-8, *Science,* 254, 99, 1991.

41. Wertheimer, S. J., Myers, C. L., Wallace, R. W., and Parks, T. P., Intercellular adhesion molecule-1 gene expression in human endothelial cells, *J. Biol. Chem.,* 267, 12030, 1992.

42. Zachariae, C., Jinquan, T., Nielsen, V., Kaltoft, K., and Thestrup-Pedersen, K., Phenotypic determination of T-lymphocytes responding to chemotactic stimulation from fMLP, IL-8, human IL-10, and epidermal lymphocyte chemotactic factor, *Arch. Dermatol. Res.,* 284, 333, 1992.

43. Jinquan, T., Larsen, C. G., Gesser, B., Matsushima, K., and Thestrup-Pedersen, K., Human interleukin 10 is a chemoattractant for CD8+ T lymphocytes and an inhibitor of CD4+ T lymphocyte migration, *J. Immunol.,* submitted.

44. Malefyt, R. W., Yssel, H., Roncarolo, M.-G., Spits, H., and de Vriets, J. E., Interleukin-10, *Curr. Opin. Immunol.,* 4, 314, 1992.

3

Chemical Skin Burns

Magnus Bruze and Sigfrid Fregert

CONTENTS

0-8493-7355-7/94/$0.00 + $.50

I. INTRODUCTION

Chemical burns are common, particularly in the industries, but they occur also in the nonworking environment. Occupationally induced chemical burns are frequently seen when visiting and examining workers at their work sites. Corrosive chemicals used in hobbies are an increasing cause of skin burns. Disinfectants and cleansers are examples of household products that can cause chemical burns. However, in most cases with a chemical burn the cause is obvious to the affected persons and the damage is minimal and heals without medical care, so medical attention is not seeked. Sometimes the chemical burns are severe and extensive with the risk of complications and long-term disability. In the acute stage there is a varying risk of systemic effects, including a fatal outcome, depending on exposure conditions and incriminating agent.[1-14] For these reasons it is important for the physician to have knowledge of corrosive chemicals as well as of chemical burns with regard to their clinical manifestations, specific medical treatments, and preventive measures.

II. DEFINITION

A chemical burn, or synonymously caustic burn, is an acute, severe irritant reaction in which the cells have been damaged to a point where there is no return to viability, i.e., a necrosis develops. One single skin exposure to certain chemicals can result in a chemical burn. These chemicals react with intracellular and intercellular components in the skin. However, the action of toxic (irritant) chemicals varies, giving partly different irritant reactions morphologically. They can damage, among other things, the horny layer, cell membranes, lysosomes, mast cells, leukocytes, DNA synthesis, blood vessels, enzyme systems, and metabolism.[15] The corrosive action of chemicals depends on chemical properties of the chemicals, concentration, pH, alkalinity, acidity, temperature of the chemicals, lipid/water solubility, interaction with other substances, and duration and type (e.g., occlusion) of skin contact.[16-20] It also depends on the body region, previous skin damage, and possibly on individual resistance capacity.

Many substances cause chemical burn only when they are applied under occlusion from, for example, gloves, boots, shoes, clothes, caps, face masks, adhesive plasters, and rings.[16,18,19] Skin folds may be formed and act occlusively in certain body regions, e.g., under breasts and in the axillae. Many products, which under ordinary skin exposure conditions cause weak irritant reactions or irritant contact dermatitis, can under occlusion give chemical burns, e.g., detergents, emulsifiers, solvents, plants, woods, topical medicaments, toiletries, insecticides, pesticides, preservatives, cleansers, polishes, plastic monomers, and portland cement.[16,18,19,21-23] For example, white spirit gives only slight dryness at open application but causes blisters under occlusion.[16] Wet cement can usually be handled without giving a chemical burn, but when present under occluding clothes for some hours, it can cause severe skin damage, e.g., on knees.[26-33]

Besides the different mechanisms for reactions with skin components for agents causing chemical and thermal burns, there is also another principal difference between them. The chemical agent causes progressive damage until no more chemical remains unreacted in the tissue or inactivated by treatment, whereas the thermal damaging effect ceases shortly after removal of the heat source.[34]

There are several thousand chemicals that can cause chemical burns and the most commonly reported are listed in Table 1.[1,9] Acids and alkalis have been grouped separately as the corrosive effect within the respective group is excerted through the same mechanism. These groups contain both strong and weak acids and alkalis, respectively. The other compounds are listed together, although their corrosive effects are mediated through different mechanisms. Most of these compounds are neutral. However, some are weak acids or alkalis, but they are considered to be corrosive due to properties other than acidity and alkalinity, respectively.

III. DIAGNOSIS

To arrive at a diagnosis of chemical burn is usually easy because the symptoms are easily recognized and the exposure to a corrosive agent is obvious. However, sometimes the exposure is concealed, at least initially.[18] For example, hospital personnel may be exposed to ethylene oxide, which may remain in gowns and straps after sterilization,[35] and cleaners may occasionally be exposed to a

TABLE 1   Agents Causing Chemical Burns

Acids	Alkalis	Miscellaneous
Acetic acid	Amines	Acetyl chloride
Acrylic acid	Ammonia	Acrolein
Benzoic acid	Barium hydroxide	Acrylonitril
Boric acid	Calcium carbonate	Alkali ethoxides
Bromoacetic acid	Calcium hydroxide	Alkali methoxides
Chloroacetic acids	Calcium oxide	Allyl diiodine
Chlorosulfuric acid	Hydrazine	Aluminium bromide
Fluorophosphoric acid	Lithium hydroxide	Aluminium chloride
Fluorosilicic acid	Lye	Aluminium trichloride
Fluorosulfonic acid	Potassium hydroxide	Ammonium difluoride
Formic acid	Sodium carbonate	Ammonium persulfate
Fumaric acid	Sodium hydroxide	Ammonium sulfide
Hydrobromic acid	Sodium metasilicate	Antimone trioxide
Hydrochloric acid		Aromatic hydrocarbons
Hydrofluoric acid		Arsenic oxides
Lactic acid		Benzene
Nitric acid		Benzoyl chloride
Perchloric acid		Benzoyl chlorodimethyl hydantoin
Peroxyacetic acid		Benzoyl chloroformiate
Phosphonic acids		Borax
Phosphoric acids		Boron tribromide
Phtalic acids		Bromine
Picric acid		Bromotrifluoride
Propionic acid		Calcium carbide
Salicylic acid		Cantharides
Sulfonic acids		Carbon disulfide
Sulfuric acid		Carbon tetrachloride
Tartaric acid		Chlorobenzene
Toluenesulfonic acid		Chlorinated acetophenons (tear gas)
Tungstic acid		Chlorinated solvents
		Chloroform
		Chlorocresols
		Chlorophenols
		Chromates
		Chromium oxichloride
		Chromium trioxide
		Creosote
		Cresolic compounds
		Croton aldehyde
		Dichloroacetyl chloride
		Dichromates
		Dimethyl acetamide
		Dimethyl formamide
		Dimethyl sulfoxide (DMSO)
		Dioxane
		Dipentene
		Dithranol
		Epichlorohydrine
		Epoxy reactive diluents
		Ethylene oxide
		Ferric chloride hexahydrate
		Fluorides
		Fluorine
		Fluorosilicate
		Formaldehyde
		Gasoline
		Gentian violet
		Glutaraldehyde
		Halogenated solvents

TABLE 1   Agents Causing Chemical Burns (continued)

Acids	Alkalis	Miscellaneous
		Hexylresorcinol
		Iodine
		Isocyanates
		Kerosene fuel
		Limonene
		Lithium
		Lithium chloride
		Mercury compounds
		Methylchloroisothiazolinone
		Methylenedichloride
		Methylisothiazolinone
		Morpholine
		Perchloroethylene
		Peroxides
		Benzoyl
		Cumene
		Cyclohexanone
		Hydrogen
		Methylethylketone
		Potassium
		Sodium
		Tetrahydronaphth
		Phenolic compounds
		Phosphorus
		Phosphorus bromides
		Phosphorus chlorides
		Phosphorus oxychloride
		Phosphorus oxides
		Piperazine
		Potassium
		Potassium cyanide
		Potassium difluoride
		Potassium hypochlorite
		Potassium permanganate
		Propionic oxide
		Propylene oxide
		Quaternary ammonium compounds
		Reactive diluents
		Sodium
		Sodium borohydride
		Sodium difluoride
		Sodium hypochlorite
		Sodium sulfite
		Sodium thiosulfate
		Styrene
		Sulfur dichloride
		Sulfur dioxide
		Sulfur mustard
		Thioglycollates
		Thionyl chloride
		Tributyltin oxide
		Trichloroethylene
		Turpentine
		White spirit
		Zinc chloride

Note: The chemicals listed are the most common reported to cause chemical burns in industries, hobbies, and households. The list contains strong corrosive substances and also less irritating compounds that require special conditions, for example, occlusion, to give chemical burns.

corrosive agent contaminating nonhazardous objects in a laboratory. Corrosive substances under occlusion may also, at least initially, confuse and delay the diagnosis.[18] Occasionally, a chemical burn can mimic other dermatoses.[23,35]

IV. CLINICAL FEATURES

Besides skin, eyes, lips, mouth, esophagus, nose septum, glottis, and lungs can also be directly affected. By resorption the toxic chemicals can damage the blood, bone marrow, liver, kidneys, nerves, brain, and other organs.

The most common localization on skin are the hands and face/neck, but the whole body can be affected. The exposure occurs usually by accidents. However, occasionally a chemical burn is the result of malingering. The major symptoms are burning and pain. Morphologically, chemical burns are characterized by erythema, blisters, erosions, ulcers, and necrosis with surrounding erythema. Usually, the symptoms develop immediately or in close connection to exposure, but certain chemicals, such as phenols, weak hydrofluoric acid, and sulfur mustard gas, can give delayed reactions, which first appear several hours, or even a day, after the exposure.[8,27] Occasionally a chemical burn can mimic other skin diseases; for example, ethylene oxide can mimic bullous impetigo and Lyell's disease.[35]

Some common toxic chemicals affect the skin in a special way. Strong acids coagulate skin proteins and by the barrier formed further penetration is decreased. Principally, all strong acids give the same symptoms and major features, including erythema, blisters, and necrosis. Some acids discolor the skin, e.g., a yellow color from nitric acid. The action of hydrofluoric acid in the skin differs from other strong acids.[3-7,9,10] It causes liquefaction necrosis and the penetration may continue for days. When an area above 1% of the total body surface is affected, systemic effects can arise. In the skin this acid causes much stronger pain than other acids. Diluted hydrofluoric acid can cause pain starting several hours or even a day after the exposure. For example, when bricklayers use this acid at a concentration of 10 to 30% for rinsing brick walls, it may penetrate into their nail beds and cause severe pain thereafter several hours.[4,6,36] The strong pain is due to the capacity of fluorine ions to bind calcium in the tissue, which affects the nerve system. Hydrofluoric acid can penetrate to the bone and there cause decalcification.[5,7] Also, fluorides and fluorosilicic acid can give the same type of symptoms.

Alkalis often give more severe damage than acids, except from hydrofluoric acid. The necrotic skin first appears dark brown and then changes to black.[37] Later skin becomes hard, dry, and cracked. Generally, no blisters appear in the skin. Alkalis split proteins and lipids, and there is a saponification of the released fatty acids. The emulsifying effect of the soap formed facilitates further penetration of the alkali into deeper layers of the skin. Chemical burns from alkaline chemicals are more painful than from acids, except from hydrofluoric acid. Because of its alkalinity, cement mixed with water can cause an acute ulcerative damage.[26-33] Severe skin damage has involved the lower limbs, often after kneeling on wet concrete or when it gets inside boots or shoes. Sometimes, necrotic skin appears 8 to 12 h after exposure. Rarely, hands can also be affected, particularly when the insides of gloves have been contaminated. The alkalinity can vary considerably between batches also from the same cement factory.[38]

Phenolic compounds,[9,11] such as phenol, cresol, and chlorocresol, penetrate the skin easily and can damage periferic nerves, resulting in insensibility. Sometimes periferic nerves can be affected without a visible damage in the skin. After exposure to phenolic compounds, the local blood vessels become constricted, which can contribute to the development of the necrosis. Shock and renal damage can appear after absorption of phenolic compounds.

Sulfur mustard, 2,2′dichlorodiethyl sulfide, is a chemical warfare agent.[8,13] It has been dumped into the sea and fishermen have been damaged when getting leaking containers in their nets. The chemical is a viscous liquid below 14°C and a gas above. In the skin the liquid causes blisters and necrosis 10 to 12 h after skin exposure. The gas attacks mainly the eyes and the respiratory organs. Sometimes the skin is also affected by direct contact with the gas and the chemical burn appears then clinically 3 to 6 h after exposure; initial redness is followed by blisters and ulcers.

Ethylene oxide gas used for sterilization of surgical instruments, textile, and plastic material can remain in these objects for several days if not ventilated enough.[35,39] Thus, when hospital personnel handle such objects, there is a possible exposure to ethylene oxide, which is not obvious, and the symptoms with erythema, edema, and large bullae may therefore be misdiagnosed as other skin diseases.[35]

Accidental skin exposure to chemicals under high pressure, for example, hydraulic oil, can result in deep penetration into the skin where a chemical burn with necrosis can develop.

V. TREATMENT

Patients with severe and extensive skin damage and/or with systemic symptoms after exposure to corrosive agents should be treated in intensive care units.[9] It should be noted that hydrofluoric acid or chromic acid exposure affecting only 1% of the total body surface of a person means risk of severe systemic effects.[2,7] Hospitalization is also recommended for persons having concurrent illnesses, implying that they are high-risk patients as well as for persons with chemical burns on the hands, foot, and perineum.[9]

Clothes, watches, rings, shoes, and so on, can be contaminated with the corrosive agent, so they should be taken off. Rinsing with water is the first aid treatment. Preferably tepid running tap water should be used. Irrigation should not be done at high pressure, as the corrosive agent may be splashed on other parts of the body or on the persons treating the burn. It is important that the treatment starts immediately after exposure and that copious volumes of water are supplied, sometimes for hours. Occasionally, chemical burns are caused by corrosive substances insoluble in water; thus, a solution of water and soap should be frequently used instead. However, sometimes specific antidotes for certain types of chemical burns are required.

Theoretically, neutralizing solutions should be an alternative treatment to water after exposure to acids and alkalis. However, neutralization of the corrosive agent with weak acid-base opposites is not recommended for two reasons:[9] (1) irrigation should not be delayed while waiting for a specific antidote (immediate irrigation provides the best removal of the agent), and (2) neutralization of the corrosive agent may produce an exothermic reaction and the heat can cause further damage.

Heat is generated when strong sulfuric acid and phosphorus acid are exposed to water; a thermal burn can thus add to the chemical burn. To prevent this, it is important that copious volumes of running water are applied. Water is contraindicated in extinguishing burning metal fragments of sodium, potassium, and lithium because a chemical burn can be caused by hydroxides formed when water is added to hot metals.[9] These metals spontaneously ignite when exposed to water. Sand can be used to extinguish the burning metal. The burn is then covered with cooking or mineral oil to isolate the metal from water. Metal pieces shall then be mechanically removed. Embedded pieces should be removed surgically. Then the area is irrigated with water to prevent an alkali burn from the hydroxides already formed from the metal and water naturally present in the skin.

Skin exposed to hydrofluoric acid should be carefully irrigated with copious volumes of running tap water and then treated with calcium gluconate gel (2.5%) by massage into the burned skin for at least 30 min (K-Y Jelly, Johnson & Johnson Products, Inc., New Brunswick, NJ[6]).[3-7,9,10] The calcium gluconate gel can also be made by mixing 3.5 g calcium gluconate with 150 g of a water-soluble lubricant.[6] Recently a variation of this treatment was suggested: ten 10 g tablets of calcium carbonate (648 mg) are crushed to a fine powder.[7] The powder is mixed with 20 ml of a water-soluble lubricant to create a slurry. This calcium preparation should be applied repeatedly to the skin until the pain has disappeared. Necrotic tissue should be excised, blisters debrided, and the underlying tissue treated with the calcium preparation. Nails should be removed if the acid penetrates to the nail bed and matrix and causes severe pain there.[6,7,9,10] If there is no effect of the topical treatment within 2 hours, calcium gluconate (10%) should be injected into and under the lesions, 0.5 ml/cm^2. No anesthetics should be given because the disappearance of pain is a sign of successful treatment. Without treatment the burn can continue in depth for several weeks.

Superficial chemical burn from chromic acid with an area greater than 1% of the total body surface implies a high risk of systemic damage to many organs, including erythrocytes.[2] Therefore, immediate irrigation of the burn with copious volumes of water is necessary. Thereafter and within 2 h after the exposure, all burn tissue must be excised.[2] To remove circulating chromium, peritoneal dialysis has to be carried out in the first 24 h.[2] Solid particles of lime, cement, and phosphorus, for example, tend to fix to the skin and should be mechanically removed before or during irrigation.

Among various types of phosphorus, above all white phosphorus is oxidized in air and can ignite spontaneously and thus cause a thermal burn.[9,40,41] Oxidized phosphorus is in water transformed into phosphoric acid, which can cause a chemical burn, so it is important to remove particles mechanically before washing with soap and water. The skin is then washed with copper (II) sulfate in water at 1%, which reacts with phosphorus forming black copper phosphide, which makes remaining phosphorous visible and thus easily removable.[9,40] Wet dressings of copper sulfate should never be applied on wounds because of the risk of systemic copper poisoning.[9] To minimize the cooper absorption a water solution of 5% sodium bicarbonate and 3% copper sulfate suspended in 1% hydroxyethyl cellulose can be used for irrigation instead of the 1% copper sulfate solution.[9] However, copper is a potential toxic substance, which can give systemic effects.[9,40] Copper sulfate must therefore be used only for a few minutes to visualize phosphorus and after mechanical removal of the phosphide, it is important to irrigate the skin with water.

Skin contaminated with bromine or iodine should be washed frequently with soap and water and then treated with 5% sodium thiosulfate, which reacts with bromine and iodine forming ions less hazardous to the skin. Skin contaminated with phenolic compounds can initially be washed with soap and water and as early as possible treated with undiluted polyethylene glycol 300 or 400, or with 10% ethanol, which all dissolve phenolic compounds.[9] Tissue with a deep damage from phenolic compounds should be excised immediately because they easily penetrate further with subsequent nerve damage. Skin contaminated with sulfur mustard liquid should be treated with a mixture of 75% calcium hypochlorite and 25% magnesium sulfate for some minutes before washing with soap and water. Also, contaminated objects should be treated with this mixture. Hot tar, pitch, and asphalt cause a burn mainly due to the heat. They stick to the skin and should not be mechanically removed, as the skin can be more damaged and thus increase the risk of secondary infection. The material will fall off spontaneously in due time.

Generally, an antibacterial cream should be given to chemical skin burns to protect the surface and to prevent secondary infection. If there is a significant element of inflammation in non-necrotic areas, a mild topical corticosteroid preparation can be used. Frequent examinations are advisable also of primarily superficial and limited burns because they can become deeper in a few days.

Surgical treatments, such as excision, debridation of blisters, transplantation, and removal of nails, can be of great value. When a limb is affected circumferentially, there is a risk of blood vessel compression. The best method for treating the black adherent necrotic tissue caused by cement and other toxic compounds is excision. For example, the healing time of cement burns on knees can be diminished from 8 to 10 weeks to 3 weeks.[42] Several chemicals, e.g., phenolic compounds, hydrofluoric acid, chromic acid, sulfur mustard, and gasoline, can also give systemic effects without severe skin injury.[1-13] When the chemical burn is not minimal, there is a risk of systemic damage, and an analysis, including hematological screening, and liver and kidney function, should be made at the first examination and then later in the course governed by the intensity and extension of the chemical burn as well as by the results of the laboratory investigations mainly to enable necessary precautions and measures to prevent and diminish damage on internal organs but also partly for legal reasons.

VI. COMPLICATIONS

Any damage of the skin involving inflammatory processes can cause hyperpigmentation or hypopigmentation. Chemical burns involving deeper parts of the skin heal with scarring. Tumors of both malignant and benign type may rarely develop in scars.[7,43] In the acute stage of chemical burns from, for instance, phenolic compounds and hydrofluoric acid/fluorides, the sensory nerve system is frequently affected. However, long-term hypoesthesia and chronic pain in scarred areas have also been reported.[10]

Many contact sensitizers also have irritant properties. Path testing with such sensitizers at too high concentrations can give an irritant reaction or a chemical burn, which seems to facilitate active sensitization. However, only a few sensitizers can cause chemical burns without occlusion, including formaldehyde, chromic acid, amines, chloroacetophenone, some plastic monomers, and methylisothiazolinones.[2,25,44,45] Even one single contact with these chemicals can both cause a chemical burn and induce sensitization with a subsequent possible development of an allergic contact dermatitis.[25] Therefore, when a potential sensitizer has caused a chemical burn, the patient should be patch tested with the sensitizer after healing of the burn, independent of whether there is subsequent development of an eczema.

Another type of eczematous dermatitis that can follow after a chemical burn is "post-traumatic eczema".[46] It can present as discoid eczema and is a poorly understood complication of skin injuries.[47] It can appear after both physical and chemical skin injuries, including chemical burns and always unrelated to infection and topical treatment.

VII. PREVENTION

Employees should be informed of the risks with exposure to corrosive agents and be well trained to handle the chemicals as well as to act when they have been exposed. Facilities for rapid irrigation with tepid tap water should be easily accessible. A copper sulfate solution at 1%, polyethylene glycol 300 or 400, sodium thiosulfate solution at 5%, and a proper calcium preparation should be present in the first aid kit. A calcium preparation for topical treatment should also be present near the employee's work site with hydrofluoric acid or fluorides. Workers at risk should wear proper protective equipment, which may include eye glasses, face masks, gloves, boots, and safety dresses.

In industries in which corrosive chemicals are handled, certain procedures are frequently encountered in accidents resulting in exposure to the chemicals. Such procedures are repairing as well as charging and discharging of procedure vessels, when chemicals can be spilled and splashed. Accidents can be caused by breakage of hoses or connections with snap couplings.[48] A nonaccidental but unintended exposure may occur to material sterilized with ethylene oxide; the material should thus be well ventilated and not used until a week after the sterilization procedure. For these reasons it is important to maintain careful planning and supervision of the work environment to prevent chemical burns.

VIII. SUMMARY

Many thousands of chemicals and products can cause chemical skin burns, some only under special circumstances, for example, occlusion. Most chemical burns are due to accidents and the majority are occupationally induced, but chemical burns also frequently occur in hobbies and households. Clinically a chemical burn is characterized by erythema, blisters, and necrotic skin. Some corrosive chemicals, such as phenolic compounds, sulfur mustard, chromic acid, hydrofluoric acid, and gasoline, may cause systemic effects that require hospitalization. Other chemical burns, particularly those affecting the hands, feet, and perineum, may also require hospitalization. To prevent and diminish the damage after exposure to corrosive agents, immediate treatment is important. Irrigation with copious volumes of water is a universal remedy, except for treatment of burning metal fragments of sodium, potassium, and lithium. First aid treatment after exposure to water-insoluble corrosive agents is washing with soap and water. Sometimes specific antidotes are needed as for chemical burns from hydrofluoric acid, phenolic compounds, phosphorus, iodine, bromine, and sulfur mustard. Surgical intervention may be required for certain chemical burns. A few corrosive compounds are potential sensitizers and one single exposure to such a compound may both give a chemical burn and induce sensitization with a subsequent allergic contact dermatitis. To prevent chemical burns, it is important to use as few corrosive agents as possible, and when unreplaceable, to use as weak ones as possible, particularly in hobbies and households. In the working environment well-informed workers, access to first aid treatment, and careful planning and supervision are required to prevent chemical burns.

REFERENCES

1. Moran, K. D., O'Reilly, T. O., and Münster, A. M., Chemical burns: a ten-year experience, *Am. Surg.*, 53, 652, 1987.
2. Terrill, P. J. and Gowar, J. P., Chromic acid burns; beware, be aggressive, be watchful, *Br. J. Plast. Surg.*, 43, 699, 1990.
3. Von Dieterle, R., Zur Therapie der Flusssäureverätzung, *Dermatosen*, 37, 26, 1989.
4. MacKinnon, M. A., Hydrofluoric acid burns, *Dermatol. Clin.*, 6, 67, 1988.
5. Tremel, H., Brunier, A., and Weilemann, L. S., Flusssäureverätzungen: Vorkommen, Häufigkeit sowie aktueller Stand der Therapie, *Med. Klin.*, 86, 71, 1991.
6. Anderson, W. I. and Anderson, J. R., Hydrofluoric acid burns of the hand: mechanism of injury and treatment, *J. Hand Surg.*, 13A, 52, 1988.
7. Chick, L. R. and Borah, G., Calcium carbonate gel therapy for hydrofluoric acid burns of the hand, *Plast. Reconstr. Surg.*, 86, 935, 1990.
8. Smith, W. J. and Dunn, M. A., Medical defense against blistering chemical warfare agents, *Arch. Dermatol.*, 127, 1207, 1991.
9. Stewart, C. E., Chemical skin burns, *Am. Fam. Physician*, 31, 149, 1985.
10. Vance, M. V., Hydrofluoric acid (HF) burns, in *Occupational Skin Disease*, 2nd ed., Adams, R. M., Ed., W. B. Saunders, Philadelphia, 1990, 18.
11. Anderson, K. E., Systemic toxicity from percutaneous absorption of industrial chemicals, in *Occupational Skin Disease*, 2nd ed., Adams, R. M., Ed., W. B. Saunders, Philadelphia, 1990, 73.
12. Schneider, M. S., Mani, M. M., and Masters, F. W., Gasoline-induced contact burns, *J. Burn Care Rehab.*, 12, 140, 1991.
13. Newman-Taylor, A. J. and Morris, A. J. R., Experience with mustard gas casualties, *Lancet*, 337, 242, 1991.
14. Sykes, R. A., Mani, M. M., and Hiebert, J. M., Chemical burns: retrospective review, *J. Burn Care Rehab.*, 7, 343, 1986.
15. Björnberg, A., *Skin Reactions to Primary Irritants in Patients with Hand Eczema*, Thesis, Göteborg, Sweden, 1968.
16. Fregert, S., Chemical burns, in *Manual of Contact Dermatitis*, 2nd ed., Munksgaard, Copenhagen, 1981, 61.
17. Berner, B., Wilson, D. R., Guy, R. H., Mazzenga, G. C., Clarke, F. H., and Maibach, H. I., The relationship of primary skin irritation and pK_a in man, in *Exogenous Dermatoses*, Menné, T. and Maibach, H. I., Eds., CRC Press, Boca Raton, FL, 1991, 37.
18. Dickinson, J. C. and Bailey, B. N., Chemical burns beneath tourniquets, *Br. Med. J.*, 297, 1513, 1988.
19. White, A. and Joseet, M., Burns from iodine, *Anaethesia*, 45, 75, 1990.
20. Farkas, J., Caustic ulcers from lime dust, *Contact Dermatitis*, 7, 59, 1981.
21. Hausen, B. M., Primary irritant skin lesions, in *Woods Injurious to Human Health: A Manual*, Hausen, B. M., Ed., Walter de Gruyter, Berlin, 1981, 7.
22. Kynaston, J. A., Patrick, M. K., Shepherd, R. W., Raivadera, P. V., and Cleghorn, G. J., The hazards of automatic-dishwasher detergent, *Med. J. Austr.*, 151, 5, 1989.
23. Mosconi, G., Migliori, M., Greco, V., and Valsecchi, R., Kerosene "burns": a new case, *Contact Dermatitis*, 19, 314, 1988.
24. Larsen, J., Jörgensen, J., Weismann, K., and Thomsen, H. K., Petroleum burns: toxic contact dermatitis (in Danish, summary in English), *Ugeskr. Laeg.*, 151, 3490, 1989.
25. Bruze, M., Dahlquist, I., and Gruvberger, B., Chemical burns and allergic contact dermatitis due to Kathon WT, *Am. J. Contact Dermatitis*, 1, 91, 1990.
26. Fisher, A. A., Chromate dermatitis and cement burns, in *Contact Dermatitis*, 3rd ed., Fisher, A. A., Ed., Lea & Febiger, Philadelphia, 1986, 762.
27. Adams, R. M., Cement burns, in *Occupational Skin Disease*, 2nd ed., Adams, R. M., Ed., W. B. Saunders, Philadelphia, 1990, 15.
28. Lane, P. R. and Hogan, D. J., Chronic pain and scarring from cement burns, *Arch. Dermatol.*, 121, 368, 1985.

29. Vickers, H. R. and Edwards, D. H., Cement burns, *Contact Dermatitis,* 2, 73, 1976.

30. Stoermer, D. and Wolz, G., Cement burns, *Contact Dermatitis,* 9, 421, 1983.

31. McGeown, G., Cement burns of the hands, *Contact Dermatitis,* 10, 246, 1984.

32. Tosti, A., Peluso, A. M., and Varotti, C., Skin burns due to transit-mixed Portland cement, *Contact Dermatitis,* 21, 58, 1989.

33. Onuba, O. and Essiet, A., Cement burns of the heels, *Contact Dermatitis,* 14, 325, 1986.

34. Curreri, P. W., Burns, in *Principles of Surgery,* 3rd ed., Schwartz, S. I., Ed., McGraw-Hill, New York, 1979, 285.

35. Biro, L., Fisher, A. A., and Price, E., Ethylene oxide burns, *Arch. Dermatol.,* 110, 924, 1974.

36. Baran, R. L., Occupational nail disorders, in *Occupational Skin Disease,* 2nd ed., Adams, R. M., Ed., W. B. Saunders, Philadelphia, 1990, 160.

37. Sawhney, C. P. and Kaushish, R., Acid and alkali burns: considerations in management, *Burns,* 15, 132, 1989.

38. Fregert, S. and Gruvberger, B., Chemical properties of cement, *Berufs-Dermatosen,* 20, 238, 1972.

39. Fisher, A. A., Ethylene oxide (EO) burns, in *Occupational Skin Disease,* 2nd ed., Adams, R. M., Ed., W. B. Saunders, Philadelphia, 1990, 17.

40. Eldad, A. and Simon, G. A., The phosphorous burn: a preliminary comparative experimental study of various forms of treatment, *Burns,* 17, 198, 1991.

41. Kaufman, T., Ullmann, Y., and Har-Shai, Y., Phosphorus burns: a practical approach to local treatment, *J. Burn Care Rehabil.,* 9, 474, 1988.

42. Fregert, S. and Dahlquist, I., Letter to the editor, *Contact Dermatitis,* 9, 243, 1983.

43. Kennedy, C. T. C., Reactions to mechanical and thermal injury, in *Textbook of Dermatology,* 5th ed., Champion, R. H., Burton, J. L., and Ebling, F. J. G., Eds., Blackwell Scientific, Oxford, 1992, 777.

44. Sagi, A., Bibi, C., and Ben Meir, P., Skin injury following contact with a complex amine, *Burns,* 14, 495, 1988.

45. Fisher, A. A., Dermatitis due to gases and propellants, in *Contact Dermatitis,* 3rd ed., Fisher, A. A., Ed., Lea & Febiger, Philadelphia, 1986, 470.

46. Mathias, C. G. T., Post-traumatic eczema, *Dermatol. Clin.,* 6, 35, 1988.

47. Wilkinson, D. S., Discoid eczema as a consequence of contact with irritants, *Contact Dermatitis,* 5, 118, 1979.

48. Hansen, T. B., Occupational accidents resulting from breakages of connections on hoses (in Danish, summary in English), *Ugeskr. Laeg.,* 153, 715, 1991.

4

Mechanical Trauma and Hand Eczema

Klaus E. Andersen

CONTENTS

I. INTRODUCTION

Eczema patients may explain that their eczema appeared after an injury to the skin. It may be a casual coincidence in some cases. However, mechanical trauma may also precipitate eczema.[1-4] Further, patients with a preexisting skin disease may experience localized aggravation of the disorder as a consequence of mechanical trauma to the site. If a dynamic relationship between trauma and the development of hand eczema is made probable, and no other cause can be found, then it has important medicolegal implications when the injury is job-related. This chapter describes aspects of hand eczema related to mechanical injury and repeated friction.

II. INDIVIDUAL FACTORS

It is likely that genetic conditions play a role in determining the response of the skin to mechanical strain. Exacerbation of atopic dermatitis and psoriasis (both partly inheritable skin diseases) may occur after mechanical trauma. Physiological factors, such as the hydration of the skin, are important. Moderate sweating hydrates the corneal layer and increases the coefficient of friction, whereas very dry or very wet skin diminishes the frictional resistance.[5] Neurological diseases may impair the withdrawal response to mechanical stimuli and lead to injury of the skin.

III. CAUSES AND FREQUENCY OF OCCUPATIONAL SKIN INJURIES

By convention, traumatic injuries result from single and brief episodes of cutaneous exposure and a subsequently rapid onset of skin ailment, whereas irritant cutaneous reactions require multiple and prolonged exposures and show a relatively delayed onset of the disorder. Table 1 lists the leading causes of job-related skin injuries in the U.S. The National Institute for Occupational Safety and Health (NIOSH) has estimated that the annual rate of occupational skin injury is 1.4 to 2.2 per 100 full-time workers.[2] In most cases the hands are probably involved, but exact figures are missing. Common complications of skin injuries include scar formation, infection, persistent pain, and contact dermatitis from topical drugs used for treatment. However, local eczema may also appear.

IV. HAND ECZEMA FOLLOWING A MECHANICAL INJURY

Post-traumatic eczema is a poorly understood complication of skin injuries caused by thermal or chemical burns, lacerations, punctures, abrasions, or chemical injury.[2] The interval between the trauma and the development of eczema is usually a few weeks. Mathias[2] divided post-traumatic

TABLE 1   Leading Causes of Occupational Skin Injuries in the U.S.

Injury type	% of total skin injuries
Lacerations, punctures	86.2
Burns, nonchemical	8.3
Foreign bodies	3.5
Burns, chemical	1.9
Radiation	0.1

Note: The percentages are based on estimates from cases reported to the National Electronic Injury Surveillance System (NEISS) by selected hospital emergency rooms in 1985.

Adapted from Mathias, C. G. T., Post-traumatic eczema, *Dermatol. Clin.*, 6, 35, 1988.

TABLE 2   Classification of Post-Traumatic Eczema

Isomorphic reaction
    Primary, precedes endogenous eczema
    Secondary, follows endogenous eczema
Idiopathic reaction, endogenous eczema absent

Adapted from Mathias, C. G. T., Post-traumatic eczema, *Dermatol. Clin.*, 6, 35, 1988.

eczema into two types. It may occur in association with an underlying endogenous eczema (isomorphic reaction or Koebner's phenomenon) or occur as an isolated idiopathic reaction, when longtime follow-up shows that no new lesions develop on nontraumatized skin (Table 2).

Koebner's phenomenon is the term applied when a dermatosis develops at the site of trauma.[6] It is well known in relation to psoriasis but also occurs in other conditions, such as lichen planus, vitiligo, Darier's disease, and discoid lupus erythematosus. Isomorphic reactions may also be seen in patients with eczema during its active phases.[7] The isomorphic reaction may be the primary manifestation of an endogenous eczema, and probably more frequently it occurs as a secondary eczema at the site of trauma. The clinical features of post-traumatic eczema are indistinguishable from typical eczema. Often, it presents within a few weeks of the acute injury as a discoid or nummular eczema with or without vesicles around the site of trauma. The trauma itself causes obvious damage accompanied by inflammation and regeneration. The post-traumatic eczema may persist or recur for a long time. The differential diagnoses include noneczematous skin diseases associated with Koebner's phenomenon, foreign body reactions, bacterial infections, herpes simplex recidivans, and a secondary allergic contact dermatitis to topical preparations.

V.   HAND ECZEMA FOLLOWING REPEATED FRICTION

Repeated minor mechanical trauma to the skin, such as friction, pressure, abrasion, punctures, and shearing forces, can cause a variety of skin changes including dermatitis.[8,9] Callosities and corns are in certain occupations regarded as a ''badge of the trade'' not leading to physical impairment affecting job function or quality of life. They rarely evoke complaints and affect the majority of persons engaged in the same work. Dermatitis from friction affects only a small proportion of exposed individuals, depending on constitutional factors and special patterns of exposure. The effects of mechanical forces may be accentuated by other physical agents, such as heat and cold.

In a few cases frictional dermatitis may develop into a dermatological problem requiring medical attention.[10-13] An acute frictional dermatitis (when repeated several times) can develop into a chronic hand dermatitis.[14] The frictional dermatitis may be elicited by carbonless copy paper paper, bus tickets,[13] artificial fur,[14] pantyhose,[15] and other items with a rough surface handled frequently over long periods of time.[12] The scarcity of reports in the literature suggests that hand eczema from repeated mechanical trauma is often mild and that the patients solve the problems themselves by the trial-and-error method. However, frictional dermatitis may go unrecognized. Mechanical injuries may be an aggravating factor, which in addition to constitutional factors, irritants, and allergens may intensify the degree of hand eczema. Meneghini[16] reported that contact allergy was more prevalent among workers who had sustained cuts, abrasions, and other mechanical injuries compared with those who had not.

REFERENCES

1. Cronin, E., Hand eczema, in *Textbook of Contact Dermatitis,* Rycroft, R. J. G., Menné, T., Frosch, P. J., and Benezra, C., Eds., Springer-Verlag, Berlin, 1992, 207.
2. Mathias, C. G. T., Post-traumatic eczema, *Dermatol. Clin.,* 6, 35, 1988.
3. Calnan, C., Eczema for me, *Trans. St. John's Hosp. Dermatol. Soc.,* 54, 54, 1968.
4. Wilkinson, D. S., Letter to the editor, *Contact Dermatitis,* 5, 118, 1979.
5. Naylor, P. F. D., The skin surface and friction, *Br. J. Dermatol.,* 67, 239, 1955.

6. Kennedy, C. T. C., Reactions to mechanical and thermal injury, in *Textbook of Dermatology,* 5th ed., Champion, R. H., Burton, J. L., and Ebling, F. J. G., Eds., Blackwell Scientific, Oxford, 1992, 777.

7. Rook, A. and Wilkinson, D. S., The principles of diagnosis, in *Textbook of Dermatology,* 3rd ed., Rook, A., Wilkinson, D. S., and Ebling, F. J. G., Eds., Blackwell Scientific, Oxford, 1979, 47.

8. Susten, A. S., The chronic effects of mechanical trauma to the skin: a review of the literature, *Am. J. Ind. Med.,* 8, 281, 1985.

9. Schwartz, L., Tulipan, L., and Birmingham, D. J., Dermatoses caused by physical and mechanical agents, in *Occupational Diseases of the Skin,* 3rd ed., Henry Kimpton, London, 1957, 126.

10. Grimalt, F. and Romaguera, C., Dry and fissured skin limited to the index finger of the right hand as a unique manifestation of housewife dermatitis, *Contact Dermatitis,* 3, 54, 1977.

11. Malten, K. E., Thoughts on irritant contact dermatitis, *Contact Dermatitis,* 7, 238, 1981.

12. Menné, T., Friction dermatitis in post-office workers, *Contact Dermatitis,* 9, 172, 1983.

13. Menné, T. and Hjorth, N., Frictional contact dermatitis, *Am. J. Ind. Med.,* 8, 401, 1985.

14. Paulsen, E. and Andersen, K. E., Irritant contact dermatitis of a gardener's hands caused by handling of fur-covered plant ornaments, *Am. J. Contact Dermatitis,* 2, 113, 1991.

15. Gould, W. M., Friction dermatitis of the thumbs caused by pantyhose, *Arch. Dermatol.,* 127, 1740, 1991.

16. Meneghini, C. L., Sensitization in traumatized skin, *Am. J. Ind. Med.,* 8, 319, 1985.

5

Irritant Contact Dermatitis

Henk B. van der Walle

CONTENTS

0-8493-7355-7/94/$0.00 + $.50
© 1994 by CRC Press, Inc.

I. DEFINITION

Irritant contact dermatitis is a localized nonimmunological inflammatory response to one or more external agents. These agents are called irritants. Any agent that produces damage is an irritant. Damage is caused by the chemical, physical, or mechanical properties of the agent. The dermatitis may be caused just by one agent, by repetition of the same agent in time, or as the cumulative effect of minor damage caused by a wide variety of different agents to which the skin is exposed simultaneously or one after the other.

II. INTRODUCTION

In the general population the incidence of hand eczema varies between 2 and 10%.[1-3] In high-risk occupations, such as hairdressing, cleaning, agriculture, construction, and steelworkers, the incidence may occasionally increase to 40%. Dermatological disorders are responsible for 30 to 40% of all occupational diseases. Scientific reports gradually show an increase of interest in irritant contact dermatitis, but most reports are still dealing with allergic contact dermatitis. In the 1970s Malten[4,5] stimulated the development and application of noninvasive techniques to investigate the damaging effects of irritants on the human skin. With water vapor loss measurements he was able to prove the concept of the cumulative irritant contact dermatitis (Plate 1*).

Irritant contact dermatitis is caused by an overbalance of irritant factors in relation to the defense and repairing capacity of the skin. The clinical picture of contact dermatitis of the hands shows a variety of expressions, which ranges from the typical oligomorphic picture of dermatitis to the classic polymorphic picture of eczema. Both pictures may be an expression of an irritant or allergic contact dermatitis. The final diagnosis is based on a combination of history, clinical picture, and patch test results. The diagnosis is the starting point for the management and treatment of the individual patient and, if necessary, for adaptations in the work environment.

III. CLINICAL PICTURE

The clinical picture is the visual outcome of the dynamic interaction between the chemical, physical, and mechanical characteristics of the irritant and the biological make-up of the exposed skin. A great variety of factors, either belonging to the irritant and/or the involved skin of the individual, is responsible for the degree of damage. The spectrum of irritant contact dermatitis varies from invisible sensations, such as stinging, burning, pain, and itching, to clinical signs, such as erythema, vesicles, blisters, necrosis, papules, scaling and fissures. In other words, the clinical picture varies from monomorph with one typical lesion, for example, a blister, to a clear polymorphic picture, clinically indistinguishable from a classic eczema.[5] The clinical picture shows a variation in time, strongly influenced by the repairing capacity of the skin, the variation in exposure to the irritants, and the applied treatment.

Hand dermatitis may show a course with improvements and exacerbations, which implies that the dermatologist is often not confronted with the dermatitis in its most active phase. In some cases it is useful to request the patient to return when the dermatitis is relapsing. An allergic eczematous contact dermatitis may show an oligomorphic aspect in its healing phase when the exposure to the allergen is omitted, or the reaction is suppressed by local corticosteroids.

Acute contact dermatitis develops after a single exposure to an irritant, the damaging force of which immediately overwhelms the defense capacity of the exposed skin. The skin may react with erythema, blisters, pustules, and necrosis, accompanied by a stinging, burning, or painful sensation. The lesions are sharply demarcated and often restricted to small spots or to a certain area of the hands. The most severe damage is seen at those places where the concentration or intensity of the offending agent was the highest or the defense capacity of the skin the lowest. The clinical picture depends strongly on the characteristics of the involved skin and the properties of the irritant. For example, a droplet of a strong alkaline solution may cause necrosis when spilled on the dorsum of the hand, but the thick stratum corneum of the palmar side may restrict the damage to a painful sensation, with erythema or a small blister.

---

* All color plates follow p. 48.

Cumulative irritant contact dermatitis is caused by the repetition of the same damaging factor or the cumulative effect of a variety of minor damaging factors. In many wet work occupations the clinical normal skin is damaged on subclinical level by exposure to water, soap, and detergents. A slight erythema with fine scaling is the first visible sign of damage. A sudden change in occupational exposure or in climate conditions[6] may push the damage from the subclinical level over the edge to a clearly visible contact dermatitis with redness, edema, scaling, chapping (fissures in the horny layer), erythema craquelé (fissures into the epidermis), or even to hemorrhagic fissures caused by cracks into the dermis. In long-standing cases of cumulative irritant contact dermatitis the clinical picture may vary from a dry palmar dermatitis with erythema, fine scaling, chapping, and shiny fingertips, in "wear and tear" dermatitis, as seen in cleaning and housekeeping, to a more ezcematous dermatitis with erythema, edema, itch and lichenification.

Any part of the hands may be involved in cumulative irritant contact dermatitis, but there are general characteristics. Chapping, for example, is predominantly seen on the back of the hands, whereas fissures and cracks are seen on the dorsal bending parts of the fingers and in the palm of the hand. Fissures and cracks at the fingertips often occur in occupations with prolonged exposure to organic solvents as in painters and offset printers. Finger-web dermatitis occurs in wet work occupations and may spread to the back of the hands, a scenario often seen in hairdressers and restaurant workers. The localization of contact dermatitis may be determined by the use of the right or left hand in certain occupations. If the dominant hand is exposed to the irritant, the dermatitis will occur on this hand, but in many occupations the dominant hand is used for handling tools or instruments and the nondominant hand is exposed to wet work and irritants. A classic example is a cumulative irritant contact dermatitis on the fingertips of the "wet hand" or "working hand" of the hairdresser, which is the nondominant hand. In occupations with wear and tear irritants, as in agriculture, the dermatitis often occurs on the first three fingers of the hands. Sometimes a contact dermatitis occurs on one or two fingers while all fingers are exposed in the same way to the same irritants. Obviously the barrier function or defense capacity of the individual fingers varies in the same patient.

Nails and fingertips are often involved in cumulative irritant contact dermatitis. The nail may show onycholysis, subungual hyperkeratosis, and textural irregularities of the nail plate with pitting and transverse depressions. Painful fissures and cracks occur at the transition of nail plate to fingertip. Wear and tear and chemical exposure may damage the fingertips with painful cracks, lamellar scaling, and abrasion of the epidermis.

IV. DIAGNOSIS

The diagnosis is based on the combination of data, obtained in history, with clinical investigation, and patch testing and, if necessary, with information or the results of investigation at the workplace. In general, histology of skin biopsy and monoclonal analysis of dermal infiltrates offer no typical clues to establish the diagnosis of irritant contact dermatitis.[7] The clinical picture should be carefully examined, and one should keep in mind that in general there is no single characteristic in the clinical picture of cumulative irritant contact dermatitis that makes the diagnosis certain. The examination should focus on localization, demarcation, and morphological expressions, such as redness, vesicles, blisters, necrosis, papules, scaling, fissures, or eczema. Besides the lesions on the hands, other skin parts should also be examined and special attention must be paid to the skin of the face and neck because many occupational dermatoses occur on both the hands and the face. Finally, the patient should be examined for minor and major signs of atopy, psoriasis, and active eczema.

The characteristics of the clinical picture are important facts to guide the questioning. An extensive history of the patient's daily activities at work, in hobbies, and at home is essential. A thorough knowledge of a variety of occupations is important; sometimes it is necessary to visit the workplace or to consult the occupational hygienist to obtain a good impression of the exposure in the occupation. Attention should be paid to the use of gloves, skin care products at work and at home, and the use of medications, both by prescription and over the counter. The course of the dermatitis may offer important clues for the final diagnosis. The dermatologist must search for a relation between improvements and relapses of the dermatitis and activities in occupation, the home environment, within weekends, holidays, sick leave, the use of gloves, and so on. The healing time of a cumulative irritant contact dermatitis after omitting the exposure to irritants is rather slow, in contrary to an allergic contact dermatitis, where avoidance of the allergen may lead to a rapid reduction of symptoms. Reexposure to the allergen aggravates the symptoms within 1 or 2 days while reexposure to minor irritants gradually aggravates the dermatitis in 1 or 2 weeks.

Patch testing is obligatory in all cases of hand dermatitis. The testing should focus on exposure to allergens in the occupation, the home environment, and to skin care products and cosmetics. Screening series of standardized allergens, related to the occupation of the patient, should be, if necessary, supplemented with materials from the work environment of the patient. The reliability of positive reactions to own materials should always be checked in patch testing of control persons and, if necessary, repeated with a dilution series. The information obtained in history, clinical examination, and patch testing will make the diagnosis cumulative irritant contact dermatitis very likely, likely, or uncertain. The interpretation of positive patch test reactions should be made carefully. A negative reaction may support the diagnosis of an irritant contact dermatitis, but it may be a false-negative reaction or an important allergen may simply be missed. In the same careful way a positive reaction should be interpreted. The reaction may be either false-positive or have no relevance to the dermatitis on the hands. In many cases the dermatologist deals with a combination of allergic and irritant contact dermatitis, aggravated by endogenous factors.

V. DIFFERENTIAL DIAGNOSIS

The differentiation of cumulative irritant contact dermatitis from another dermatitis or eczematous lesion of the skin is a challenge for the dermatologist with a moderate success rate. Atopic dermatitis often occurs on the hands in young adults and is provoked and aggravated in occupations with a high exposure to water and irritants, such as hairdressing, cleaning, and housekeeping.[8,9] It is often difficult to weight the individual role of irritants and atopic consitution. In many cases it is the atopic disorder of the skin that is primarily responsible for the development of a cumulative irritant contact dermatitis. Psoriasis of the hands can imitate an eczema or an irritant contact dermatitis.[10] Careful examination of the whole skin to look for minor signs of psoriasis is important. In the follow-up of these patients a psoriasis may be developed in other areas. Somtimes a combination of atopy and psoriasis occurs on the hands with itchy vesicles. Some of these patients experience a sudden aggravation of the dermatitis after exposure to water. Tinea of the hands may simulate a dry palmar dermatitis. A unilateral localization and involvement of the nails are important clues to diagnose a tinea. Prolonged exposure to organic solvents may cause a scaly, fissured, hyper- keratotic skin on the palmar side of the hands, which has to be differentiated from the hyperkeratotic palmar eczema (tylotic eczema).

The differentiation between a cumulative irritant and an allergic contact dermatitis is a great challenge but not often possible (Figure 1). In general, an allergic contact dermatitis is more polymorphic with an unsharp demarcation, a tendency for spreading, with sometimes localizations at wrist, forearm, and the face, especially on the eyelids. The course is often relapsing with improvement during weekends and holidays. In the work environment only one or a few persons are affected and a relevant positive patch test makes the diagnosis definite. Especially in cases of fingertip dermatitis and eczema is it impossible to differentiate an allergic contact dermatitis from a cumulative irritant contact dermatitis or psoriasis. Long-standing cases of allergic contact der- matitis with a lichenified character (nickel and chromate allergies) may change in character from eczematous to more psoriasis-like.

A typical Type I allergy causes a contact urticaria lesion, but daily exposure to allergens in patients with Type I allergies may cause a persistent dermatitis with eczematous aspects. This frequently occurs in occupations with intense exposure to biological materials, for example, exposure to vegetables, fish, and meat in kitchens, wheat, flavors, and fruits in bakeries, and meat in slaughterhouses. Pompholyx (dyshidrotic eczema) may be caused by irritants as is described in metalworkers.[11] In many cases the combination of constitutional, irritant, and allergic factors is the cause of a chronic hand dermatitis. The start is often an irritant or allergic contact dermatitis, but the dermatitis may continue after avoiding irritants and allergens as a constitutional post-insult form of eczema.[12]

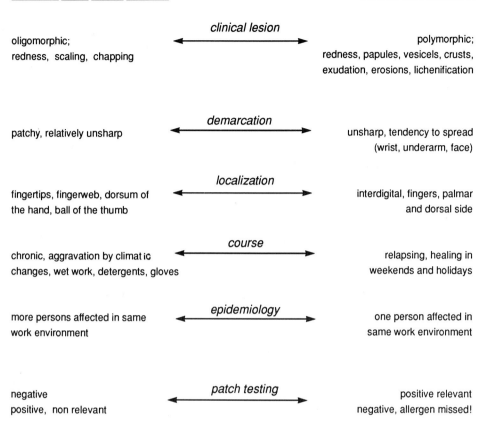

cumulative irritant contact dermatitis | | allergic contact dermatitis

clinical lesion

oligomorphic; redness, scaling, chapping ←————→ polymorphic; redness, papules, vesicels, crusts, exudation, erosions, lichenification

demarcation

patchy, relatively unsharp ←————→ unsharp, tendency to spread (wrist, underarm, face)

localization

fingertips, fingerweb, dorsum of the hand, ball of the thumb ←————→ interdigital, fingers, palmar and dorsal side

course

chronic, aggravation by climatic changes, wet work, detergents, gloves ←————→ relapsing, healing in weekends and holidays

epidemiology

more persons affected in same work environment ←————→ one person affected in same work environment

patch testing

negative positive, non relevant ←————→ positive relevant negative, allergen missed!

FIGURE 1. Characteristics of occupational hand dermatitis; cumulative irritant versus allergic contact dermatitis.

VI. PATHOPHYSIOLOGY

The chemical, physical, or mechanical properties of an irritant may damage a variety of intercellular and cellular structures and molecules, which for each individual has their own characteristics. The interaction between these components of the skin and the characteristics of the irritant may lead to a disturbance in the metabolism and histological or anatomical structures of the skin. Gradually the different ways of action of irritants are unraveled.[13,14] Detergents are damaging the horny layer and cellular membranes and stimulate DNA synthesis and epidermal metabolism, leading to acanthosis. Others, including phorbol esters and croton oil, stimulate the activity of leukocytes and their migration. Organic solvents quickly penetrate the epidermis and directly attack the blood vessels in the dermis, causing hyperemia.

The irritant effect of water is an intriguing phenomenon. The overhydration of the skin in wet work occupations not only enhances the penetration of many irritants but may release inflammatory mediators and their inhibitors from the stratum corneum, the mechanism of which may lead to a gradual damage of the skin. Irritants cause in first instance damage on the subclinical level, which is demonstrated by noninvasive methods, such as transepidermal water loss and laser Doppler flowmetry. These methods have shown that the skin reacts in different ways to the exposure of irritants.[15] First, there is a strong repairing and hardening mechanism that limits the progression to a visible contact dermatitis and enables the skin to withstand the daily exposure to a great variety of low-grade irritants. If the cumulative effect of the repeated exposure to one irritant or to a variety of different irritants gradually breaches the stratum corneum skin barrier, the defense and repairing capacity of the skin is overwhelmed and a visible cumulative irritant contact dermatitis develops. In its most classic form there is a slight erythema with fine scales, a tendency to chapping, some itch, and ill-defined dermarcation. This scenario is often seen in wet work occupations, such as hairdressing, housekeeping, and cleaning work. In these occupations the daily exposure to water, soap, detergents, and other irritants gradually causes an irritant contact dermatitis, which is often suddenly provoked by an increase in work load, for example, in hairdressing in the weeks before Christmas, or by a sudden change in climate, often from humid with low pressure to days with high pressure and dry wind.[6] A fully developed cumulative contact dermatitis is often maintained by the exposure to low-grade irritants, which normally are innocuous to the skin.

Several exogenous and endogenous factors may influence the development or course of a cumulative irritant contact dermatitis. An increase in temperature, a low environmental humidity, and exposure under occlusion, which causes hyperhydration of the skin, make the skin more susceptible for irritation.[16] Atopy is the most imporatant endogenous factor that negatively influences the response of the skin to an irritant. Individuals with a hyperirritable skin do exist without relation to race or atopy. There seems to be an association with light skin type I and II and with a high baseline transepidermal water loss.[17] Increased susceptibility to some irritants occurs in eczematous patients or in patients with an active skin ulceration (e.g., leg ulcer).[18]

VII.   MANAGEMENT AND TREATMENT

Because cumulative irritant contact dermatitis is caused by an overbalance of irritant exogenous factors in relation to the defense and repairing capacity of the skin, which in some patients is influenced by endogenous factors such as atopy and hyperirritable skin, management and treatment should be directed to restoring this balance by the following:

1. A reduction of the irritant factors
2. Protection of the skin
3. Enhancement of the defense and repairing capacity of the skin

This implies that for every patient a tailored treatment and management plan should be made. If the patient is a representative of a profession with a high incidence of irritant contact dermatitis, initiatives should be taken to change working conditions by consultancy and cooperation with occupational hygienists, management of the factory, and producers of materials involved. The basis for action is reduction of the possibilities to expose the skin to a wide variety of irritants and water. It is often necessary to change work procedures, to introduce instruments and tools, to modify the application form of products, and to supply adequate protective materials (e.g., gloves). In the meantime the individual patient has to be treated, which is directed to protection and local treatment of the skin. Protection can sometimes be obtained by using the right gloves on the right place. It is important to select the adequate type of glove and to instruct the patient on how and when to use the gloves. The choice of gloves should be based on the requirements of the occupation. Some chemicals degrade the polymer of the glove or penetrate the glove material easily.[19] The elasticity, thickness, and type of glove polymer greatly determines the acceptability of a certain type of glove for a certain task. Damaging factors at home and with hobbies should not be overlooked. The patient has to be instructed to take care with dish washing, hair washing, and all other activities at home in which contact with water, detergents, or organic solvents may occur. In severe cases the patient may be instructed to use a simple polyethylene glove when washing hair, buy a dishwasher, and use gloves when doing dirty work to avoid the use of strong detergents to clean the skin afterwards.

Barrier creams do not really exist, but some ointments show some protective effect, especially to the exposure of water and water-soluble irritants. The acceptability of this "barrier cream" depends strongly on the cosmetic acceptance of the product. Ointments that stay sticky are not accepted. Some glycerine-containing ointments are not sticky or greasy a few minutes after the application and may be beneficial to a certain degree in the protection of the skin in wet work professions.[20] Special attention should be given to the cleaning of the skin. It should be as mild as possible, and the patient should avoid the use of hard brushes or other abrasives.

Medical treatment is based on the severity of the contact dermatitis and occurrence of endogenous factors. No medication should be chosen that contains ingredients that irritate the skin and/or have a negative effect on the defense capacity of the skin. This means that application of potent corticosteroids should be avoided, if possible, because they impair the thickness of the stratum corneum. Local UVB treatment may be considered to enhance the defense capacity of the skin. In severe cases, especially in combination with allergic contact dermatitis or psoriasis, PUVA treatment of the hands should be considered.[21,22] It may be beneficial in the chronic forms, ingenuity, and with some equipment can be arranged for home treatment.[23]

REFERENCES

1. Lantinga, H., Nater, J. P., and Coenraads, P. J., Prevalence, incidence and course of eczema on the hands and forearms in a sample of the general population, *Contact Dermatitis,* 10, 135, 1984.
2. Agrup, G., Hand eczema and other hand dermatoses in South Sweden, *Acta Derm. Venereol.,* 49, (Suppl. 61), 1969.
3. Meding, B., *Epidemiology of Hand Eczema in an Industrial City,* University of Göteborg, Göteborg, Sweden, 1990.
4. Malten, K. E. and den Arend, J. A. C. J., Irritant contact dermatitis: traumiterative and cumulative impairment by cosmetics, climate, and other daily loads, *Dermatosen,* 33, 125, 1985.
5. Malten, K. E., Thoughts on irritant contact dermatitis, *Contact Dermatitis,* 7, 435, 1981.
6. Gaul, L. E. and Underwood, G. R., Relation of dew point and barometer pressure to chapping of normal skin, *J. Invest. Dermatol.,* 19, 9, 1952.
7. Brasch, J., Burgard, J., and Wolfram, S., Common pathogenetic pathways in allergic and irritant contact dermatitis, *J. Invest. Dermatol.,* 98, 166, 1992.
8. Rystedt, I., Factors influencing the recurrence of hand eczema in adults with a history of atopic dermatitis in childhood, *Contact Dermatitis,* 12, 247, 1985.
9. Bäurle, G., Hornstein, O. P., and Diepgen, T. L., Professionelle Handekzeme und Atopie, *Dermatosen,* 33, 161, 1985.
10. Maibach, H. I. and Epstein, E., Eczematous psoriasis, *Semin. Dermatol.,* 2, 45, 1983.
11. Boer de, E. M., Bruynzeel, D. P., and Ketel van, W. G., Dyshidrotic eczema as an occupational dermatitis in metal works, *Contact Dermatitis,* 19, 184, 1988.
12. Wilkinson, J. D. and Rycroft, R. J. G., *Textbook of Dermatology,* 5th ed., Blackwell Scientific, Oxford, 1992, 611.
13. Frosch, P., *Hautirritation und empfindliche Haut,* Grosse Verlag, Berlin, 1985.
14. Frosch, P. J., Dooms-Goossens, A., Lachapelle, J. M., Rycroft, R. J. G., and Scheper, R. J., *Current Topics in Contact Dermatitis,* Springer-Verlag, Berlin, 1989, 385.
15. Marzulli, F. N. and Maibach, H. I., *Dermatotoxicology,* 3rd ed., Hemisphere, Washington, D.C., 1987.
16. Rothenberg, H. W., Menné, T., and Sjölin, K. E., Temperature dependent primary irritant dermatitis from lemon perfume, *Contact Dermatitis,* 3, 37, 1977.
17. Pinnagoda, J., Tupker, R. A., Coenraads, P. J., et al., Prediction of susceptibility to an irritant response by transepidermal water loss, *Contact Dermatitis,* 20, 341, 1989.
18. Björnberg, A., *Skin Reactions to Primary Irritants in Patients with Hand Eczema,* Isacsons, Göteborg, Sweden, 1968.
19. Mellström, G., Protective gloves of polymeric materials, *Acta Derm. Venereol.,* Suppl. 163, 1991.
20. Kurte, A., Zylka, M., and Frosch, P. J., New text model for evaluating the efficacy of barrier creams, *International Symposium on Irritant Contact Dermatitis,* final program and abstract book, Stichting Milieu-en Arbeidsdermatologie, Groningen, Holland, October 3-5, 1991, 45.

21. Taube, K. M. and Lubbe, D., UV-radiation suppresses irritative and allergic skin reactions, *International Symposium on Irritant Contact Dermatitis,* final program and abstract book, Stichting Milieu-en Arbeidsdermatologie, Groningen, Holland, October 3-5, 1991, 29.

22. Rosén, K., Mobacken, H., and Swanbeck, G., Chronic eczematous dermatitis of the hands: a comparison of PUVA and UVB treatment, *Acta Derm. Venereol.,* 67, 48, 1987.

23. Epstein, E., Home PUVA treatment for chronic hand and foot dermatoses, *Cutis,* 44, 423, 1989.

6

The Atopic Hand Eczema

Halvor Möller

CONTENTS

I. INCIDENCE

The incidence of atopic hand eczema differs greatly in published reports depending on differences in the populations studied or, probably more importantly, on different criteria for atopy. In a large epidemiological study on hand eczema, Meding and Swanbeck[1] found 22% atopic hand eczema using the criteria "a history of previous atopic dermatitis or present atopic dermatitis at other sites on the body." In a patient material of hand eczema, Svensson[2] found an atopic background of 33% if the criteria were previous or present flexural dermatitis; if an elaborate point system were used, atopic hand eczema was diagnosed in 49%. Similarly high figures were obtained in occupational as well as nonoccupational patients in a German hand eczema material.[3]

II. CLINICAL PROFILE

The atopic hand eczema has no uniform clinical picture. Still the experienced dermatologist, supported by some anamnestic information, recognizes the entity and establishes the diagnosis. The distribution is almost always symmetric. In many cases, however, the picture is obscured by one or several exogenous factors. It should always be kept in mind that a patient with a previous atopic skin disease is prone to develop an irritant, traumiterative dermatitis of the hands or, vice versa, that a majority of patients with an irritant hand eczema have an atopic background.

The most frequent type of atopic hand eczema involves the dorsal aspects of the hands and fingers with no sharp delineation of affected areas. Dryness, weak erythema, and lichenification predominate (Plate 42*). The patient has a long history, half a year or more, of periodic itching and decreasing mobility of the fingers, with increasing thickness of the knuckles in particular. Erosions from scratching and fissures imply painful episodes with disturbed function of the hands. Infectious and noninfectious inflammation contributes to dermal edema, some of which may remain and get organized. The result is a continuously or periodically itching and thickened skin with decreased mobility of the fingers.

Another dorsal type of atopic hand eczema has a less homogenous distribution, occurring rather in nummular irregular patches (Plate 43). (Therefore, a genuine nummular eczema confined to the hands may be a differential diagnosis.) This variant is usually more active with bouts of vesicular eruptions intermingled with crusted infiltrates. Summertime usually implies a period of less disease activity with diminished itching and erythema, but dryness and lichenification are permanent features. By fall, the eczematous activity may start again, often triggered by exogenous factors including a low environmental humidity because of central heating at home or the workplace, a low outdoor temperature, and contact irritants. Because of inflammatory damage to the nail matrix, corresponding fingernails eventually become involved. The nail plates are thickened and disfigured by transverse ridges and furrows, and paronychias may be a recurring problem.

Some atopic patients have a chronic palmar eczema with a disease pattern that is usually individual. Thus, it may take the form of a clear-cut pompholyx, i.e., symmetric vesicular eruptions of the palms, sometimes also involving the soles. Pompholyx is an eczematous manifestation of several etiologies, such as a systemically administered contact allergen (e.g., nickel), dermatophytide from a focal mycosis, dyshidrosis (rare in temperate climates), and nummular eczema. It is, however, frequently an expression of atopy. Itching as well as pinpoint size intraepidermal vesicles occur primarily in the central parts of the palms, do not disrupt but are absorbed, leaving a slightly scaling skin. Bouts of vesicular eruptions occur irregularly, from a few times per year to a couple of times per month.

Another palmar type, also centrally located, has a profound chronic character with a dry, lichenified thickening and periodic itching (Plate 44). Presumably, the atopic pompholyx and this lichenified variant are extremes of the same eczematous pattern because features of one of them sometimes occur in the other. A clinical variant of hand eczema, not uncommon in childhood, is characterized by fissuring and painful fingerpulps, pulpite digitale (Plate 45). It probably constitutes a disease entity analogous to "atopic winter feet" (why not "atopic winter hands"?) and occurs in 25% of those afflicted with this plantar dermatitis.[4]

---

* Color plates follow p. 48.

TABLE 1   The Most Frequent Positive
         Patch Test Reactions to
         Standard Allergens in 101
         Patients with Atopic Hand
         Eczema

	No.	%
Nickel	45	14
Colophony	17	5
Cobalt	15	5
Fragrances	14	4
Ethylene diamine	9	3
Balsam of Peru	8	2
Neomycin	6	2
Chromium	5	2
Amerchol (lanolin)	5	2

III.   DIAGNOSIS

It is essential to establish the diagnosis of atopic skin disease among all patients with hand eczema. With this diagnosis the prognosis is less promising with regard to a long-term cure. It is also important for therapeutic reasons (e.g., occupational counseling, ultraviolet radiation treatment). Although many experienced dermatologists believe that they can diagnose atopic hand eczema at a glance, this is not corroborated by careful studies on the type and distribution of eczematous lesions.[2,5,6] The diagnosis is usually secured after supplementing inspection with a few questions on atopic disease in self and close relatives. Today, there is no laboratory test, not even serum immunoglobulin E (IgE), that is diagnostically helpful for atopic skin disease of limited extension. However, an elaborate point system based on history and cutaneous lesions has proved valuable.[7] The need for established clinical criteria in diagnosing atopic skin disease has recently been confirmed using a similar point system.[8]

Among exogenous complicating factors, contact allergy may be added to the patient's constitutional problems. This occurs despite the well-known decreased capacity to mount T cell-mediated immunologic reactions. Thus, the incidence of contact allergy among atopic patients is lowered in comparison with nonatopics but still comprises about one third of tested patients.[9,11]

During the years 1984 to 1990, all patients patch tested in the Departmant of Dermatology, Malmö, because of suspected contact allergy, were also questioned on an atopic background. This history was taken before the application of skin tests. Atopy was defined as a personal, previous or present flexural dermatitis and/or allergic mucous membrane disease, such as asthma and/or hayfever. The test methods have been described elsewhere.[11] Particular caution was observed when reading test reactions from metal allergens, notoriously difficult to assess in atopic patients.[12] During the 7 year period there were 780 tested patients with atopic skin disease, 331 of whom (42%) had hand eczema. One or more positive patch tests were obtained in 101 patients (31%) with atopic hand eczema. The frequency of different contact allergies is presented in Table 1. The outcome is similar to that for atopic dermatitis in general. The frequency of contact allergy to nickel, the leading allergen, was only 13.6%, which is significantly lower ($p < 0.001$) than that for nickel allergy in nonatopic patients with hand eczema (267 of 1167, 22.9%). This finding underlines the lacking correlation between nickel allergy and the atopic state.

The possibility of a protein contact dermatitis should also be considered in an atopic subject. The patient reports rapid flare-ups of his/her hand eczema in a matter of minutes after contact with certain foods, particularly fish, shellfish, and other animal proteins. The disease was first described in Danish "smørrebrødsjomfruer" (sandwich makers).[13] Despite its nature of immediate reaction, the flare-up contains macroscopic vesicles and histologic spongiosis. The protein contact dermatitis is presumed to be IgE-mediated and is not detected by conventional epicutaneous testing. Rather, a scratch chamber or similar test with a 20-min reading should be exercised.[14] It is also presumed that a prerequisite for a high-molecular protein allergen to penetrate the skin barrier is an (at least low-grade) irritant dermatitis.

A secondary infection of the hand eczema should be suspected when ache is substituting itch in the patient's complaints, when fingers are edematous and their mobility inhibited, and if the serous exudation becomes purulent. A positive culture for *Staphylococcus aureus* may not be relevant because the atopic skin in general is often inhabited by this microbe without clinical consequences.[15] However, in many cases adequate eczema treatment will not be successful until antistaphylococcal treatment is added. A cultural finding of β-hemolytic streptococci should, however, always be considered pathogenic and the patient given proper antibiotic.

The pathogenetic importance of *P. ovale* in atopic dermatitis is being discussed,[16] mainly, however, for localizations other than the hands. Nor has conclusive evidence been brought forward of a causal role for house dust mites in this disease.[17]

IV. TREATMENT

The introduction of hydrocortisone for topical treatment of eczematous disorders in the 1950s was clearly a major breakthrough in dermatology. It is, however, recognized today that this drug is insufficient in many cases of atopic dermatitis, particularly when itch and lichenification predominate. This also holds true for atopic hand eczema, which often needs to be treated with stronger corticosteroids, always as an introduction, usually for bouts of eczema, and sometimes for maintenance therapy. Therefore, betamethasone valerate (group 3) has long been the drug of choice for treating an active atopic hand eczema. An initial schedule of 2 or 3 applications per day is usually appropriate. With yielding eczematous activity, the treatment should be tapered down by increasing the intervals or by substituting a lower-grade corticosteroid, such as hydrocortisone-17α butyrate (group 2), or plain hydrocortisone (group 1).

An even stronger corticosteroid, clobetasol propionate (group 4), may be used successfully in atopic hand eczema. Atrophy and tachyphylaxis are avoided if the drug is given intermittently under supervision.[18] There is a widespread fear among the general public of the side effects of corticosteroids. The experience, consequently, of most dermatologists[19] when taking care of patients with atopic dermatitis is that the greatest problem is not those patients using too much of these drugs but those using too little. Oral corticosteroids are sometimes needed to quench an eruption of atopic hand eczema. A vesicular or oozing dermatitis responds rapidly even to a moderate dose of prednisolone, e.g., 30 mg/day, which should be tapered down after 1 week. The pompholyx variant in particular is usually resistant to topical therapy and goes nicely in remission by a short prednisolone course.

In topical treatment the vehicle for the hands should be an oil-in-water emulsion cream, this being less messy than the ointment. Also, paradoxically, the atopic patient with dry skin usually prefers the cream bases to the ointments. Some, however, choose a compromise, "the fat cream". Emollients are cornerstones in the skin care of the atopic patient who is also particular in the preference of emollients, and various creams or lotions should be tried. The water-binding effect of carbamide (urea) (5 to 10%) is often helpful in improving the elasticity of dry and fissuring fingers. The emollient may be used intermittently when tapering down the corticosteroid treatment and later frequently as a prophylaxis. Perfumed preparations should be avoided because of the risk of sensitization.

When secondary infection is suspected or demonstrated, a systemic antibiotic is preferable to a topical one, again because of the risk of sensitization. For a streptococcal infection the patient should be given oral phenoxymethyl penicillin for 10 days. When the target is *S. aureus*, a penicillinase-resistant penicillin is preferred. Often a patient with corticosteroid-resistant eczema turns into a responder after such a course. It has, however, been demonstrated that staphylococcal colonization of atopic skin may be diminished by topical mupirocin treatment with a satisfactory effect on the eczematous activity.[20] It has also been shown that atopic hand eczema contaminated with *S. aureus* can be treated successfully with the strong clobetasol propionate, in which case the bacterial flora will decrease.[21]

Good results have been obtained by using ultraviolet radiation of different modalities in atopic dermatitis;[22] this also holds true for the atopic hand eczema. UVB, alone or in combination with UVA, is usually effective. In stubborn cases even PUVA may be tried. The reader is referred to Chapter 28 for a detailed text.

Antihistamines lack anti-inflammatory, antieczematous, and antripruritic effects and should not be used. If there is need for a sedative, a traditional antihistamine might be chosen because of the well-known side effect. Topical antihistamines or anesthetics should not be prescribed because of the risk of sensitization. Sodium cromoglycate, systemically or topically administered, has proven worthless in atopic dermatitis despite its effect in atopic mucous membrane disease. Dietary addition of essential fatty acids (from evening primrose oil or fish oil) has given promising results[23] in generalized atopic dermatitis, but no study on atopic hand eczema has been published.

REFERENCES

1. Meding, B. and Swanbeck, G., Epidemiology of different types of hand eczema in an industrial city, *Acta Derm. Venereol.*, 69, 227, 1989.
2. Svensson, Å, Hand eczema: an evaluation of the frequency of atopic background and the difference in clinical pattern between patients with and without atopic dermatitis, *Acta Derm. Venereol.*, 68, 509, 1988.
3. Bäurle, G., Hornstein, O. P., and Diepgen, Th. L., Professionelle Handekzeme und Atopie: Eine klinische Prospektivstudie zur Frage des Zusammenhangs, *Derm. Beruf Umwelt*, 33, 161, 1985.
4. Svensson, Å, Prognosis and atopic background of juvenile plantar dermatosis and gluteo-femoral eczema, *Acta Derm. Venereol.*, 68, 336, 1988.
5. Bandmann, H.- J. and Agathos, M., Die atopische Handdermatitis, *Derm. Beruf Umwelt*, 28, 110, 1980.
6. Cronin, E., Clinical patterns of hand eczema in women, *Contact Dermatitis*, 13, 153, 1985.
7. Svensson, Å, Edman, B., and Möller, H., A diagnostic tool for atopic dermatitis based on clinical criteria, *Acta Derm. Venereol. Suppl.*, 114, 33, 1985.
8. Diepgen, T. L., Fartasch, M., and Hornstein, O. P., Kriterien zur Beurteilung der atopischen Hautdiathese, *Derm. Beruf Umwelt*, 39, 79, 1991.
9. Blondeel, A., Achten, G., Dooms-Goossens, A., et al., Atopie et allergie de contact, *Ann. Dermatol. Venereol.*, 114, 203, 1987.
10. de Groot, A. C., The frequency of contact allergy in atopic patients with dermatitis, *Contact Dermatitis*, 22, 273, 1990.
11. Edman, B. and Möller, H., Contact allergy and contact allergens in atopic skin disease, *Am. J. Contact Dermatitis*, 3, 27, 1992.
12. Möller, H., Intradermal testing in doubtful cases of contact allergy to metals, *Contact Dermatitis*, 20, 120, 1989.
13. Hjorth, N. and Roed-Petersen, J., Occupational protein contact dermatitis in food handlers, *Contact Dermatitis*, 2, 28, 1976.
14. Kanerva, L., Estlander, T., and Jolanki, R., Skin testing for immediate hypersensitivity in occupational allergology, in *Exogenous Dermatoses: Environmental Dermatitis*, Menné, T. and Maibach, H., Eds., CRC Press, Boca Raton, FL, 1991, 103.
15. Leyden, J. J., Marples, R. R., and Kligman, A. M., *Staphylococcus aureus* in the lesions of atopic dermatitis, *Br. J. Dermatol.*, 90, 525, 1974.
16. Kieffer, M., Bergbrant, I.- M., Faergemann, J., et al., Immune reactions to Pityrosporum ovale in adult patients with atopic and seborrheic dermatitis, *J. Am. Acad. Dermatol.*, 22, 739, 1990.
17. de Groot, A. C. and Young, E., The role of contact allergy to aeroallergens in atopic dermatitis, *Contact Dermatitis*, 21, 209, 1989.
18. Möller, H., Svartholm, H., and Dahl, G., Intermittent maintenance therapy in chronic hand eczema with clobetasol propionate and flupredniden acetate, *Curr. Med. Res. Opin.*, 8, 640, 1983.
19. Vickers, C. F., The management of the problem atopic child in 1988, *Acta Derm. Venereol. Suppl.*, 144, 23, 1989.
20. Lever, R., Hadley, K., Downey, D., and Mackie, R., Staphylococcal colonization in atopic dermatitis and the effect of topical mupirocin therapy, *Br. J. Dermatol.*, 119, 189, 1988.

21. Nilsson, E., Henning, C., and Hjörleifsson, M.- L., Density of the microflora in hand eczema before and after topical treatment with a potent corticosteroid, *J. Am. Acad. Dermatol.*, 15, 192, 1986.

22. Jekler, J., Phototherapy of atopic dermatitis with ultraviolet radiation, *Acta Derm. Venereol. Suppl.*, 72, 171, 1992.

23. Horrobin, D. F., Essential fatty acids in clinical dermatology, *J. Am. Acad. Dermatol.*, 20, 1045, 1989.

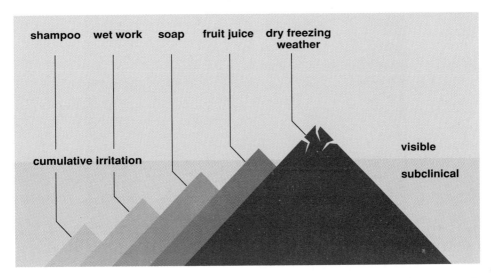

PLATE 1. Cumulative irritant contact dermatitis. A free interpretation of the concept as described by Malten.[5]

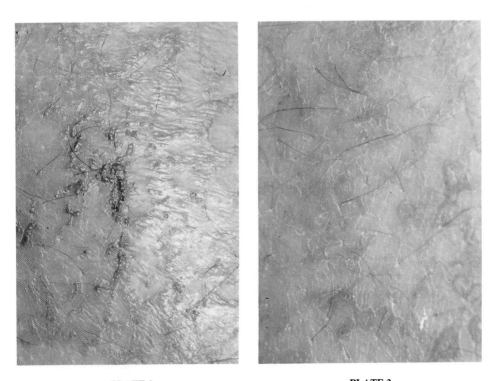

PLATE 2   **PLATE 3**

PLATE 2. Experimentally induced chapping with hemorrhagic fissures caused by daily repeated short exposure to alkaline cement solutions.

PLATE 3. Healing phase of Plate 2.

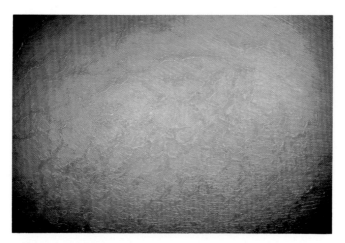

PLATE 4. Chapping.

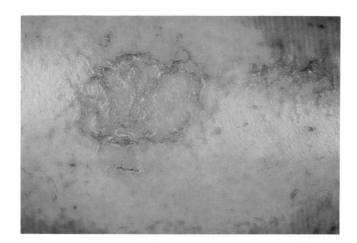

PLATE 5. Erythema craquele with fissures.

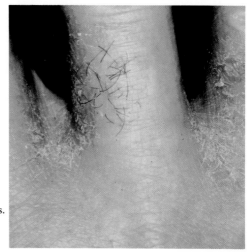

PLATE 6. Finger web dermatitis.

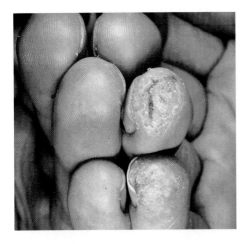

PLATE 7. Cumulative irritant contact dermatitis on the fingertips of the"wet hand" of a hairdresser.

PLATES 8, 9. Shiny fingertips with erythema and fine scaling in wet work occupations.

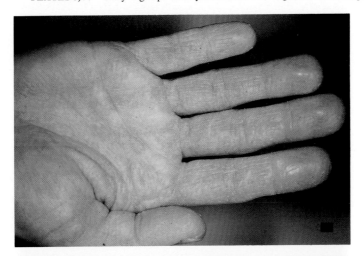

PLATE 8

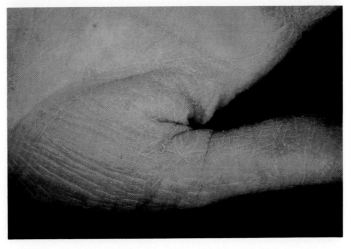

PLATE 9

PLATES 10-13.   Cumulative irritant contact dermatitis; from chapping to more lichenified, eczematous forms.

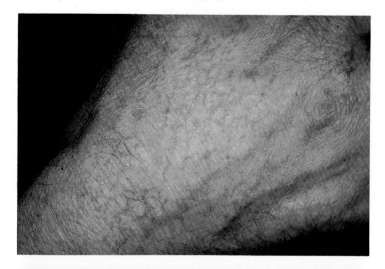

PLATE 10

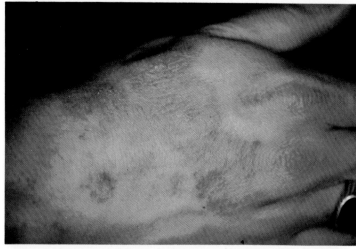

PLATE 11

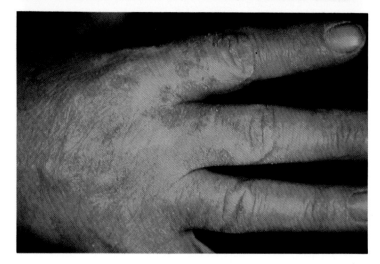

PLATE 12

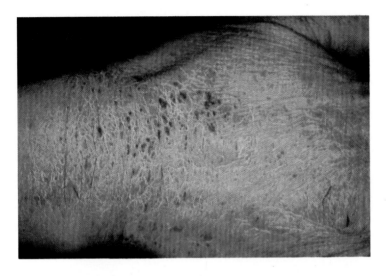

PLATE 13

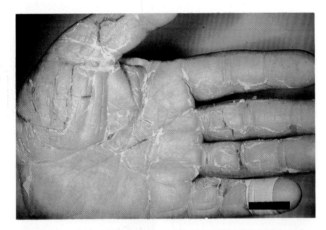

PLATE 14. Cumulative irritant contact dermatitis of a metal worker caused by daily exposure to organic solvents.

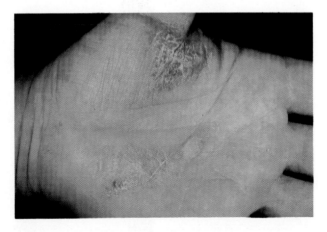

PLATE 15. Cumulative irritant contact dermatitis with vesicles caused by mechanical traction of a dog lead.

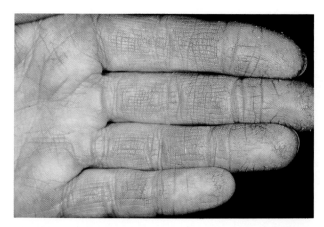

PLATE 16.   Cumulative irritant contact dermatitis caused by wear, tear, and soil in a farmer.

PLATES 17, 18.   Cumulative irritant contact dermatitis caused by the chemomechanical irritation of cement powder. No dichromate allergy present.

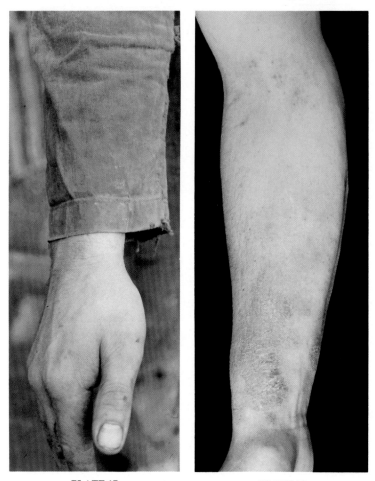

PLATE 17   PLATE 18

PLATES 19, 20. Cumulative irritant contact dermatitis caused by daily small paper handling in an office worker.

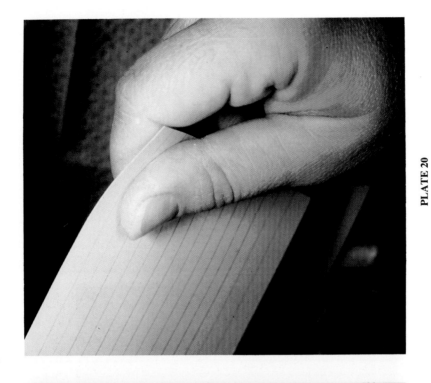

PLATE 20

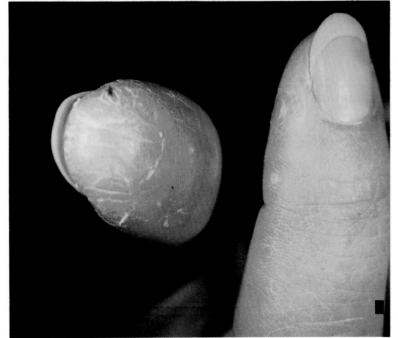

PLATE 19

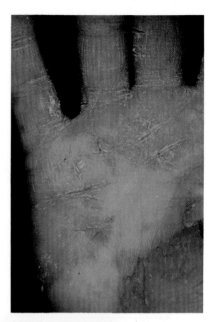

PLATE 21. Psoriasis with irritant contact dermatitis in a housewife.

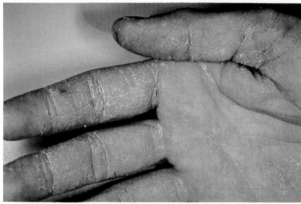

PLATE 22. Allergy to colophony in a storehouse worker (cardboard boxes).

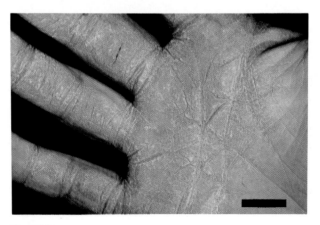

PLATE 23. Mycotic infection.

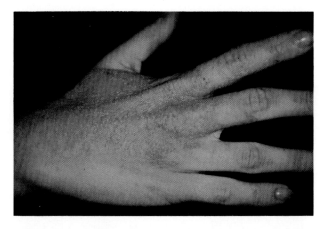

PLATE 24. Cumulative irritant contact dermatitis in a nurse caused by overexposure to detergents in wintertime.

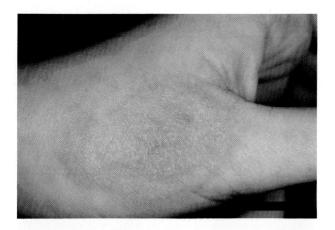

PLATE 25. Allergy to balsam of Peru and colophony.

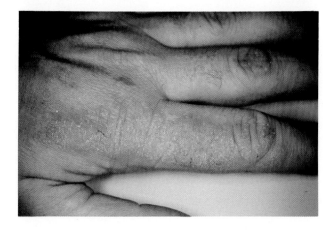

PLATE 26. Neurodermatitis circumscripta.

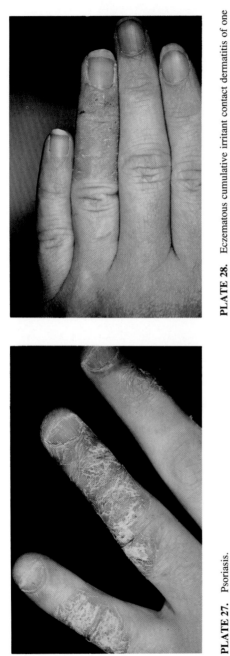

PLATE 27. Psoriasis.

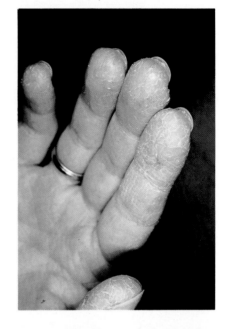

PLATE 28. Eczematous cumulative irritant contact dermatitis of one finger of a baker.

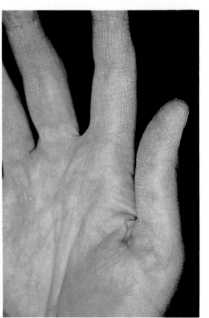

PLATE 29. Cumulative irritant contact dermatitis in cleaning work.

PLATE 30. Psoriasis.

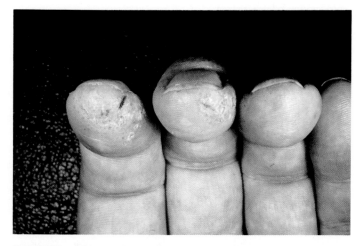

PLATE 31. Allergy to glycerylthioglycolate in a hairdresser.

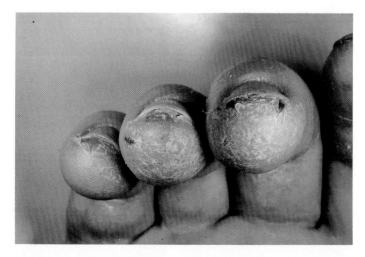

PLATE 32. Allergy to components in animal food in a farmer.

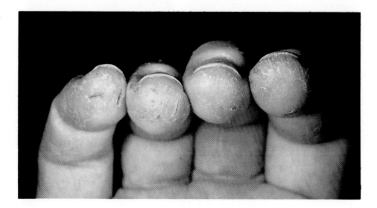

PLATE 33. Type I allergy to salmon and tomatoes in a restaurant worker.

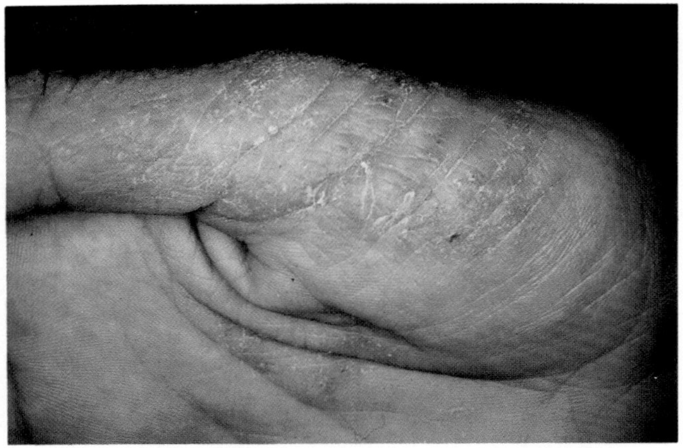

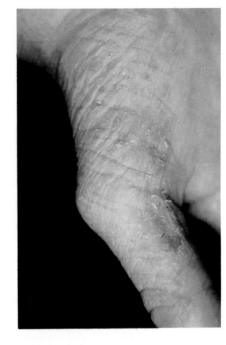

PLATE 36. Fragrance allergy in a hairdresser.

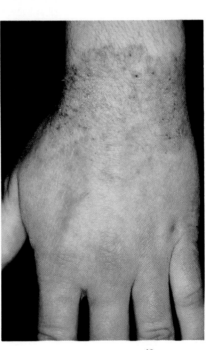

PLATE 37. Cumulative irritant contact dermatitis in a hairdresser.

PLATES 34, 35. Dermatitis in a slaughterhouse worker caused by a combination of mechanical friction and Type I allergy to pork.

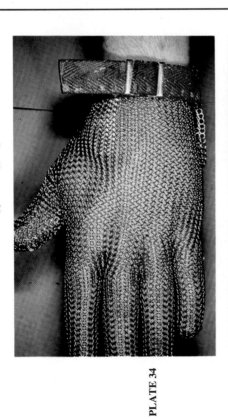

PLATE 34

PLATE 35

PLATES 38, 39. Dermatits caused by Type I allergy to tomato and chicken in a kitchen worker.

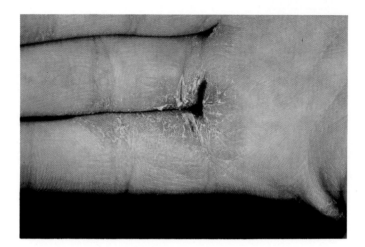

PLATE 38

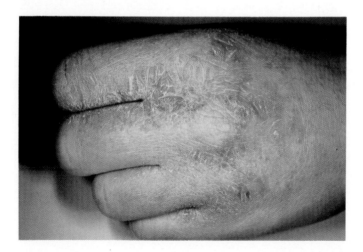

PLATE 39

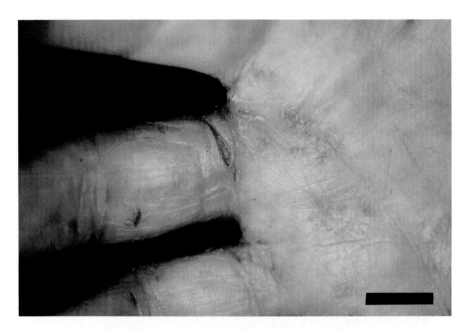

PLATE 40. Dermatitis caused by Type I allergy to chestnuts and kiwi in a baker.

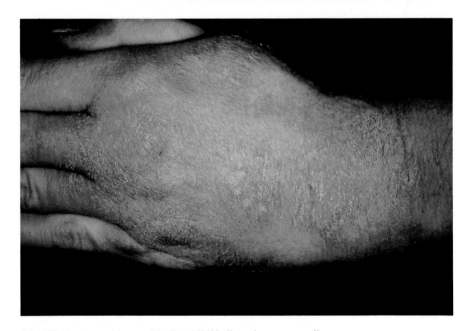

PLATE 41. Dermatitis caused by Euxyl K400 allergy in a massage oil.

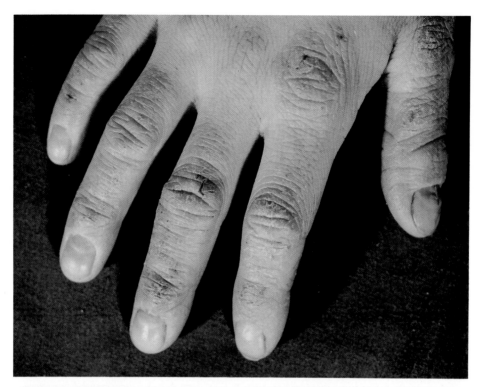

PLATE 42. Atopic hand eczema, dorsal type. Lichenification and fissuring, particularly over the knuckles. Note disfigured thumbnail while others are polished from scratching.

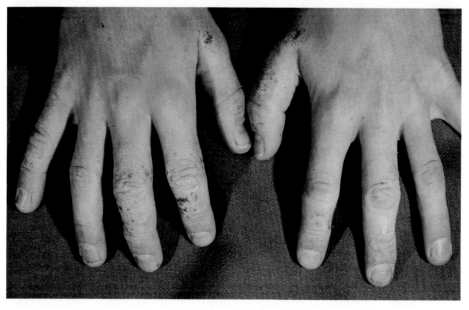

PLATE 43. Atopic hand eczema, dorsal type. Symmetric nummular infiltrates, chronic (lichenified) as well as acute (vesicular, crusted).

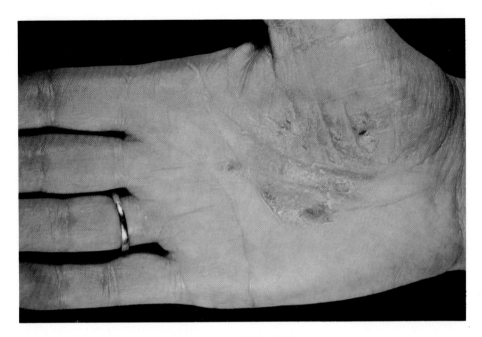

PLATE 44. Atopic hand eczema, volar type. Central, lichenified.

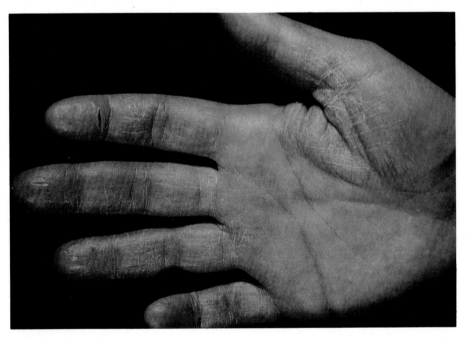

PLATE 45. Atopic hand eczema, volar type, with erythema and fissures. "Pulpite digitale", "atopic winter hands".

7

Palmar Eczema in Atopics

Hans J. Schwanitz

CONTENTS

I. INTRODUCTION

"Dyshidrosis" is a palmo-plantar dermatosis that manifests itself in the form of itching vesicles along the sides of the fingers. The disease has a high incidence and causes significant psychological problems, which may in turn results in excessive absenteeism from work. On the basis of a variety of clinical and experimental tests, we defined in 1985 the pathogenesis of dyshidrosis as an "atopic palmo-plantar eczema".[1] The disease is thus a variant form of atopic dermatitis, which can be provoked from without through irritants or from within through various factors, including stress. This hypothesis was controlled and verified later by other authors.[2,3] Lodi et al.[3] studied a group of 104 patients with pompholyx and found familiar and personal atopic diathesis in 50% of patients versus 11.5% of controls (control group included 208 subjects). Diepgen et al.[2] saw the symptom pompholyx in 30% of a group of patients with atopic dermatitis (control group, 6%).

The next section considers the evolution of the respective explanations for dyshidrosis and cheiropompholyx without extensive recapitulation of the theories involved. A condensed presentation of clinical aspects and causes and effects follows in Sections III and IV.

II. HISTORY OF "DYSHIDROSIS"

Tilbury Fox described in 1873 a blistering disease of the palms and soles, "dyshidrosis".[4] He stated, "the origin of the eruption was in the sweat apparatus . . . ". The sweat is retained, leading to swelling and kinking of the ducts, and stopping further excretion. At this stage a small vesicle becomes visible macroscopically. Second, the epidermis becomes macerated, and an "inflammatory erythema" is seen in the periphery of the blister.[5] Fox developed his theory of dyshidrosis in analogy to the contemporary concept of acne, which viewed the pathological process as an obstruction of the follicular infundibulum, resulting in an accumulation of sebaceous material. In 1876, Hutchinson[6] rejected Fox's theory. He used a term that he had employed in lectures since 1871 and published a description of the same disease as cheiropompholyx, i.e., blisters in the hand. The etiological theories of both Fox and Hutchinson were different. The controversy has lasted up to the present time. In 1966, Simons reviewed 10,000 serial sections from 26 patients and concluded that there was usually no connection between the blisters and the sweat glands, although occasional coincidental exceptions were found.[7]

In the past 25 years most authors agree with Hutchinson's opinion that the pathogenesis of an extretion of a serous fluid develops at deeper levels of the horny layer because this hypothesis is in accordance with the classification of dyshidrosis as an eczema.[6,8] In 1983, Wurzel and Kutzner reported on the ultrastructural features that the spongiosis develops as a result of microacantholysis, after an intercellular edema led to a rupture of the desmosomes.[9]

In summary, the occurrence of blisters on the palms (dyshidrosis or cheiropompholyx) is caused by the anatomy of these areas, i.e., a thick epidermis and thicker overlying stratum corneum.[10] When classifying dyshidrosis as an eczema, it may seen disturbing that clinically the vesicles seem to erupt in a macroscopically unaltered skin. One often observes no initial redness, even though histologically a perivascular infiltrate can be seen along with vascular dilation, especially in the dermal papillae.

At the end of the nineteenth century, dermatological microbiology gained more importance. This influenced the theories regarding dyshidrosis from fungi or, in other words, that it is a dermatomycosis. The criticism of this theory is based on the following points:

1. Mycological proof was found only in some cases, mainly on the feet and not on the hands.[11-14]
2. Clinically, dyshidrosis was insufficiently or not at all differentiated from tinea pedum.[7,11,15]
3. Saprophytes or only facultatively pathogenic fungi were often found.[16,17]
4. The damage of the barrier functions of the skin in dyshidrosis facilitates secondary fungal infections.[11]

In 1911, Jadassohn developed the theory of id reactions to dermatophytes.[18,19] This new theory was teleologically necessary when it became evident that dyshidrosis could not just be reduced to a mycotic infection of the hands and feet. Many investigators, indeed, successfully demonstrated ringworm of the feet but agreed that the lesions of the hands, especially the dyshidrotic blisters, were sterile.[20,21]

These observations can be explained within the id theory. The fungus would gain access to the vascular system by chemical or mechanical alterations, spreading thereafter throughout the body. The allergic reaction in the skin that follows the presentation of the antigen would destroy the fungi. The clinical manifestation of this allergic reaction would be the epidermophytid.[21] The hypothesis that dyshidrosis is an id reaction to fungi had not been proven up until today. Simons stated in 1966 that this concept is more accepted as a dogma by textbook tradition than as an academically proven fact.[7]

In recent years metal allergies received great interest, especially nickel. In the 1950s, dyshidrotic eczema occurred in 3% of occupational dermatoses, and the environmental exacerbation of the disease by working with metal was recognized.[22] Nickel and chrome are the allergens most frequently involved in occupational dermatoses.[23]

Nickel allergy manifests itself on the hands up to 77% of the time as dyshydrosis.[24] The majority of patients with nickel allergy are women. In Denmark, about 10% of all women have been found to have a nickel allergy.[25,26] Of 222 patients seeking disability pensions for acquired occupational contact allergy, 99 women had a nickel allergy and approximately one half of these were recognized as due to their occupation.[27] There is a strong correlation between nickel allergy and the presence of eczema on the hands. Eczema of the hands promotes the development of nickel allergies, and existing nickel allergies are often followed by eczemas of the hands.[28,29]

Yet pompholyx cannot always be considered a contact eczema because in the course of the disease it does not necessarily heal when contact to the allergen is interrupted. There is a statistical correlation between atopy and nickel allergy. Diepgen et al.[2] integrated nickel allergy into their atopy score system. We conclude that atopy promotes a secondary sensitization, especially to metal. We would explain the frequently found sensitization in atopic eczema by the fact that the disturbed barrier function of the horny layer allows potential allergens, i.e., metal ions, to penetrate more easily.

III. CLINICAL ASPECTS

Typical clinical features can be summarized as follows:

1. The disease preferentially affects the palms and margins of the fingers.
2. Cutaneous discomfort (tension and itching) precedes the eruption of blisters.
3. Clear blisters appear symmetrically.
4. Small blisters coalesce into larger ones.
5. The blisters dry out and do not rupture.
6. Recurrence is frequent.

This allows a differential diagnosis from pustular psoriasis and the palmo-plantar pustulosis because of their morphology and location. The symmetry precludes the diagnosis of herpes simplex infection, and the location excludes consideration of hand, foot, and mouth disease. Dermatophytic infections are not preceded by cutaneous discomfort, and the distribution is usually not symmetrical. In a group of 58 patients we studied, the average age was settled to 32.2 years, i.e., atopic palmar eczema affects mainly young adults and becomes manifest after or during the professional training. In our patient group there were more women than men affected (ratio 2:1).

Figure 1 shows the time sequences of vesiculation, redness, scaling, and itching. Pompholyx begins with the eruption of vesicles and is frequently heralded by the sensation of itching or tension of the skin. The sensation of itching increases during the phase of vesiculation and persists with a lower intensity after the vesicles have disappeared. The redness usually appears when vesicles are still apparent. Scaling follows vesiculation. The entire episode calms down to either a moderate scaling or a mild persisting redness. Our model describes the symptomatic development of only one attack. For those cases in which the episodes of vesiculation follow each other at short intervals,

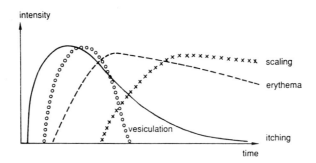

FIGURE 1.   Model demonstrating the time sequence of the intensity of vesiculation, erythema, scaling, and itching during an exacerbation of dyshidrosis.

the pattern of curves is altered by the summation of individual overlapping curves, such that the simultaneous picture of scaling and vesicles may be seen. This is particularly striking in the case mentioned by Christensen and Möller[24] with 15 attacks per year. Nail changes were noted to be relatively common. Like other eczemas, atopic palmar eczema can lead to impairments of the matrix and/or nail bed. There are slight changes (e.g., pits or transverse grooves) but also other changes (e.g., trachyonychia).

We found a familial predisposition for the dyshidrosis; 22% of the patients' parents have or have had a dyshidrosis. Nearly all patients with atopic palmar eczema feel psychologically burdened because of their illness. Using a 4-point scale (0 = none; 1 = slight; 2 = considerable; 3 = severe), the psychological strain was estimated to be considerable to severe by 75% of the patients. Most had social difficulties.

Dyshidrosis is a psychological burden for practically all patients and most are considerably or extremely hindered socially. The seriousness of the psychological consequences has not as yet been expressed to this extent, although English points out in 1949 that patients suffer and are restricted in the use of their hands.[30]

The psychosocial difficulties may have various causes. The human hand functions primarily as a mechanical instrument. These functions are impaired in the dyshidrotic patient. Contact with hard objects can be painful during acute eczematous skin changes. Contact with substances that irritate the skin is practically impossible. The sensitivity of the fingers for fine work is disturbed and altogether lost with the wearing of gloves. The movement of the finger joints is reduced. One patient had a flexure contraction of his finger joints due to chronic recurrent inflammations. These functional impairments may lead to disability and loss of one's working place. The hands also function as an organ of contact. Much of what Borelli[31] wrote concerning the face as an "organ of contact" applies to the hands as well. Neither face nor hands are concealed by clothes. The hands can disclose race, ace, and profession (clavi). They can stress verbal expressions through gesture. Shaking hands is in itself an elementary means of communication.

IV.   CAUSES AND EFFECTS

The patients mainly work in a damp environment, a causative or promoting exogenous factor. Reichenberger[32] previously published similar observations. We are under the impression, just as was Lindemayr,[33] that unlike normal persons our patients cannot react with a hardening effect to chronic skin irritation, but their efforts at compensation result in an eczema of the palms. This susceptibility of atopic patients is well known.[34] The patients are more prone than others to develop eczemas of the hands while working in moist environments.[35] In patients with atopic palmar eczema we could detect elevated transepidermal water loss in unaffected skin, as did Rajka[36] in atopic dermatitis.

These results also indicate a common reduced barrier function of the horny layer.[34,37] The reduced barrier function explains the sensitivity toward irritants and moist environments. This susceptibility leads to a more frequent affection of the palms of the hands than of the soles of the feet. In contrast to other forms of atopic dermatitis, atopic palmar eczema depends more on exogenous factors because the hand is constantly involved with different external factors because of its function as a tool and instrument of communciation.

The psychosocial consequences of their disease can be considerable for patients with dyshidrosis and should always be taken into account during therapy. During periods of extreme psychological strain, a circulus vitiosus may develop, as is also found in atopic dermatitis. The patient concentrates all his attention on the illness, the constant awareness of itching is increased, the itch is stronger, the patient scratches more, the condition worsens, and so on. This sequence often occurs at night while in bed, when the patient is at rest, or rather when he is restless.

Atopic palmar eczema enhances development of other diseases that were formerly thought to be causative factors in dyshidrosis, such as secondary infections with fungi or delayed hypersensitivity reactions. It is well known that in atopy barrier function of the horny layer is disturbed as well as skin after irritation with toxic agents and exhibits enhanced susceptibility to contact sensitization.[38,39] An indication suggesting a secondary sensitization is that when the contact allergen is avoided atopic palmo-plantar eczema does not heal. Delayed hypersensitivity is without clinical importance if there is no correlation between the worsening of the skin condition and allergen contact.[24] Nevertheless, we know that atopic palmar eczema combined with nickel allergy is of a worse prognosis than nonatopic eczema with the same sensitization.[40]

Prevention of atopic palmar eczema can be effective if all factors that exacerbate atopic dermatitis are avoided, including heat sweating and wetting, infections, dry skin, low humidity, emotional stress, irritants, and allergens.[41] In special cases there is a strict avoidance of allergenic food indicated. We observed that many patients with atopic palmar eczema were smokers. Newer studies showed smoking to be a risk factor for elevated serum immunoglobulin E levels.[42] Working in wet surroundings is the most important factor causing or aggravating atopic palmar eczema. Hairdressers with eczema often have atopic palmar eczema, and they noted an aggravation in the eczema in wet and alkaline working environments.[32,43] The importance of such surroundings is stressed by many authors. In 1991, we showed that in a population of more than 4000 hairdressers in the first year of their professional training, more than 70% developed skin problems.[44] In Germany more than 30% of all hairdressers leave their profession because of chronic hand eczema. In this group most patients have atopic palmar eczema.

REFERENCES

1. Schwanitz, H. J., *Atopic Palmoplantar Eczema,* Springer-Verlag, Berlin, 1988.
2. Diepgen, T. L., Fartasch, M., and Hornstein, O. P., Evaluation and relevance of atopic basic and minor features in patients with atopic dermatitis and in the general population, *Dermatol. Venerol. (Stockh.),* 144, 50, 1989.
3. Lodi, A., Betti, R., Chiarelli, G., Urbani, C. E., and Crosti, C., Epidemiological, clinical and allergological observations on pompholyx, *Contact Dermatitis,* 26, 17, 1992.
4. Fox, T., Clinical lecture on dyshidrosis (an undescribed eruption), *Br. Med. J.,* 1, 365, 1873.
5. Hebra, H. V., *Veränderungen der Haut und ihrer Anhangsgebilde,* Friedrich Wreden, Braunschweig, 1884, 425.
6. Hutchinson, J., Cheiro-pompholyx, *Lancet,* 1, 630, 1876.
7. Simons, R. D. G. P., Dyshidrosiform eruptions, *Excerpta Medica,* 17, 107, 1966.
8. Musger, A., Zur Ätiologie und Pathogenese der Cheiropompholyx (Dyshidrosis), *Dermatol. Wochenschr.,* 153, 111, 1967.
9. Wurzel, R. M. and Kutzner, H., Zur Ultrastruktur dyshidrosiformer Bläschen, *Hautarzt,* 34 (Suppl. 4), 323, 1983.
10. Marks, R., The pathology and pathogenesis of the eczematous reaction, in *Eczema,* Marks, R., Ed., Martin Dunitz, London, 1992, 21.
11. Grund, W., Beitrag zur Frage der interdigitalen Mykosen nebst einer Übersicht über den jetzigen Stand der Frage, *Dermatol. Z.,* 45, 175, 1925.
12. Taniguchi, Y., Beiträge zur Studie der Dyshidrosis, *Jpn. J. Med. Sci. Trans.,* 13, 1, 43, 1927.

13. Griff, F. and Itkin, M. M., Zur Atiologie der Dyshidrosen, *Acta Derm. Venerol.*, 11, 508, 1930.

14. Vilanova, X. and Casanovas, M., Dermatitie dyshidrosiforme des mains et des pieds, causée par un aspergillus, *Ann. Dermatol. Syphiligr.*, 78, 292, 1951.

15. McLachlain, A. D. and Brown, W. H., Cheiropompholyx, *Br. J. Dermatol.*, 46, 457, 1934.

16. Schramek, M., Befunde bei Pilzerkrankungen der Hände und Füße, *Arch. Dermatol. Syphilol.*, 121, 630, 1916.

17. Graffenried, C. V., Beitrag zur Frage der mykotischen Dyshidrosis (Kaufmann-Wolf), *Dermatol. Wochenschr.*, 66, 361, 1918.

18. Jadassohn, W. and Peck, S. M., Epidermophytide der Hände, *Arch. Dermatol. Syphilol.*, 158, 16, 1929.

19. Bloch, B., Die Trichophytide, in *Handbuch der Haut- und Geschlechtskrankheiten*, Jadassohn, J., Ed., Springer-Verlag, Berlin, 1928, 564.

20. Miescher, G., Trichophytien und Epidermophytien, in *Handbuch der Haut- und Geschlechts krakheiten*, Jadassohn, J., Ed., Springer-Verlag, Berlin, 1928, 378.

21. Walthard, B., Zur Pathogenese des dyshidrotischen Symptomenkomplexes: Über ein unter dem Bilde einer Dyshidrosis verlaufendes Epidermophytid, *Dermatol. Z.*, 53, 692, 1928.

22. Bory, R., Guyotjeannin, Ch., and Negri, R., Etude clinique et pathogénetique de la dyshidrose professionnelle, *Arch. Mal. Prof.*, 15, 26, 1954.

23. Hjorth, N., Geschichte der Kontaktdermatitis und ihr Einfluß auf die heutigue Arbeitsdermatologie, *Hautarzt*, 31, 621, 1980.

24. Christensen, O. B. and Möller, H., Nickel allergy and hand eczema, *Contact Dermatitis*, 1, 129, 1975.

25. Menné, T., The prevalence of nickel allergy among women: an epidemiological study in hospitalized female patients, *Dermatosen*, 26, 123, 1978.

26. Hjorth, N., Fregert, S., and Magnusson, B., Einige Berufe und ihre Kontaktallergene, *Allergologie*, 2, 296, 1979.

27. Menné, T. and Bachmann, E., Permanent disability from hand dermatitis in females sensitive to nickel, chromium and cobalt, *Dermatosen*, 27, 129, 1979.

28. Meneghini, C. L. and Angelini, G., Contact and microbial allergy in pompholyx, *Contact Dermatitis*, 5, 46, 1979.

29. Menné, T., Borgan, O., and Green, A., Nickel allergy and hand dermatitis in a stratified sample of the Danish female population: an epidemiological study including a statistical appendix, *Acta Derm. Venerol.*, 62, 35, 1982.

30. English, O. S., Role of emotion in disorders of the skin, *AMA Arch. Dermatol.*, 60, 1063, 1949.

31. Borelli, S., Haut und Psyche, *Parfum Kosmetik*, 42, 427, 1961.

32. Reichenberger, M., Befunde bei Erstuntersuchungen von Hautkrankheiten im Friseurgewebe unter besonderer Berücksichtigung der Dyshidrosis, *Berufs-Dermatosen*, 20, 124, 1972.

33. Lindemayr, H., Das Friseurekzem, *Dermatosen*, 32, 5, 1984.

34. Frosch, P. J., *Hautirritation und empfindliche Haut*, Gross, Berlin, 1985.

35. Lammintausta, K., Hand dermatitis in different hospital workers, who perform wet work, *Dermatosen*, 31, 14, 1983.

36. Rajka, G., Transepidermal water loss on the hands in atopic dermatitis, *Arch. Dermatol. Forsch.*, 251, 111, 1974.

37. Grosshans, E., Physiopathologie de l'eczéma constitutionnel, 1st Congress of the European Society of Pediatric Dermatology, Münster, 1984.

38. Stüttgen, G., Die Ekzemgenese in pathophysiologischer Sicht, *Z. Hautkr.*, 52 (Suppl. 2), 8, 1977.

39. Foussereau, J. and Cavelier, C., Toxische Dermatitis und Pseudo-Kontaktallergie, *Dermatosen*, 26, 156, 1978.

40. Christensen, O. B., Pronosis in nickel allergy and hand eczema, *Contact Dermatitis*, 8, 7, 1982.

41. Schwanitz, H. J., Prävention chronischer Friseurekzeme, *Allergologie*, in press.

42. Björkstén, B., IgE und Lmyphozytenfunktion bei Kleinkindern als Vorhersager einer Allergie, *Z. Hautkr.*, 59, 817, 1984.

43. Fredericks, M. G. and Becker, F. T., Vesicular eruptions of the hands and feet of dyhidrotic type, *AMA Arch. Dermatol.*, 70, 107, 1954.

44. Budde, U. and Schwanitz, H. J., Kontaktdermatitiden bei Auszubildenden des Friseurhandwerks in Niedersachsen, *Dermatosen*, 39, 41, 1991.

8

Acute and Recurrent Vesicular Hand Dermatitis (Pompholyx)

Niels K. Veien and Torkil Menné

CONTENTS

I. INTRODUCTION AND DEFINITION

Acute or recurrent vesicular hand dermatitis, or pompholyx, is an eruptive, pruritic, vesicular dermatitis seen on the palmar aspects of the hands and fingers, the interdigital spaces, and the periungual area. The deep-seated, sago grain-like vesicles contain a clear fluid and often occur in clusters. Vesicles may coalesce to form small bullae. There is usually little or no inflammation, but frequent recurrences may lead to inflammation, making the distinction between this dermatitis and chronic hand eczema difficult. Repeated eruptions are characteristic and may eventually damage the matrices of the nails. Transverse ridging of the nails is a characteristic feature of recurrent vesicular hand dermatitis.[1] Some patients have pompholyx-like lesions on the soles of the feet and/ or in the interdigital spaces of the feet with no involvement of the hands.

The morphology of contact dermatitis of, for example, some nickel-allergic patients may be identical to pompholyx, but nickel eczema is usually also seen at sites other than the hands and feet. The current review includes patients with pompholyx who may also have eczema at other sites.

The terms "dyshidrosis" and "dyshidrotic eczema" in referring to pompholyx should be abandoned because no relationship between sweating or the sweat glands and pompholyx has ever been demonstrated. These terms are used only when they have appeared in the studies cited.

When making a diagnosis of recurrent vesicular, palmar dermatitis (pompholyx), with or without lesions in other areas of the skin, it is important to keep in mind that pompholyx is a nonspecific reaction pattern. An attempt should therefore always be made to identify the cause of the dermatitis. Cuases that should be considered are listed in Table 1.

II. EPIDEMIOLOGY

Hand eczema is common among adults. An epidemiological study performed in Gothenburg, Sweden, showed a 5.4% prevalence of hand eczema among adults and also that twice as many women as men had hand eczema;[2] 5% of the 1457 patients who participated in this study had pompholyx, a diagnosis that excluded allergic and irritant dermatitis, atopic hand eczema, nummular hand eczema, hyperkeratotic hand eczema, and unclassified variants.

In a study of 1659 patients with various hand dermatoses, 827 were found to have hand eczema; 51 had eczema of a recurrent, vesicular morphology.[3] Edman[4] found vesicular, palmar eczema in 153 of 425 patch-tested patients; 10% of these had eczema at sites other than the palms. This study

TABLE 1   Possible Causes of Dermatitis

Allergic contact dermatitis
External contactants
Systemic aggravating factors
Medicaments
Implanted or ingested metals
Nickel
Cobalt
Chromate
Fragrances and flavorings
Preservatives
Other haptens that may be ingested
Foodstuffs (in connection with mechanisms other than delayed-type hypersensitivity)
id reactions
Dermatophytids
Other infections
Severe eczemas
Parasitoses, such as scabies
Psychosomatic factors
Smoking
Drugs other than those causing systemic contact dermatitis

also showed vesicular, palmar eczema to be far more common among women than among men. A total of 1% of all patients appearing for first consultations in a hospital department of dermatology in Lund, Sweden, had pompholyx, and the prevalence in the Swedish population was estimated to be 1 per 1000. Seasonal variation was seen in only 18% of the patients. These patients had eruptions of dermatitis in the spring and fall.[5]

III. HISTORY AND REVIEW

Pompholyx was first described more than 100 years ago when Fox[6] and Hutchinson[7] wrote of vesicular, palmar eruptions. In 1953, Shelley[8] reviewed the condition known as dyshidrosis or pompholyx and stressed that it is a nonspecific reaction pattern of the palmar and plantar skin. He listed anatomical, physiological, biochemical, and experimental reasons for believing there was no association between pompholyx and the sweat glands or sweat ducts. Although in his series the cause of pompholyx in most cases remained unknown, most eruptions occurred during the warmest months of the year. Psychosomatic factors were seen to precipitate attacks of pompholyx, and id reactions and drug reactions were also seen.

Castelain[9] described 145 patients with dyshidrotic eczema. Seventy-one of these had lesions on their hands, 15 had lesions on the feet, and 39 had lesions on both hands and feet. Twenty patients had lesions on the hands, feet, and elsewhere. Most patients in this study experienced aggravation during the warmest months. Although 38 patients had positive patch tests, the reactions were considered to be relevant for no more than 8 of them. Forty patients were found to be atopic, and 10 patients reacted to oral challenge with metals: 4 reacted to nickel, 2 to chromate, 3 to nickel and cobalt, and 1 to nickel and chromate. Five patients in the study were considered to have id reactions, and for 11 patients, a psychosomatic cause was considered of importance. For 46 patients no cause of the eczema could be determined.

Lodi et al.[10] determined the cause of pompholyx in 104 patients through the use of patch tests, prick tests, and intradermal tests with aeroallergens, as well as with microbial and food allergens, oral challenge tests, blood tests, and histopathology. These patients were compared with 208 age- and sex-matched control persons. Patch testing revealed nickel allergy in 21 of the patients. Eighty-three patch test-negative patients were subjected to a placebo-controlled, oral challenge procedure, and in this way six were shown to have nickel allergy. Thus, 26% of 104 patients were shown to be nickel sensitive compared with 6% of the control persons. The eczema patients also had more positive prick tests to inhalant allergens than did control persons; 34% of the patients reacted to *Dermatophagoides farinae* compared with 6% of the controls.

The eczema of 41% of these patients showed seasonal variation; 80% of the patients experienced flares when temperatures were high, 37% had hyperhidrosis, and 17% experienced flares at times of emotional stress. Histopathology regularly disclosed spongiosis and lymphocyte exocytosis regardless of the cause of the pompholyx. These authors concluded that pompholyx is a nonspecific reaction pattern seen in predisposed individuals.

Menné and Hjorth[1] reviewed the literature of pompholyx up until the early 1980s and concluded that, in those cases in which it is possible to determine an etiology, pompholyx is an allergic reaction to epicutaneous or systematic exposure to haptens or proteins. They also concluded that available diagnostic methods are insufficient, in part, perhaps because no animal model is available for further study.

IV. CLINICAL FEATURES

An eruption of vesicular hand eczema is usually preceded by severe itching, occasionally accompanied by a burning sensation. Vesicles appears within 24 h. They may appear on otherwise uninvolved skin as individual, tiny blisters or as clusters of vesicles imbedded in or protruding from the palmar skin of the fingers and hands (Figure 1). Bullae are occasionally seen in severe eruptions, and tiny vesicles can sometimes be seen on the lid of the bullae. A symmetrical distribution of recurrent vesicular dermatitis is typical. Pruritis usually persists throughout the eruption. Some patients find relief if the lids of the vesicles are scratched open.

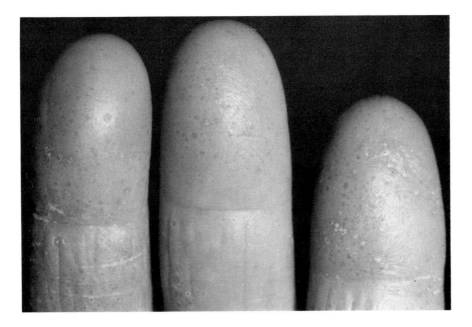

FIGURE 1.   An eruption of vesicles embedded in the skin.

Inflammation may occur, particularly if there are repeated vesicular eruptions. Repeated eruptions with inflammation commonly occur interdigitally but may also involve the entire palm of the hand. Frequent eruptions in the same area may also be followed by scaling (Figure 2), and if there are frequent recurrences of both inflammation and scaling, recurrent vesicular hand eczema may be clinically indistinguishable from other types of chronic hand eczema.

Inflammation of single lesions may be so severe as to resemble vasculitis. Transverse furrows in the nails may accompany a vesicular eruption of the periungual area and the nail matrix. A careful inspection of the nails may alert the dermatologist to the previous occurrence of eruptions (Figure 3).

Some patients experience concurrent, symmetrical vesicular eruptions on plantar and palmar skin or interdigitally on the toes and fingers. Plantar eruptions may also occur when there are no palmar eruptions.

V.   HISTOPATHOLOGY

In early studies of recurrent vesicular hand dermatitis, it was presumed that the sweat ducts were involved and that the occlusion of pores was an important aspect of the pathogenesis.[6] More recent studies of the histopathology have shown no such association. Simons[11] studied 10,000 histopathological sections from 26 cases of dyshidrotic eczema and found no connection between sweat ducts and vesicles.

Similarly, Kutzner et al.[12] studied the vesicular palmar and plantar eruptions of patients for whom all other diagnoses had been excluded. The authors made use of both light microscopy and electron microscopy, and they concluded that the acrosyringium is not involved in pompholyx and that this clinical entity represents a spongiotic dermatitis modified by the distinctive characteristics of palmar and plantar skin (Figure 4). These authors and Ackerman[13] declared that due to the lack of involvement of the sweat ducts and the acrosyringium, dyshidrosis was a misnomer.

Christensen et al.[14] examined biopsies of test sites as well as the palmar skin of five nickel-sensitive patients before and after flares of their usual vesicular palmar dermatitis induced by oral challenge with nickel. Twenty-four hours after the challenge marked dermal edema and epidermal spongiosis were seen. A dense lymphocytic infiltrate was seen around the superficial dermal vessels. Immunofluorescence disclosed no deposits of immunoglobulins.

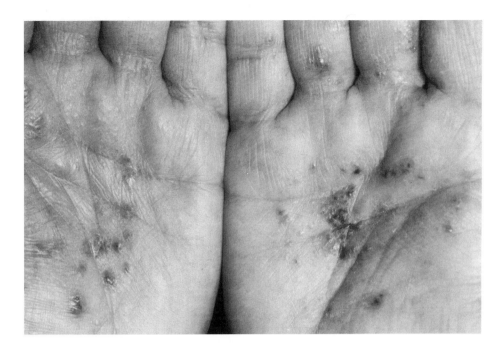

FIGURE 2. Recurrent vesicular dermatitis with features of chronic hand eczema.

VI. RECURRENT VESICULAR HAND ECZEMA AND ALLERGIC CONTACT DERMATITIS

Although pompholyx is usually thought of as an endogenous dermatitis, a morphologically identical pattern of dermatitis resulting from contact with pesticides has been described.[15] In another study, 21 of 286 metalworkers had dyshidrotic eczema. Three had one or more positive patch tests, and one patient was considered to be atopic. The predominant cause of the vesicular dermatitis in this series was considered to be a primary irritant dermatitis from soluble oil.[16]

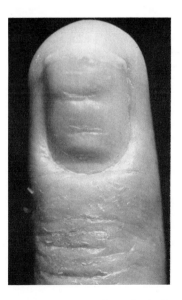

FIGURE 3. Transverse furrows on a nail associated with recurrent vesicular dermatitis of the fingers.

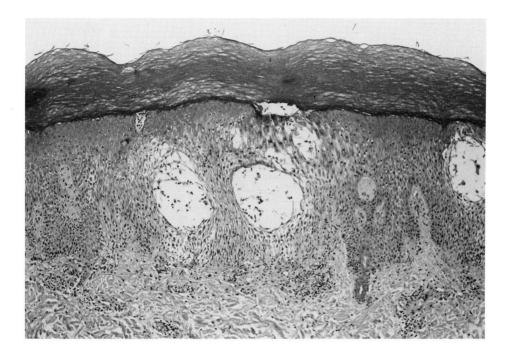

FIGURE 4. Histological changes in a biopsy specimen from palmar vesicular dermatitis. There is spongiotic dermatitis with three distinct vesicles (original magnification x 63). (Courtesy of Annelise Krogdahl, M.D., Institute of Pathology, Aalborg Sygehus, Aalborg, Denmark.)

Meneghini and Angelini[17] patch tested 364 patients who had pompholyx. Most of the patients were also tested intradermally with various microbial antigens; 9.3% were sensitized to paraphenylenediamine, 7.4% reacted to potassium dichromate, 3% reacted to cobalt chloride, and 2.2% to parabens. Six (2.8%) of 213 patients compared with none of 182 control persons had positive reactions to intradermal testing with epidermophytin.

Hjorth and Roed-Petersen[18] described hand eczema in food handlers and stressed the fact that vesicles appeared within 20 min of contact with the offending food. Tosti et al.[19] also saw the rapid devleopment of spongiotic vesicles after contact with foods. The reactions in this latter study occurred only on previously involved skin on the fingers, but not when testing was carried out on the back. These authors concluded that what they were observing was probably a nonimmunological mechanism that occurred when mediators were liberated by the foods used for testing. In another study, one occluded patch test with nickel left for 24 h on the fingers of a nickel-sensitive patient with pompholyx produced a vesicular response.[1]

In patients with allergic contact dermatitis, pompholyx has been described as a *de novo* eruption when the hapten is given orally. Ekelund and Möller[20] gave 12 patients known to be sensitive to neomycin an oral challenge with the hapten and saw pompholyx in 3 patients, 5 experienced a flare of the original dermatitis, and 6 had flares at previous patch test sites. Menné and Weismann[21] described similar *de novo* vesicular hand eczema in a neomycin-sensitive patient.

Roed-Petersen and Hjorth[22] described two patients sensitive to the antioxidants butylhydroxyanisole and butylhydroxytoluene who developed vesicular dermatitis on the fingers after open oral challenge with the same substances. Both patients remained free of symptoms when they avoided these antioxidants in food.

A vesicular flare-up reaction with hemorrhagic lesions was seen in a patient sensitized to pyrazinobutazone when a dose of 300 mg pyrazinobutazone was given orally twice daily for 3 days. A flare at a previously positive patch test site was also seen.[23] Similar reactions have been seen when attempts to hyposensitive with rhus antigen have been carried out in patients sensitive to poison ivy.[24,25]

A. Implanted Metals

In persons who are sensitive to nickel, cobalt, and/or chromate, the implantation of metals to repair fractures, the metal casings of pacemakers, the metal parts of artificial replacement joints, and metals used in corrective dental procedures may cause systemic contact dermatitis. Recurrent vesicular palmar dermatitis may be a clinical manifestation of this type of hypersensitivity.

Hubler and Hubler[26] described in detail a chromate-sensitive patient who developed widespread dermatitis, including a vesicular eruption on the palms and soles, shortly after the insertion of a metal dental plate. The dermatitis disappeared when the dental plate was removed and recurred when it was reinserted.

A nickel-sensitive woman who had previously had hand eczema developed a pompholyx-like eruption on both legs 2 days after the implantation of a pacemaker.[27] A woman with positive patch tests to nickel and cobalt developed severe dermatitis of the palms and forearms after the insertion of a plate made of vitallium (a cobalt-chromium alloy) after suffering a fracture of the distal forearm. The dermatitis was most severe directly over the site of the inserted plate. Patch testing with the plate itself produced a positive reaction.[28]

Two of six nickel-sensitive patients developed systemic contact dermatitis, including vesicular palmar dermatitis, after the use of infusion needles shown to release nickel.[29]

Similarly, three of four nickel-sensitive patients described by Oakley et al.[30] developed pompholyx-type hand eczema shortly after skin clips were used for wound closure. Three of the patients were patch tested with the skin clips and all had positive reactions.

On the whole, the general population runs little risk of developing the aforementioned side effects after implantation of metals. Staerkjaer and Menné[31] reviewed the risk of developing such dermatological side effects among 1085 girls with orthodontic braces and found no increased risk in this particular group. Neither did Spiechowicz et al.[32] see any increased risk in a similar study conducted in Poland. Hensten-Pettersen[33] reviewed dermatological complications from orthodontic treatment and concluded that, although nickel allergy is of concern in orthodontic treatment, most patients, even those who are nickel sensitive, suffer no adverse dermatological effects.

Wilkinson[34] reviewed the subject on nickel allergy and orthopedic prostheses and concluded that prosthetic loosening was most commonly associated with sensitivity to metals other than nickel and that cutaneous side effects were most often caused by nickel in the prostheses. Modern prostheses with a metal-on-plastic or metal-on-ceramic construction do not generally cause dermatological problems.

B. Nickel Eczema and Antabuse®

Drugs that interfere with nickel and cobalt metabolism may cause flare-up reactions in patients who are sensitive to these metals. Veien[35] described four nickel-sensitive patients who experienced flares of dermatitis after the initiation of Antabuse® (disulfiram) therapy for alcoholism. Disulfiram chelates nickel. Two of the patients in this study developed vesciular hand eczema (Figure 5).

Case studies of patients who inadvertently developed dermatitis while being treated with Antabuse for chronic alcoholism are paralleled by studies of the deliberate use of Antabuse as a chelating agent in the treatment of nickel-allergic patients. When a daily dose of 300 mg Antabuse® was used in the treatment of 11 nickel-allergic patients, 9 of the patients experienced flares of dermatitis. One patient had a persistently marked increase of nickel levels in serum and urine and developed transient vasculitis after 4 to 8 weeks of treatment. The treatment did not benefit this patient, whereas the dermatitis of seven other patients in this study healed during Antabuse® treatment.[36] Similarly, Christensen and Kristensen[37] found Antabuse® to be useful in treating nickel-sensitive patients with pompholyx hand eczema. They also noticed that flares of dermatitis occurred about 1 week after the initiation of treatment with 100 mg of Antabuse® taken twice daily. Nine of 11 patients in this study also had secondary eruptions at previous sites of nickel contact dermatitis or nickel patch tests. All the patients relapsed upon discontinuation of the treatment.

A placebo-controlled trial in which 24 patients with nickel allergy and vesicular hand eczema received Antabuse® or a placebo showed that Antabuse® had a marginally better effect. Five of 11 patients treated with Antabuse healed compared with 2 of 13 patients who received a placebo.[38]

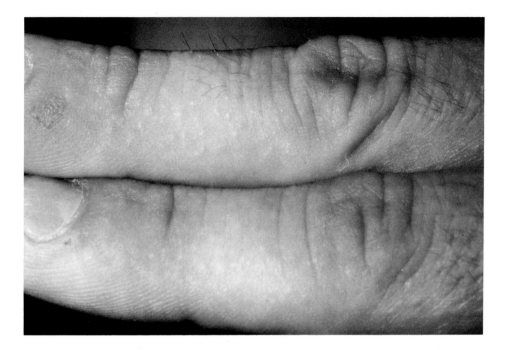

FIGURE 5. A *de novo* eruption of vesicular dermatitis on the fingers of a nickel-sensitive man seen after the initiation of Antabuse® therapy for the treatment of chronic alcoholism.

Nickel levels in the plasma and urine of alcoholics treated with disulfiram remained high during the treatment period.[39] The aforedescribed experience indicates that nickel may cause systemic contact dermatitis and that recurrent vesicular hand eczema may be one of the clinical features of this type of dermatitis.

C. Nickel Allergy and Hand Eczema

Menné[40] found an association between nickel allergy and hand eczema in an omnibus study of 1961 women. In this study, the eczema of half of the nickel-sensitive patients with hand eczema was of a pompholyx morphology. Christensen[41] and Edman[4] found an association between nickel allergy and interdigital as well as palmar eczema. In a study of the association between the course of atopic dermatitis in adults and nickel allergy, Lammintausta et al.[42] did not find an overrepresentation of pompholyx among their nickel-allergic, atopic patients.

In a detailed study of the available literature on the association between nickel allergy and hand eczema, Wilkinson and Wilkinson[43] discussed many unsolved problems, some of which are due to differences in methods of patient selection.

D. Oral Ingestion of Nickel

The assumption that there is an association between nickel allergy and recurrent vesicular hand eczema is supported by several trials of placebo-controlled oral challenge with doses of nickel ranging from 0.5 to 5.6 mg. These studies indicate that an oral dose of nickel may reactivate vesicular hand eczema in nickel-sensitive patients and that the response is dose-dependent. A dose of 0.5 mg nickel will reactivate vesicular hand eczema in only a small proportion of nickel-sensitive patients. Oral challenge with 2.5 mg nickel will cause a flare of dermatitis in approximately 50% of such patients, and a majority of nickel-sensitive patients will experience a flare-up reaction after a dose of 5.6 mg nickel.[44] Foods rich in nickel content caused flares of vesicular hand eczema in 11 of 14 nickel-sensitive patients.[45]

Nickel-sensitive persons with delayed type hypersensitivity to nickel characteristically appear to experience aggravation of palmar and interdigital vesicular eczema after oral challenge with nickel. Some patch test-negative persons with recurrent vesicular hand eczema experience flares of this eczema after oral challenge with salts of nickel, cobalt, or dichromate. Women appear more likely to react to nickel, whereas men more typically react to chromate.[46] Careful questioning of some of the women in the study who reacted to nickel disclosed that some of them had a history of intolerance to metal items in close contact with the skin, thus indicating that these women had false-negative patch tests.

A vesicular eruption seen as the result of oral challenge with nickel appears to be characteristic for patients who present with vesicular eczema as a part of their clinical disease. In one study, none of 299 patients with negative patch tests and eczema other than vesicular hand eczema experienced flares of vesicular hand eczema after oral challenge with nickel. Seven of 61 patients with hyperkeratotic hand eczema reacted to oral challenge to nickel with pruritus and fissures, and 3 of 28 women with other than keratotic and vesicular hand eczema experienced flares of dermatitis.[47]

None of 27 persons intoxicated with nickel released from a heater used for dialysis developed vesicular hand eczema.[48] Two days after dialysis, these persons were shown to have nickel levels in plasma of up to 4.7 mg/l, indicating that there were levels of up to 9 mg/l immediately after dialysis. The characteristic symptoms of intoxication included nausea, vomiting, general weakness, headache, and palpitation.

Twenty workers who accidentally ingested up to 2.5 g nickel in drinking water experienced nausea, abdominal pain, headache, diarrhea, vomiting, coughing, and shortness of breath. All these symptoms disappeared within 3 days. No mention was made of the appearance of hand dermatitis.[49]

E. Low-Nickel Diets

One implication of the flares of dermatitis seen after oral challenge with nickel is that nickel-sensitive patients with vesicular hand eczema might benefit from following a nickel-restricted diet. This is a somewhat controversial issue, and due to the difficulties inherent in carrying out well-controlled diet trials, no properly controlled trials have thus far been conducted. The issue is further complicated by the fact that the doses of nickel used in oral challenge experiments are much higher than the amounts of nickel naturally ingested in food. The challenge experiments with foods rich in nickel indicate that certain foods containing significant amounts of nickel may aggravate the vesicular hand eczema of nickel-sensitive patients.

In one open diet trial,[50] the vesicular hand eczema of 9 of 17 nickel-sensitive patients who had followed a low nickel diet showed improvement. All the patients experienced flares of dermatitis after oral challenge with 2.5 mg nickel. In 11 of 14 of these patients there was a decrease in the nickel excreted in the urine during the diet period. Gawkrodger et al.[51] had a similar experience with one extremely nickel-sensitive patient.

In another study, 204 nickel-sensitive patients, approximately half of whom had recurrent vesicular hand and/or foot eczema, were asked to follow a low-nickel diet.[52] The dermatitis of 121 of these patients improved after a period of 1 to 2 months. One-hundred fifty of the patients responded to a questionnaire 1 to 5 years later, and 88 of those who responded maintained that diet treatment helped to control their nickel dermatitis.

Pigatto[53] saw no benefit of diet treatment of eight nickel-sensitive patients with vesicular hand eczema. In the same study, the vesicular eczema of eight other patients improved after treatment with disodium chromoglycate.

It is likely that moderately nickel-sensitive patients respond better to a reduction in nickel intake than do very sensitive patients. This may be because it is difficult to reduce nickel intake in food to less than half of normal, prediet levels,[54] which is probably not sufficient to bring very nickel-sensitive patients under their reactivity-to-nickel threshold.

The real value of diet treatment cannot be determined until an effective, safe nickel-chelating agent has been found or until more is known about the metabolism of nickel. Thus far, little is known about the amounts of nickel that reach the target organ, i.e., the skin, after ingestion or absorption of nickel from various sources.

F. Cobalt

Contact allergy to cobalt is commonly associated with hand eczema, and concomitant nickel and cobalt allergy appears to be linked to severe hand eczema.[55] Cobalt allergy appears, likewise, to be associated with the morphology of dermatitis known as recurrent vesicular hand eczema. Fifty-three of 146 patients who were challenged orally with nickel, cobalt, and a placebo had recurrent vesicular hand eczema. Thirteen of these patients had positive patch tests to cobalt, and seven of them experienced flares of their dermatitis after challenge with 1 mg cobalt given as cobalt chloride, but not after a placebo. Three of six patients who had cobalt allergy and recurrent vesicular hand eczema reacted to cobalt.[56]

A cobalt-sensitive man who was treated for chronic alcoholism with a daily dose of 800 mg disulfiram developed vesicular-bullous hand eczema 1 to 2 days after initiation of this therapy. Treatment was continued, and the hand eczema faded when the dose of disulfiram was reduced to 200 mg/day. Disulfiram chelates both nickel and cobalt, and this reaction pattern supports the hypothesis that endogenous cobalt dermatitis is a clinical entity.[57]

G. Chromium

Chromate-sensitive patients may develop occupational hand eczema that persists even after the work during which they were sensitized is discontinued.[58] Some of these patients have recurrent vesicular hand eczema, and a group of 19 such patients took part in a placebo-controlled oral challenge with 2.5 mg chromium given as potassium dichromate. Nine of the patients reacted to chromate, but not to the placebo, with a flare of their usual vesicular hand eczema.[59] Goitre et al.[60] also described a patient with recurrent vesicular hand eczema who experienced a flare after oral challenge with 2.5 mg chromium given as potassium dichromate. Fregert[61] saw vesicular hand eczema in all five of the patients he challenged with just 50 μg potassium dichromate. In another placebo-controlled study, Sertoli et al.[62] carried out an oral challenge with 50 μg potassium dichromate, and 1 of 3 patients had a flare of vesicular hand eczema. Mali[63] described a patient with vesicular hand eczema who had a positive reaction to an intradermal test with potassium dichromate. He suspected that the dermatitis was caused by the inhalation of chromate.

H. Balsam of Peru

In a classic study by Hjorth,[64] the vesicular hand eczema of a balsam-sensitive patient flared after the ingestion of a large quantity of orange marmelade. Veien et al.[65] challenged 17 balsam-sensitive patients with 1 g balsam of Peru. Four of four patients with recurrent vesicular hand eczema had flare-up reactions after oral challenge with balsam but not after challenge with a placebo. Dooms-Goossens et al.[66] studied reactions to spices and described three patients who had dyshidrotic hand eczema that flared after the ingestion of various spices.

VII. DOES FOOD PLAY A ROLE?

Recurrent vesicular eruptions on the hands of 30 patients improved after they had followed a strict diet regimen, eliminating certain foods.[67] The foods ascertained to be most likely to cause a recurrence of dermatitis were tuna fish, wheat, milk, tomato, pork, pineapple, American cheese, eggs, lamb, chocolate, and chicken.

One-hundred thirteen patients with various types of eczema took part in an open study of the effects of an elimination diet. Thirty-eight of the patients had recurrent vesicular eczema on the fingers and/or the palms. The dermatitis of approximately 50% of all the patients improved after diet treatment. The foods most commonly implicated in repeated open oral challenges were egg, milk, tomato, cheese, and food additives.[68] In a study of 21 patients with various types of eczema who consumed excessive quantities of coffee, the same authors found 9 patients with recurrent vesicular hand eczema. The eczema of all patients in this latter group improved when coffee intake was reduced. None of three patients challenged orally with caffeine showed any reaction.[69]

VIII. "ID" REACTION ON THE HANDS

The classical example of the "id" reaction is a dermatophytid, a symmetrical vesicular eruption on the hands caused by dermatophytosis of the feet. Sulzberger and Baer[70] provided a clear description of this entity and suggested that four requirements must be met before the diagnosis of an id reaction can be made: (1) there must be a demonstrable focus of primary fungus infection on the feet or elsewhere; (2) the onset of the eruption on the hands must follow activation or irritation of the primary focus; (3) the eruption on the hands must be symmetrically distributed and be found primarily on the thenar and hypothenar eminences, the palms, and the sides of the fingers; and (4) the eruption on the hands must subside within a reasonable period after the primary focus of the fungus infection has cleared or has at least been brought under control. These authors also suggested that id eruptions on the hands may follow eczematous eruptions on the feet and possibly elsewhere. Haxthausen[71] described widespread id reactions in 88 of 235 patients with stasis eczema. An autoimmune, cellular immune reaction has been suggested as the cause of id-like reactions from hypostatic eczema.[72] In temperate climates, dermatophytids are most common in the summer months. Most dermatophytids are caused by the zoophilic variant of *T. mentagrophytes* and are associated with inflammatory tinea pedis.[73] Vesicular eruptions of the palms and fingers may also be seen in connection with scabies. In such cases, immediate-type hypersensitivity to the infestation may be responsible.[74]

IX. THE RELATIONSHIP BETWEEN RECURRENT VESICULAR HAND ECZEMA AND ATOPY

Approximately 50% of those who have severe atopic dermatitis in childhood will develop hand eczema as adults.[75] In a study of 58 patients, Schwanitz[76] considered recurrent vesicular palmoplantar dermatitis to be a varient of atopic dermatitis.

Bäurle[77] found that 44% of 350 patients with dyshidrotic hand eczema were atopics and found a correlation between dyshidrotic hand eczema, total plasma immunoglobulin E (IgE), and smoking. In this study, patients with recurrent vesicular hand eczema were more likely to have contact sensitivity than patients with other types of hand eczema.

Lodi et al.[10] found personal and familial atopy in 50% of their patients with pompholyx compared with 11.5% of control persons.

Schuppli[78] performed extensive allergy testing in 68 patients with dyshidrosis and found many positive stratch tests to house dust and pollens. Based on elimination and challenge tests, Schuppli[78] considered a number of these reactions to be relevant and suggested that the inhalation of flour could cause dyshidrosis in bakers.

Young[79] examined 75 patients with dyshidrotic eczema and, after excluding cases caused by fungus, compared the results of intracutaneous tests performed on these patients with results obtained in a control group of 55 persons. He found positive reactions to one or more allergens among 34 of the 75 patients (45%) compared with 3 of 55 (5.5%) of the control persons. Twenty-one of the 75 patients (28%) had positive reactions to one or more allergens and a family history of atopy compared with 2 of 55 control persons (3.5%). Twenty-five of the patients had seasonal eruptions, usually in the spring and/or summer. Fourteen of the 34 patients with positive scratch tests experienced seasonal aggravation of their dermatitis, whereas 11 of 41 with negative scratch tests had such aggravation. Using both the intracutaneous test and the radioallergosorbent test, Van Ketel et al.[80] found a reaction to human dander in 12 of 30 patients with pompholyx. Ten of 30 reacted to house dust mites.

Edman[4] found no relationship between vesicular palmar eczema and atopy in 153 patients. Eight of 50 patients with atopic dermatitis admitted to a dermatology ward developed pompholyx 4 to 12 days after admission. No explanation was found[81]

X. ARE PSYCHOLOGICAL FACTORS OF SIGNIFICANCE?

Some patients with recurrent vesicular hand dermatitis report eruptions or aggravation of their dermatitis when experiencing emotional stress. In one study, 20 patients with dyshidrotic eczema were seen to have less aggressive and more permissive personalities than a control population.[82] Kellum[83] reported great success in using psychotherapy in the treatment of patients with pompholyx.

Miller and Coger[84] studied 33 patients with dyshidrotic eczema who were randomly assigned to either increase or decrease the electrical conductivity of their skin using a biofeedback technique. The dermatitis of those patients who demonstrated a decrease in conductivity showed improvement, whereas patients with no change in conductivity had no change in the activity of their dermatitis. In an uncontrolled study,[85] in which relaxation was encouraged by means of a biofeedback technique, the severe pompholyx of five patients showed substantial improvement after this therapy.

XI. RECURRENT PALMO-PLANTAR DERMATITIS AS A MANIFESTATION OF OTHER DERMATOSES

Vesicular palmar and plantar dermatitis is associated with a variety of disorders. Several authors[86-88] have described hemorrhagic vesicular lesions in patients with bullous pemphigoid, but other patients in these same studies presented with vesicular eczema indistinguishable from classical pompholyx. A joint study carried out in the bullous disease clinic at the Oxford and St. John's Hospitals showed vesicular palmo-plantar lesions in patients with pemphigoid and linear IgA disease as well in patients with herpes gestationis.[89] In another study,[90] hemorrhagic pompholyx was seen in a 29-year-old man with linear IgA disease. Lichen planus may also present with vesicular palmar and plantar lesions,[91] and one of various clinical manifestations of scabies is vesicular palmar and plantar dermatitis, probably caused by an immune reaction to the scabies mite.[74]

The clinical features of autoimmune progesterone dermatitis may include a palmar vesicular eruption in addition to more pleomorphic, widespread skin lesions. Two patients with positive immediate-type skin tests to progesterone and clinical features, which included vesicular palmar dermatitis, were described by Miura et al.[92]

XII. DIFFERENTIAL DIAGNOSIS

Certain pustular diseases are seen in the same sites as recurrent vesicular palmo and/or plantar dermatitis. Palmo-plantar pustulosis characteristically presents with crops of 1- to 4-mm tense pustules in the central part of the palms and/or soles. The lesions dry out leaving a brown scale. Although there is normally little or no pruritus, the condition can be pruritic, and initial lesions may appear as vesicles. On close inspection, the content of the early vesicles is seen to be cloudy, and the lesions soon take on the appearance of pustules. A transition from purely vesicular to pustular eruptions is also occasionally seen.[93] Pustular bacterid is a pustular palmo-plantar eruption, which appears suddenly and is more widespread on the palmar and plantar surfaces than palmo-plantar pustolosis. Lesions may also appear around the nails and on the dorsal aspects of the fingers. Acrodermatitis continua is a painful, severely inflamed pustular eruption, usually appearing on the fingers and toes. The condition results in nail dystrophy, and dystrophy of the involved digits may occur. Infantile acropustulosis is intensely pruritic vesicular and pustular eruptions on the hands and feet seen in infancy. This condition fades spontaneously.[94,95]

Some scaly and/or hyperkeratotic palmo-plantar dermatoses may resemble recurrent vesicular palmar and/or plantar dermatitis. Dyshidrosis lamellosa sicca appears more superficially in the palmar epidermis than vesicular eruptions. A tiny desquamation of the stratum corneum is initially seen. The lesion expands to become a superficial annular scale before gradually disappearing (Figure 6). There is no pruritus, and this disease rarely evolves into actual hand eczema. Repeated eruptions may make the stratum corneum so thin that the palmar surface itself becomes thin and sensitive. Hyperkeratotic palmar and/or plantar dermatitis characteristically appears with well-demarcated patches of hyperkeratosis with fissures in the palms and/or soles. Although this dermatosis may be eruptive, there is normally no pruritus. Flares, however, manifest themselves as pruritus and new fissures with no vesicles.[96]

Repeated eruptions of vesicular hand eczema may lead to hyperkeratosis, and it is not unusual for the two conditions to resemble each other. If there are vesicles at the outer edge of an eruption, it should be classified as vesicular eczema. Psoriasis of the palms usually presents as well-demar-

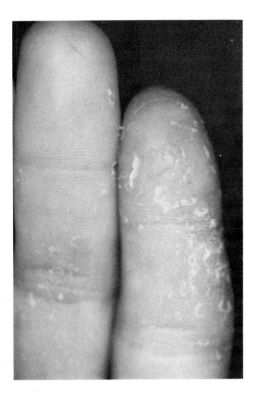

FIGURE 6. Dyshidrosis lamellosa sicca.

cated plaques that exhibit psoriasiform scaling. If palmar pustules are present in the area affected by psoriasis, it can be difficult to make the differential diagnosis to vesicular palmar dermatitis. Psoriasis is usually non-pruritic, and vesicles are rarely seen.

XIII. CONCLUSIONS

This review is based on a broad definition of pompholyx as an acute or recurrent pruritic vesicular eruption of the palms, palmar aspects, and/or sides of the fingers, possibly with an accompanying, similar plantar dermatitis. Patients with pompholyx who may have dermatitis at other sites as well as pompholyx have also been included.

This broad definition would make pompholyx more common than previously cited studies[2,3] indicate. In these studies pompholyx was the diagnosis made when allergic contact dermatitis, atopic hand eczema, and nummular eczema had been excluded.

Keeping the broad definition in mind, pompholyx is best viewed as a nonspecific reaction pattern. Once a diagnosis of pompholyx has been made, the search for an etiology should begin along the lines given in the introduction to this chapter. If no etiology can be determined, aggravating factors should be sought.

Patients should be trained to recognize the eruption of vesicles. Experience in the use of the oral challenge procedure in which patients with allergic contact dermatitis are challenged with the hapten indicate that flares appear within 3 days of the challenge. Some patients can detect aggravating factors by systematically recording possible aggravating factors with which they have been in contact during the days immediately preceding a vesicular eruption.

REFERENCES

1. Menné, T. and Hjorth, N., Pompholyx: dyshidrotic eczema, *Semin. Dermatol.*, 2, 75, 1983.
2. Meding, B. and Swanbeck, G., Epidemiology of different types of hand eczema in an industrial city, *Acta Derm. Venereol.*, 69, 227, 1989.
3. Agrup, G., Hand Eczema and Other Hand Dermatoses in South Sweden, Ph.D. thesis, University of Lund, Lund, Sweden, 1969.
4. Edman, B., Palmar eczema: a pathogenetic role for acetylsalicylic acid, contraceptives and smoking?, *Acta Derm. Venereol.*, 68, 402, 1988.
5. Thelin, I. and Agrup, G., Pompholyx: a one year series, *Acta Derm. Venereol.*, 65, 214, 1985.
6. Fox, T., on dyshidrosis, *Am. J. Syphilol. Dermatol.*, 4, 1, 1873.
7. Hutchinson, J., Cheiro-pompholyx: notes of a clinical lecture, *Lancet*, 1, 630, 1876.
8. Shelley, W. B., Dyshydrosis (pompholyx), *Arch. Dermatol.*, 68 (Suppl.), 314, 1953.
9. Castelain, P.-Y., Les Dysidroses, *Ann. Dermatol. Venereol.*, 114, 579, 1987.
10. Lodi, A., Betti, R., Chiarelli, G., Urbani, C. E., and Crosti, C., Epidemiological, clinical and allergological observations on pompholyx, *Contact Dermatitis*, 26, 17, 1992.
11. Simons, R. D. G. Ph., *Eczema of the Hands*, S. Karger, Basel, Switzerland, 1966, 26.
12. Kutzner, H., Wurzel, R. M., and Wolff, H. H., Are acrosyringia involved in the pathogenesis of "dyshidrosis"?, *Am. J. Dermatopathol.*, 8, 109, 1986.
13. Ackerman, A. B., *Histological Diagnosis of Inflammatory Skin Diseases*, Lea & Febiger, Philadelphia, 1978.
14. Christensen, O. B., Lindström, C., Löfberg, H., and Möller, H., Micromorphology and specificity of orally induced flare-up reactions in nickel-sensitive patients, *Acta Derm. Venereol.*, 61, 505, 1981.
15. Crippa, M., Misquith, L., Lonati, A., and Pasolini, G., Dyshidrotic eczema and sensitization to dithiocarbamates in a florist, *Contact Dermatitis*, 23, 203, 1990.
16. De Boer, E. M., Bruynzeel, D. P., and Van Ketel, W. G., Dyshidrotic eczema as an occupational dermatitis in metal workers, *Contact Dermatitis*, 19, 184, 1988.
17. Meneghini, C. L. and Angelini, G., Contact and microbial allergy in pompholyx, *Contact Dermatitis*, 5, 46, 1979.
18. Hjorth, N. and Roed-Petersen, J., Occupational protein contact dermatitis in food handlers, *Contact Dermatitis*, 2, 28, 1976.
19. Tosti, A., Fanti, P. A., Guerra, L., Piancastelli, E., Poggi, S., and Pileri, S., Morphological and immunohistochemical study of immediate contact dermatitis of the hands due to foods, *Contact Dermatitis*, 22, 81, 1990.
20. Ekelund, A.-G. and Möller, H., Oral provocation in eczematous contact allergy to neomycin and hydroxyquinolines, *Acta Derm. Venereol.*, 49, 422, 1969.
21. Menné, T. and Weismann, K., Hämatogenes Kontaktekzem nach oraler Gabe von Neomyzin, *Hautarzt*, 35, 319, 1984.
22. Roed-Petersen, J. and Hjorth, N., Contact dermatitis from antioxidants, *Br. J. Dermatol.*, 94, 233, 1976.
23. Dorado Bris, J. M., Aragues Montanes, M., Sols Candela, M., and Garcia Diez, A., Contact sensitivity to pyrazinobutazone (Carudol®) with positive oral provocation test, *Contact Dermatitis*, 26, 355, 1992.
24. Kligman, A., Poison ivy (rhus) dermatitis, *AMA Arch. Dermatol.*, 77, 149, 1958.
25. Shelmire, B., Cutaneous and systemic reactions observed during oral poison ivy therapy, *J. Allergy*, 12, 252, 1941.
26. Hubler, W. R., Jr. and Hubler, W. R., Sr., Dermatitis from a chromium dental plate, *Contact Dermatitis*, 9, 377, 1983.
27. Landwehr, A. J. and Van Ketel, W. G., Pompholyx after implantation of a nickel-containing pacemaker in a nickel-allergic patient, *Contact Dermatitis*, 9, 147, 1983.
28. Thomas, R. H. M., Rademaker, M., Goddard, N. J., and Munro, D. D., Severe eczema of the hands due to an orthopaedic plate made of vitallium, *Br. Med. J.*, 294, 106, 1987.
29. Smeenk, G. and Teunissen, P. C., Allergische reacties op nikkel uit infusie-toedieningssystemen, *Ned. Tijdscht. Geneeskd.*, 121, 4, 1977.

30. Oakley, A. M. M., Ive, F. A., and Carr, M. M., Skin clips are contraindicated when there is nickel allergy, *J. R. Soc. Med.,* 80, 290, 1987.
31. Staerkjaer, L. and Menné, T., Nickel allergy and orthodontic treatment, *Eur. J. Orthodontol.,* 12, 284, 1990.
32. Spiechowicz, E., Glantz, P.-O., Axéll, T., and Chmielewski, W., Oral exposure to a nickel-containing dental alloy of persons with hypersensitive skin reactions to nickel, *Contact Dermatitis,* 10, 206, 1984.
33. Hensten-Pettersen, A., Nickel allergy and dental treatment procedures, in *Nickel and the Skin: Immunology and Toxicology,* Maibach, H. I. and Menné, T., Eds., CRC Press, Boca Raton, FL, 1989, 195.
34. Wilkinson, J. D., Nickel allergy and orthopedic prosthesis, in *Nickel and the Skin: Immunology and Toxicology,* Maibach, H. I. and Menné, T., Eds., CRC Press, Boca Raton, FL, 1989, 187.
35. Veien, N. K., Cutaneous side effects of Antabuse® in nickel allergic patients treated for alcoholism, *Boll. Dermatol. Allergol. Prof.,* 2, 139, 1987.
36. Kaaber, K., Menné, T., Tjell, J. C., and Veien, N., Antabuse® treatment of nickel dermatitis: chelation — a new principle in the treatment of nickel dermatitis, *Contact Dermatitis,* 5, 221, 1979.
37. Christensen, O. B. and Kristensen, M., Treatment with disulfiram in chronic nickel hand dermatitis, *Contact Dermatitis,* 8, 59, 1982.
38. Kaaber, K., Menné, T., Veien, N., and Hougaaard, P., Treatment of nickel dermatitis with Antabuse®; a double blind study, *Contact Dermatitis,* 9, 297, 1983.
39. Hopfer, S. M., Linden, J. V., Rezuke, W. N., O'Brien, J. E., Smith, L., Watters, F., and Sunderman, F. W., Jr., Increased nickel concentrations in body fluids of patients with chronic alcoholism during disulfiram therapy, *Res. Commun. Chem. Pathol. Pharmacol.,* 55, 101, 1987.
40. Menné, T., Nickel Allergy, Ph.D. thesis, University of Copenhagen, Copenhagen, Denmark, 1983.
41. Christensen, O. B., Nickel Allergy and Hand Eczema in Females, Ph.D. thesis, University of Lund, Malmö, Sweden, 1981.
42. Lammintausta, K. and Kalimo, K., Nickel sensitivity and the course of atopic dermatitis in adulthood, *Contact Dermatitis,* 22, 144, 1990.
43. Wilkinson, D. S. and Wilkinson, J. D., Nickel allergy and hand eczema, in *Nickel and the Skin: Immunology and Toxicology,* Maibach, H. I. and Menné, T., Eds., CRC Press, Boca Raton, FL, 1989, 133.
44. Veien, N. K. and Menné, T., Nickel contact allergy and a nickel-restricted diet, *Semin. Dermatol.,* 9, 197, 1990.
45. Nielsen, G. D., Jepsen, L. V., Jørgensen, P. J., Grandjean, P., and Brandrup, F., Nickel-sensitive patients with vesicular hand eczema: oral challenge with a diet naturally high in nickel, *Br. J. Dermatol.,* 122, 299, 1990.
46. Veien, N. K., Hattel, T., Justesen, O., and Nørholm, A., Oral challenge with metal salts. I. Vesicular patch-test-negative hand eczema, *Contact Dermatitis,* 9, 402, 1983.
47. Veien, N. K., Hattel, T., Justesen, O., and Nørholm, A., Oral challenge with metal salts: II, various types of eczema, *Contact Dermatitis,* 9, 407, 1983.
48. Webster, J. D., Parker, T. F., Alfrey, A. C., Smythe, W. R., Kubo, H., Neal, G., and Hull, A. R., Acute nickel intoxication by dialysis, *Ann. Intern. Med.,* 92, 631, 1980.
49. Chromium, Nickel and Welding, IARC Monogr. on the Evaluation of Carcinogenic Risks to Humans, Vol. 49, World Health Organization, International Agency for Research on Cancer, 1990.
50. Kaaber, K., Veien, N. K., and Tjell, J. C., Low nickel diet in the treatment of patients with chronic nickel dermatitis, *Br. J. Dermatol.,* 98, 197, 1978.
51. Gawkrodger, D. J., Shuttler, I. L., and Delves, H. T., Nickel dermatitis and diet: clinical improvement and a reduction in blood and urine nickel levels with a low-nickel diet, *Acta Derm. Venereol.,* 68, 453, 1988.
52. Veien. N. K., Hattel, T., Justesen, O., and Nørholm, A., Dietary treatment of nickel dermatitis, *Acta Derm. Venereol.,* 65, 138, 1985.

53. Pigatto, P. D., Gibelli, E., Fumagalli, M., Bigardi, A., Morelli, M., and Altomare, G. F., Disodium cromoglycate versus diet in the treatment and prevention of nickel-positive pompholyx, *Contact Dermatitis*, 22, 27, 1990.

54. Veien, N. K. and Andersen, M. R., Nickel in Danish food, *Acta Derm. Venereol.*, 66, 502, 1986.

55. Rystedt, I. and Fischer, T., Relationship between nickel and cobalt sensitization in hard metal workers, *Contact Dermatitis*, 9, 195, 1983.

56. Veien, N. K., Hattel, T., Justesen, O., and Nørholm, A., Oral challenge with nickel and cobalt in patients with positive patch tests to nickel and/or cobalt, *Acta Derm. Venereol.*, 67, 321, 1987.

57. Menné, T., Flare-up of cobalt dermatitis from Antabuse® treatment, *Contact Dermatitis*, 12, 53, 1985.

58. Joensen, H. D., Thormann, J., Jespersen, N. B., and Brodthagen, H., Kromallergi, *Ugeskr. Laeg.*, 141, 1404, 1979.

59. Kaaber, K. and Veien, N. K., The significance of chromate ingestion in patients allergic to chromate, *Acta Derm. Venereol.*, 57, 321, 1977.

60. Goitre, M., Bedello, P. G., and Cane, D., Chromium dermatitis and oral administration of the metal, *Contact Dermatitis*, 8, 203, 1982.

61. Fregert, S., Sensitization to hexa- and trivalent chromium, *Proc. Congr. Hung. Derm. Soc.*, 50, 50, 1985.

62. Sertoli, A., Lombardi, P., Francalanci, S., Gola, M., Giorgini, S., and Panconesi, E., Effetto della somministrazione orale di apteni in soggetti sensibilizzati affetti da eczema allergico da contatto, *G. Ital. Dermatol. Venereol.*, 120, 213, 1985.

63. Mali, J. W. H., Über einen Fall von dyshidrotischem Ekszem durch Chromat, *Hautarzt*, 11, 27, 1960.

64. Hjorth, N., Overfølsomhed for balsam, *Spectrum*, 8, 97, 1971.

65. Veien, N. K., Hattel, T., Justesen, O., and Nørholm, A., Oral challenge with balsam or Peru, *Contact Dermatitis*, 12, 104, 1985.

66. Dooms-Goosens, A., Dubelloy, R., and Degreef, H., Contact and systemic contact-type dermatitis to spices, *Contact Dermatitis*, 8, 89, 1990.

67. Flood, J. M. and Perry, D. J., Recurrent vesicular eruption of the hands due to food allergy, *J. Invest. Dermatol.*, 7, 309, 1946.

68. Veien, N. K., Hattel, T., Justesen, O., and Nørholm, A., Dermatitis induced or aggravated by selected foodstuffs, *Acta Derm. Venereol.*, 67, 133, 1987.

69. Veien, N. K., Hattel, T., Justesen, O., and Nørholm, A., Dermatoses in coffee drinkers, *Cutis*, 40, 421, 1987.

70. Sulzberger, M. B. and Baer, R. L., Eczematous eruptions of the hands, in *The 1948 Year Book of Dermatology and Syphilology*, Sulzberger, M. B. and Baer, R. L., Eds., Year Book, Chicago, 1948, 7.

71. Haxthausen, H., Generalized "ids" ("autosensitization") in varicose eczemas, *Acta Derm. Venereol.*, 35, 271, 1955.

72. Cunningham, M. J., Zone, J. J., Petersen, M. J., and Green, J. A., Circulating activated (DR-positive) T lymphocytes in a patient with autoeczematization, *J. Am. Acad. Dermatol.*, 14, 1039, 1986.

73. Kaaman, T. and Torssander, J., Dermatophytid: a misdiagnosed entity?, *Acta Derm. Venereol.*, 63, 404, 1983.

74. Champion, R. H., Burton, J. L., and Ebling, F. J. G., Eds., *Textbook of Dermatology*, Vol. 2, 5th ed., Blackwell Scientific, Oxford, 1991, 1302.

75. Rystedt, I., Hand Eczema and Long-Term Prognosis in Atopic Dermatitis, Ph.D. thesis, Karolinska Institute, Stockholm, Sweden, 1985.

76. Schwanitz, H. J., *Das atopische Palmoplantarekzem*, Springer-Verlag, Berlin, 1986.

77. Bäurle, G., *Handekzeme*, Schattauer, Stuttgart, 1986.

78. Schuppli, R., Zur Ätiologie der Dysidrosis, *Dermatologica*, 108, 393, 1954.

79. Young, E., Dysidrotic (endogen) eczema, *Dermatologica*, 129, 306, 1964.

80. Van Ketel, W. G., Aalberse, R. C., Reerink-Brongers, E., and Woerdeman-Evenhuis, J. T., Comparative examination of the results of the RAST and intracutaneous test in eczema dyshidroticum, *Dermatologica,* 156, 304, 1978.

81. Norris, P. G. and Levene, G. M., Pompholyx occurring during hospital admission for treatment of atopic dermatitis, *Clin. Exp. Dermatol.,* 12, 189, 1987.

82. Hansen, O., Küchler, T., Lotz, G.-R., Richter, R., and Wilckens, A., Es juckt mich in den Fingern, aber mir sind die Hände gebunden, *Z. Psychosom. Med.,* 27, 275, 1981.

83. Kellum, R. E., Dyshidrotic hand eczema, *Cutis,* 16, 875, 1975.

84. Miller, R. M. and Coger, R. W., Skin conductance conditioning with dyshidrotic eczema patients, *Br. J. Dermatol.,* 101, 435, 1979.

85. Koldys, K. W. and Meyer, R. P., Biofeedback training in the therapy of dyshidrosis, *Cutis,* 24, 219, 1979.

86. Barth, J. H., Fairris, G. M., Wojnarowska, F., and White, J. E., Haemorrhagic pompholyx is a sign of bullous pemphigoid and an indication for low-dose prenisolone therapy, *Clin. Exp. Dermatol.,* 11, 409, 1986.

87. Duhra, P. and Ryatt, K. S., Haemorrhagic pompholyx in bullous pemphigoid, *Clin. Exp. Dermatol.,* 13, 342, 1988.

88. Rongioletti, F., Parodi, A., and Rebora, A., Dyshidrosiform pemphigoid, *Dermatologica,* 170, 84, 1985.

89. Barth, J. H., Venning, V. A., and Wojnarowska, F., Palmo-plantar involvement in autoimmune blistering disorders: pemphigoid, linear IgA disease and herpes gestationis, *Clin. Exp. Dermatol.,* 13, 85, 1988.

90. Duhra, P. and Charles-Holmes, R., Linear IgA disease with haemorrhagic pompholyx and dapsone-induced neutropenia, *Br. J. Dermatol.,* 125, 172, 1991.

91. Feuerman, E. J., Ingber, A., David, M., and Weissman-Katzenelson, V., Lichen ruber planus beginning as a dyshidrosiform eruption, *Cutis,* 30, 401, 1982.

92. Miura, T., Matsuda, M., Yanbe, H., and Sugiyama, S., Two cases of autoimmune progesterone dermatitis: immunohistochemical and serological studies, *Acta Derm. Venereol.,* 69, 308, 1989.

93. Uehara, M., Pustulosis palmaris et plantaris: evolutionary sequence from vesicular to pustular, *Semin. Dermatol.,* 2, 51, 1993.

94. Klein, C. E., Weber, L., and Kaufmann, R., Infantile akropustulose, *Hautarzt,* 40, 501, 1989.

95. Vignon-Pennamen, M.-D. and Wallach, D., Infantile acropustulosis, *Arch. Dermatol.,* 122, 1155, 1986.

96. Hersle, K. and Mobacken, H., Hyperkeratotic dermatitis of the palms, *Br. J. Dermatol.,* 107, 195, 1982.

9

Statistical Relations Between Hand Eczema and Contact Allergens

Björn Edman

CONTENTS

0-8493-7355-7/94/$0.00 + $.50

I. INTRODUCTION

In the literature, only few eczema sites have been correlated to different allergens. One exception is contact dermatitis of the lower leg, which has been associated with many allergens described by several authors mentioned by Cronin.[1] Many case reports have been presented regarding contact allergy and hand eczema, but no systematic survey has been presented. A computer makes it possible to correlate various contact allergens to eczema of different parts of the hand on a great number of patients. The data base DALUK[2] was set up in 1982 at the Department of Dermatology and has already been used to perform such a study.[3]

II. DALUK — THE DATA BASE OF CONTACT ALLERGY

The DALUK data base consists of two parts: a patient file and a product file. The DALUK patient file today lists information of history and patch test results on ~6000 patients starting from 1982; furthermore, during the period 1962 to 1981 patch test results are only available on an additional 11,400 patients.

The patient file includes variables, such as age, sex, residential area, occupation and former occupations, primary and secondary eczema sites, personal atopy, family atopy, childhood eczema, history of metal sensitivity, symmetry of the eczema, duration of the eczema, course of the eczema, and smoking and drug habits. All information is registered at the time of the application of the test to minimize influence from the result of the patch test reading.

The patch test results are registered by the following variables:

Morphology	Interpretation	Correlation
Negative	Doubtful	None
Doubtful	Contact allergy	Doubtful
Positive	Irritancy	Former/past
	Phototoxicity	Relevant (occupational
	Contact urticaria	or nonoccupational)

The DALUK product file now lists more than 1500 various products (e.g., pharmaceutical specialties, pharmaceutical preparations, over-the-counter [OTC] preparations, cosmetics, health skin care products) and 600 associated substances on the Swedish market as well as information on 1000 manufacturers, including addresses. The product file also generates information lists to all patients with a contact allergy, listing all known products containing the allergen.

III. MATERIALS AND METHODS

Eczema sites are recorded for all patch-tested patients. The different sites of the hand used for this purpose are presented in Table 1. During the period 1982 to 1991, we performed patch testing on ~5700 patients referred to us by the indication of suspected contact allergy. Sixty-five percent of all the patients were females, and the mean age of all patients was 40 ± 25 (SD) years. The positive outcome, defined as the number of patients with at least one contact allergy in relationship to the number of tested patients, was 40% on average. Eczema of hand and/or fingers was found in 26% of all patients positive to one or more contact allergen (Table 2).[4] Atopy was defined in three ways: (1) personal (present or previous) allergic rhinitis/asthma, (2) present or previous atopic eczema, and (3) allergic rhinitis/asthma in relatives (of the first degree). The atopy distribution according to the three categories are shown in Table 3, divided in the two groups with and without hand eczema.

IV. STATISTICS

Statistical correlations of hand eczema and all contact allergens present in all standard series were tested with Fisher's exact test. The test was performed in two steps. In the first step contact allergens

TABLE 1   Definition of Sites of the Hand

Hand
Back
Palm
Center
Peripheral
Fingers
Dorsal
Joints
Between joints
Cuticle
Palmar
Interdigital
Tip
Wrists

were correlated to the whole of the hand (except the fingers) as well as to the whole of the fingers. In the second step locations of the hand and fingers were divided according to Table 1. When testing a certain object, e.g., an occupation, the frequency of that particular occupation is compared with the frequency of all other occupations. Level of significance was first set to 5%, then adjusted by a method suggested by Eklund and Seeger.[5] The method estimates the number of significant relationships that might be random findings. If you decide on the maximal proportion of random findings among all significant correlations (k), the required level of significance could be calculated from:

$$\frac{\alpha[1 - P(\alpha)]}{(1 - \alpha)P(\alpha)} \leq k$$

where α is the level of significance, e.g., 0.05 (5%), $P(\alpha)$ is the proportion of significant relationships divided by the total number of statistical tests (e.g., 11/120), and k is the maximal proportion of random findings, e.g., 0.1 (10%). A table according to Fisher's exact test could be as follows:

	Fingers	Other sites	Σ	
Nickel-positive	140	760	900	
Nickel-negative	560	4240	4800	$p = 0.0016$
Σ	700	5000	5700	

V.   CORRELATIONS OF HAND ECZEMA AND CONTACT ALLERGENS

Twenty-four various statistical correlations were found of different contact allergens and different sites of the hand (Figures 1 and 2).

TABLE 2   Distribution of Eczema Sites in Patients with and without 1 or More Contact Allergy (CA)

Eczema site	% with CA	% without CA	Significance
Hands (except fingers)	18	18	NS
Fingers	26	21	$p < 0.001$
Face and head	24	25	NS
Arms	8	11	$p < 0.001$
Legs	10	10	NS
Trunk	5	5	NS
Feet	4	4	NS
Other sites	4	6	$p < 0.01$

TABLE 3   Distribution of Atopy in Patients with and without Hand Eczema

	Hand eczema (%)	Other eczema (%)	Total number	Significance
Flexural dermatitis	49	51	483	NS
Personal history of hay fever/asthma	42	58	495	$p < 0.001$
Family history of hay fever/asthma	41	59	1008	$p < 0.001$
No atopy at all	51	38	2824	$p < 0.001$
Tested number of patients	1770	3040	4810	

A.   Correlations of the Hand

1.   The Whole Hand

Eczema of the whole hand was correlated to five allergens: thiuram mix, PPD mix, (p-phenylene diamine (PPDA), chromate, and balsam of Peru. The chemicals included in the thiuram mix are known to be found in domestic rubber, such as gloves,[1] and most of our patients with this contact allergy are working as cleaners, nurses, etc., occupations in which gloves often are being used.[6]

The substances in PPD mix, on the contrary, are mostly found in industrial rubber products, e.g., tires and cables.[1] In our study the patients often had eczema on the feet as well, and an allergy to shoe materials seemed to be the main cause. The question must therefore be asked about whether the hand eczema is secondary to the feet dermatitis.

PPDA allergy was found mostly in patients with an additional eczema of the scalp, which indicates that the cause is the applying procedure of hair dyes using the hands. In some cases a cross-reaction with chemicals in the PPD mix is the probable explanation. Another reason could be PPDA-dyed leather gloves.[1]

Chromate is a well-known source of leather ware allergy, such as gloves and shoes, and may thereby cause dermatitis on the hands in people with this particular contact allergy.[1] Trivalent chromium compounds are used to tan the leather.

Balsam of Peru is found in many perfumes and perfumed cosmetics.[1] Because most of our patients with a contact allergy to balsam of Peru also had eczema elsewhere, it could be suspected

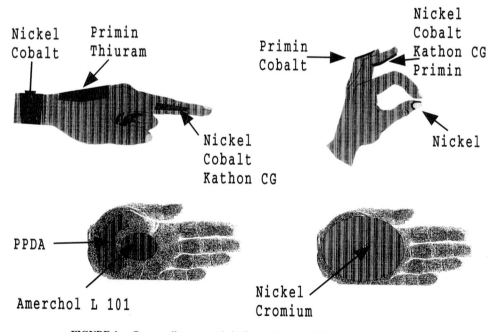

FIGURE 1.   Contact allergens statistically correlated to different sites of the hand.

FINGERS	Cobalt	INTERDIGITAL	Nickel
	Nickel		Cobalt
	Kathon CG		Kathon CG
		PALMAR	Nickel
			Kathon CG
			Cobalt
			Primin
		VOLAR	Primin
			Cobalt
		CUTICLE	Nickel
		BETWEEN JOINTS	Cobalt

HANDS	PPD-mix	BACK	Primin
	Chromium		Thiuram mix
	PPDA	CENTER OF PALM	Amerchol
	Thiuram-mix	PERIPHERAL	PPDA
	Balsam of Peru		

WRISTS	Nickel
	Cobalt

FIGURE 2.   Contact allergens correlated to different sites of the hand.

that eczema on the hands occurs when perfumed products are applied on other parts of the body using the hands.

2.   Back of Hands

Thiuram mix was correlated specifically to the back of hands, thereby confirming that use of rubber globes is the main cause considering that the skin is thinner there. However, no correlation between rubber mixes and the dorsal finger was found.

Primin was correlated to the back of hands as well as to the fingers, both being well-known sites of dermatitis due to primula obconica.[1]

3.   Palms

Amerchol L 101 was correlated only to the center of palm. So, most of these patients also had eczema on the face, lower legs, etc. The reason for this seems to be that ointments often are put in the palm to apply them on other parts of the body, i.e., some of them also had a contact allergy to products, such as Hirudoid® ointment, a common product used on the legs, which contains wood alcohols.

PPDA was correlated to the peripheral palm. Here a probable source would be PPDA-dyed leather gloves.[1] The reason why the peripheral palm is involved in particular might be that the pressure on this part is stronger than on the center of the palm.

B.   CORRELATIONS OF THE FINGERS

1.   Interdigital and Palmar

Nickel contact allergy is known to manifest as pompholyx involving the sides of fingers as well as the palmar side.[7]

Kathon CG is found in various kinds of products today: cosmetics, shampoos, washing-up liquids, cutting fluids, glues, cleaning agents, paints, and photo processing products.[8] The common denominator with most of these products is that they come in contact with the hands and especially with the fingers.

2. Volar

Cobalt allergy situated on the volar side of the finger (and especially between the joints) implies that rings made of non-golden metals could be responsible. Many so-called nickel-free jewelry contains cobalt instead, i.e., patients with concomitant contact allergy to nickel buy nickel-free jewelry and still get eczema due to the cobalt allergy. Secondary eruption, as with nickel, might be another explanation.

Primin was correlated to the volar side of the finger as well as to the back of hands, both being well-known sites of dermatitis due to primula obconica.[1]

3. Cuticle

Nickel is often present in metal balls used in nail varnish to simplify stirring, so if it contaminates the surrounding skin, the cuticles are logical sites to be involved.

C. Correlations of the Wrists

Eczema of the wrists was correlated to the metals cobalt and nickel. Both are found in metal watch bracelets and in ordinary bracelets not made of gold.

D. General Comments

As shown in Table 2, eczema on the fingers is more common in patients with contact allergy than in those without contact allergy ($p < 0.001$). Furthermore, no difference was found concerning the hand (fingers excluded). This could mean that the fingers more often are sensitized than the rest of the hand. In consequence, it was found that the fingers had 14 correlations of contact allergens, whereas the hand only had 9.

It is urgent to adjust the level of significance when performing many comparisons on the same variables. In the analysis of relationships between contact allergens and hand eczema, 275 comparisons were made and 24 of them were found to be significant. If you use a decision level of 5%, it could be calculated[5] that a maximum of 55%, i.e., 13 of the 24 relationships found, could be obtained by pure chance. If you minimize the risk and only accept a maximum of 0.5% (corresponding to one of the 24 significant findings) could be random findings, the level of significance must not be higher than 0.005 (0.5%), and this level had consequently been used in this study when looking for relationships between contact allergens and eczema sites of the hand and fingers.

Finally, it is important to decide whether the sites involved are primary, secondary, or irrelevant. Correlations of the wrist should be primary, and palmar and interdigital areas of the hand are most often secondary sites.[9] In the cases of involvement of the areas between finger joints and dorsal parts of the finger both primary and secondary sites could be discussed.

VI. OTHER CORRELATIONS OF HAND ECZEMA

Besides the correlations found between different parts of the hand and various contact allergens, another 13 correlations were detected between the hands and other registered variables. All these correlations, presented in Figure 3, are found independently from any contact allergies.

A. Fingers

1. Atopy

Patients with a present or previous history of atopic eczema (flexural dermatitis) had an overrepresentation of eczema on the fingers and especially interdigital and on the volar side compared with patients with no atopy. Furthermore, patients with a family history of hayfever and/or asthma were correlated to sides of fingers. However, as shown in Table 3, no relationship between atopic eczema and hand eczema (the whole hand including the fingers) was detectable. Only when dividing into different parts could any statistical correlation be found.

FINGERS	Occupations	INTERDIGITAL	Contraceptives
	Low age		Acetylsalicylic acid
	Flexural dermatitis		Smoking
			Family history of atopy
		PALMAR	-
		VOLAR	Flexural dermatitis
		CUTICLE	Females
		BETWEEN JOINTS	-
HANDS	Males	BACK	-
	Low age	PALM	Smoking
	Occupations		
WRISTS	Females		
	Low age		

FIGURE 3.   Different sites of the hand correlated to various factors.

2. Internal Drugs

Patients using contraceptives and/or acetylsalicylic acid had more often than expected eczema on the sides of fingers. A statistical correlation between these two drugs and pompholyx has been demonstrated before in a previous study, partly including the same cases as in this new study.[10] However, this study adds many new cases, thus increasing the reliability of this finding.

3. Smoking

Eczema on the sides of fingers was statistically correlated to smoking habits. A similar correlation was also found between the palms and smoking. This was also shown in a previous study.[10]

4. Occupations

Some occupations (e.g., cook, nurse, cleaner, waitress, cashier) were correlated to eczema on the fingers. The first four of these could be regarded as "wet" occupations, likely to cause irritant dermatitis on the fingers. Most of the cashiers in this study are allergic to nickel. Consequently, they could all be classified as risk occupations.

B. Hands (Except Fingers)

1. Occupations

A completely different group of occupations apart from those found in patients with eczema on the fingers was correlated to eczema of the whole hand: food work (e.g., cook, waitress), metalwork (e.g., metal finishing, metal machining), textile work (e.g., tailor, weaver), electrical work, store work, and teaching. All except the first two could be regarded as "dry" occupations. Furthermore, all of the occupations apart from teacher could be regarded as strenuous work for the hands, i.e., the hands are very much used and also exposed to various allergens.

2. Topical Products

No correlations were found between topical products (e.g., cosmetics, pharmaceutical specialites) and eczema of the different parts of the hand and fingers. The reason for this is probably too few cases of each tested product to detect any significant correlation.

3. Age

Both eczema of fingers and hands as well as wrists were negatively correlated to age, i.e., eczema on these sites seemed to be more common at younger age than at older age in comparison with other eczema sites. A possible explanation could be that people, as well as the skin, adapt to the situation causing the problem. The skin gets thicker with strenuous work and people may change occupation to avoid a work that develops hand eczema. Women with nickel contact allergy learn to avoid contact with nickel-containing jewelry and other metal objects.

4. Sex

Sex was significantly correlated in two cases. It was found that men more often than women had eczema on the hands (fingers excluded). Wrist and cuticle, however, were overrepresented in women. The reason why men more often have eczema on the hands could be found by penetrating the selection of patients included in this study. Women were tested twice as often as men and nickel allergy was found in about 28% of the women. According to Figure 3, nickel was only correlated to locations of the finger but not to the rest of the hand. This means that nickel allergy in women is a confounding factor, and if those women are excluded, no overrepresentation of hand eczema among men could be detected compared with women. The probable explanation of the last case is that women more often have contact allergy to nickel, and nickel is often found in watch bracelets and in nail varnish (sometimes containing a nickel ball).

5. Smoking

Eczema on the palms was statistically correlated to smoking habits. A simultaneous correlation was also found between the sides of the fingers and smoking. This has also been shown in a previous study, which partly included the same patients;[10] however, this study adds many new cases, thus increasing the reliability of this finding.

C. General Comments

The statistical error demonstrated in Section VI.B.4, where the confounding factor of nickel allergy gave a false-positive significant result about sex and hand eczema, illustrates the fact that relationships often are complex, i.e., a relationship could be dependent on other relationships, often by sex and age. A confounding factor could cause a false-negative or a false-positive correlation. Thirteen significant correlations of 72 tested relationships were found. To avoid bias due to massignificance, the level of significance was set to 1%, which implies that a maximum of 5% of all significant correlations could be random findings,[5] i.e., less than 1 of the 13 relationships.

As shown in Table 3, hand eczema (the whole hand including the fingers) was underrepresented in patients with personal atopy as well as patients with family history of atopy, and consequently, overrepresented in patients with no atopy at all. This remarkable finding might, however, be due to selection mechanisms, e.g., that most patients with an atopic dermatitis are not referred to patch testing. Furthermore, no difference between patients with and without hand eczema was seen concerning atopic eczema (flexural dermatitis); however, as mentioned in Section VI.A.1, atopy, defined as flexural dermatitis, and family history were correlated to certain parts of the fingers.

REFERENCES

1. Cronin, E., *Contact Dermatitis,* Livingston, London, 1980.
2. Edman, B., Computerised Patch Test Data in Contact Allergy, *Ph.D. thesis,* University of Lund, Malmö, Sweden, 1988.
3. Edman, B., Sites of contact dermatitis in relationship to particular allergens, *Contact Dermatitis,* 13(3), 129, 1985.
4. Von Förg, T., Bury, G., and Zirbs, S., Häuftigkeitsanalytische Untesuchungen allergischer Kontaktekzeme bei Hausfrauen, *Dermatosen,* 30(2), 48, 1982.
5. Eklund, G. and Seeger, P., Massignifikansanalys, *Statis. Tidskr.,* 5, 355, 1965.
6. Von Agathos, M. and Bernecker, H. A., Hand dermatitis bei medizinischen Personal, *Dermatosen,* 30(2), 43, 1982.

7. Christensen, O. B., Nickel Allergy and Hand Eczema in Females, Ph.D. thesis, University of Lund, Malmö, Sweden, 1982.
8. Bruze, M., Gruvberger, B., and Björkner, B., Kathon CG: an unusual contact sensitizer, in *Exogenous Dermatoses: Environmental Dermatitis,* Menné, T. and Maibach, H. I., Eds., CRC Press, Boca Raton, FL, 1991, 285.
9. Christensen, O. B. and Möller, H., External and internal exposure to the antigen in the hand eczema of nickel allergy, *Contact Dermatitis,* 1, 136, 1975.
10. Edman, B., Palmar eczema: a pathogenetic role for acetylsalicylic acid, *Acta Derm. Venereol.,* 68, 402, 1988.

10

Quantitative Aspects of Allergen Exposure in Relation to Allergic Contact Dermatitis on the Hands

David A. Basketter and C. F. Allenby

CONTENTS

I. INTRODUCTION

Although everyone recognizes that higher levels of a contact allergen and/or a greater degree of skin exposure will render both the primary induction of the allergic state and elicitation of dermatitis in a sensitized individual more likely, in very few cases is it possible to give a quantitative view of the response that will follow a certain level of exposure. Nevertheless, we are not in complete ignorance. We are aware that 2,4-dinitrochlorobenzene (DNCB) is a potent contact allergen for which a single skin contact may well be sufficient to induce an allergic status in most people.[1] In contrast, although chromates are strong sensitizers, until recently the commonest cause of chromate allergy was persistent contact with trace levels in cement.[2] Here the mean time to a clinical problem was 10 or more years. A third scenario is represented by the cetostearyl alcohols, which seem to be extremely ineffective sensitizers, partly because they are widely and safely used in skin products. However, when used on the damaged skin of a leg ulcer, even these chemicals can represent a significant problem.[3] So, in this chapter we will examine what is known of quantitative aspects of the induction of contact allergy (not much), the elicitation of a contact dermatitis (a little more), and also consider the factors that, in our view, may have a profound influence on quantitative considerations.

II. DOSE RESPONSE STUDIES WITH CONTACT ALLERGENS

A. DNCB

Since the early days of the scientific study of contact allergy, DNCB has been used as a model contact allergen.[4] In view of this and the fact that it is a chemical with which humans do not ordinarily come into contact, it is not surprising that it has been used in an ethical manner to investigate not only details of the elicitation of contact allergic responses in humans but also the characteristics of the induction of the contact allergic state.[1] In these experiments a number of key aspects of contact allergy have been demonstrated. First, the induction of dose-response to DNCB was shown to follow the classic biological sigmoid profile. From this a 50% effective sensitizing dose of 116 μg DNCB (applied as a single patch to the arm) was calculated and subsequently vindicated by experiment. Second, the overriding determinant of sensitization rate was shown to be the dose per unit area at induction. Thus, 62.5 μg applied to a 3-cm diameter area of arm skin sensitized 8% of subjects; when applied to a 1.5-cm skin area (i.e., 4 x the dose per unit area) the same quantity of DNCB sensitized 88% of subjects. Furthermore, sufficient DNCB persisted at the induction site to cause an eczematous reaction 1 to 2 weeks after the sensitizing dose had been applied. Finally, there was a dose response to challenge, with higher challenge doses being required to elicit a reaction in subjects who had received lower induction doses.

Moss et al.[5] extended their studies using a group of individuals who exhibited multiple contact sensitivities and who, on this basis, were judged to be particularly prone to the development of contact allergy. In these subjects the dose-response curves for DNCB were steeper, indicating a greater degree of allergic sensitivity. Although the cellular mechanisms that might underlie this are not known, it is tempting to speculate that they may reside in the reciprocal interactions of the two types of helper T lymphocytes, T_{H1} and T_{H2}, which mediate the development of contact allergy and respiratory allergy, respectively.[6] Thus, those individuals whose immune systems, for whatever reason, tend to favor T_{H1} activation will be more prone to the development of contact allergies. However, whatever the complexities of the immunology, the implications are clear for quantitative considerations of allergen exposure and ACD: studies of "normal" individuals may underestimate the risk.

B. Metals

Although DNCB presents the opportunity to study all phases of contact allergy, the frequency of occurrence of sensitivity to metals in the general population, especially to nickel, permits a detailed examination of the factors governing the elicitation of allergic skin responses. The most basic type of study has been the determination of the elicitation dose-response profile on normal back skin using standard patch testing techniques.[7,8] Such studies serve to demonstrate that within any group of allergic subjects, the vast majority respond upon challenge at high concentration, whereas a significant minority will still react at very much lower concentrations. The precise minimal dose capable of eliciting a response will depend on patch test type and regimen,[9] vehicle,[10] skin test site,[11] size of the test panel, and statistical considerations. However, such studies fail to take into account what are perhaps the most important factors that might be expected to affect elicitation thresholds in metal allergic subjects. These include the consideration of repeated treatment of compromised skin on "at risk" individuals and are discussed herein.

It is also noteworthy that nickel-allergic subjects in certain occupations (e.g., banking, shop work) may have prolonged hand contact with nickel-containing coins. The action of sweat can release considerable amounts of nickel (e.g., 50 μg in 4 h). However, this apparently obvious likely cause of a nickel hand eczema seems to be rather rare.[12]

In their quantitative investigations of DNCB sensitization, Moss et al.[5] considered the differences between normal subjects and those with multiple contact allergies. In essence, they asked the question, "How do at risk individuals compare to normal subjects." When investigating elicitation dose-response profiles in metal allergic subjects, we considered it essential to take into account certain factors that could have a major impact on the result: site variation in sensitivity and the presence of some eczematous reaction at the test site. The motivation was the known association of nickel and chromium allergy with chronic eczema, especially related to the hands and arms,[2,12] and the suggestion from certain quarters that trace levels of metals in household products were a key factor in the persistence of an allergic hand eczema.[13-17]

It is not necessary for the purposes of this chapter to review in detail the early results of studies in metal-allergic subjects. This earlier work, supplemented by an Italian study, served to demonstrate that under circumstances in which the skin barrier function is compromised or bypassed, a few nickel-, cobalt-, or chromium-allergic subjects will react to concentrations as low as 1 ppm.[18-20] Such results with nickel are in accord with the reported incidences of ACD on delicate skin from cosmetics containing low parts per million levels of nickel in nickel-allergic subjects.[21-23] However, how can the data be related to in-use situations and to hand eczema?

Because of potential ethical problems relating to the elicitation of allergic reactions on the hands of nickel-sensitive subjects, our studies have largely utilized forearm skin. To model the typical wet work/domestic situation that may predispose the (often female) nickel-allergic subject to chronic hand eczema, we developed a system in which the forearm was repeatedly immersed, twice per day, in a dilute surfactant solution (0.5% sodium dodecyl sulfate [SDS]) until a moderate degree of inflammation was induced.[24] This model was then employed in a panel of 20 nickel-allergic subjects in whom one forearm was surfactant treated and the other forearm acted as a control.[25] Once the surfactant treatment had induced moderate inflammation, the dorsal aspect of both forearms was patch tested, using Finn chambers applied for 48 h, with a series of dilutions of nickel in the range 0.5 to 10 ppm. The results of these patch tests are contained in Table 1 and show that there is a marked enhancement in response and a substantial lowering of the threshold for elicitation of allergic nickel reactions in skin that has been compromised by repeated surfactant treatment. Under these test conditions, 10% of the nickel-allergic panel reacted to 0.5 ppm nickel on compromised forearm skin.

The significance of this result has been discussed elsewhere,[26] but it clearly points to an area of concern in situations in which very low concentrations of nickel may have prolonged and perhaps

TABLE 1 Allergic Reactions to Nickel on Normal and Surfactant-Treated Forearm Skin

	Nickel concentration (ppm)				
	10	5	1	0.5	0
Untreated forearm skin	15	15	0	Not done	0
Treated forearm skin	60	50	15	10	0

Note: Values are percentages of test panel with positive allergic response.

occlusive contact with skin in a highly sensitive allergic individual. Nevertheless, the data still relate to largely experimental conditions and notably derive from the dorsal forearm, not the hand. This aspect may be of considerable significance because the prime problem area is the hand. It is typically a chronic hand eczema that shows an association with nickel allergy,[17] not chronic dermatitis of the forearm. However, we did not believe that ethically it was proper to try to elicit an allergic contact dermatitis on normal or eczematous hands of allergic subjects due to the possibility of a reaction become chronic. Therefore, to obtain valid and relevant data, we considered it proper, with fully informed consent, to use a representative section of hand skin with open and repetitive, rather than occluded single, treatment.[27]

A protocol was designed such that it incorporated increasing repetitive surfactant and nickel insult to the thumb and thenar region of one hand of a nickel-allergic subject. The opposite thumb and thenar region received an identical insult except that the nickel was omitted. The thumb and thenar region were considered to be a reasonable and representative selection of hand skin sites on which it would be ethical to induce a possibly allergic, but certainly an irritant, dermatitis with an acceptably low risk of precipitating a more widespread hand eczema. The test sites were immersed in 40°C SDS solutions for 10 min twice daily on weekdays, for a total period of 23 days. The SDS concentration was increased from 0.1 to 0.3% for the last 9 days to ensure a moderate degree of persistent skin irritation. In each of the four nickel-allergic subjects, one thumb and thenar region was also treated via the SDS solution with nickel at 0.1 ppm (week 1), 0.5 ppm (week 2), and 1.0 ppm (final 9 days). Two of the four nickel-allergic subjects were individuals in whom we had obtained positive patch test results at 1 ppm.

Figure 1 from one panelist at one test site presents typical results. Over the time course of the experiment both redness/erythema (subjective scale 0 to 4) and dryness (subjective scale 0 to 3) tended to increase. By the end of the experiment (48 h score after final treatment) both erythema and dryness scores were elevated, consistent with the development of inflammation. As shown in the particular case in Figure 1, the degree of redness or dryness on the nickel-treated sites was not different from control in any of the four panelists at any thumb or thenar site. There were no other clinical signs of an allergic reaction on the nickel-treated sites that were monitored for several days after the final treatment. The implications (and imperfections) of these results are discussed in Section IV.

C. Kathon CG

The last contact allergen for which there is a significant body of quantitative dose-response data is the preservative Kathon CG. This particular preservative has been the subject of a substantial number of human repeat insult patch tests (HRIPTs) and of well-controlled use tests.[28,29] Diagnostic patch testing with a range of concentrations of Kathon CG in nine allergic subjects suggested that the minimal eliciting level was 25 ppm.[28] Interestingly, in threshold prophetic patch testing, in which much larger groups of nonallergic subjects were treated with a range of products containing low levels of Kathon CG, one subject reacted to 12.5 ppm and two reacted to 20 ppm.[29] The total panel size was 1450. Such results demonstrate that to determine true minimal eliciting levels for an allergen, it is necessary to use a large panel size. The significant outbreak of Kathon CG-related ACD in the 1980s further served to demonstrate the dangers of too literal an interpretation patch test dose response and HRIPT data. Subsequently, the clinical evidence has suggested that the minimal eliciting concentration may be as low as 7 ppm,[30] and this is reflected in the current recommended maximal concentration of 7.5 ppm for products with prolonged skin contact.[31]

D. Other Allergens

There are numerous contact allergens that have been the subject of elicitation dose-response studies, but it would not be helpful to catalog them here. Many are details of only one patient, such as that for propylgallate.[32] Other studies have examined small groups of subjects and may consequently provide more valuable data, such as those for colophony[33] and formaldehyde, showing that the minimal eliciting levels for these contact allergens are in the range of 10 to 100 ppm.[34,35] However,

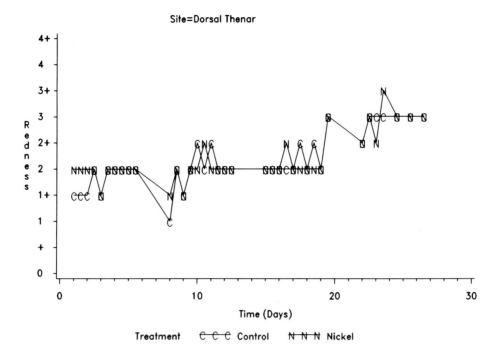

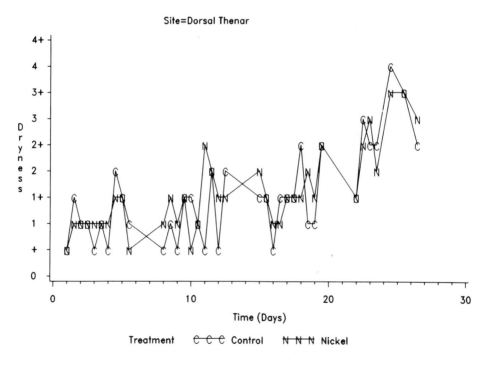

FIGURE 1. Reactions to repeated surfactant treatment, with and without nickel on the thumb and thenar region of nickel allergic subjects. The development of erythema (top) and the development of dryness (bottom) in a typical subject/site during the course of the study.

they serve to emphasize one important point: at least some individuals with allergy to a chemical will be capable of reacting to surprisingly low concentrations of that chemical.

III.   IN USE TESTS WITH CONTACT ALLERGENS

In use tests have typically been employed to demonstrate that even though a person is allergic to a chemical, he/she can use products that contain it with impunity.[36,37] Given the obvious differences between patch test conditions and use conditions for some products, e.g., a shampoo, this seems hardly surprising. In addition, it is the experience of most dermatologists that some patients have positive patch test results that seem irrelevant to their dermatitis even though the offending substance is a common one with which the patient would be expected to come into contact.

Nevertheless, it is possible to view in use tests in another manner. They frequently use small numbers of subjects, often those in whom an allergy has been "artificially induced" via an HRIPT (see Weaver et al.,[28] for example). These individuals, who by the nature of their original selection are not eczema prone, then undertake use tests on normal skin sites, e.g., volar forearm. This approach does not have a direct one-to-one relationship with the individual who may have, or be prone to, the development of eczema and/or contact allergies. In other words, in-use tests may tell us little about the at-risk population unless they are both well conducted and appropriately interpreted.

IV.   CONCLUSIONS — THE RELATIONSHIP TO THE HANDS

The work reviewed thus far has attempted to combine our own data with those of others to demonstrate the range of knowledge regarding quantitative relationships for contact allergens and how these data might be related to more normal modes of exposure to contact allergens. In this final section, we will draw on all this information (but make no apology for concentrating on our own data) as we consider the implications in the context of hand eczema.

Between an allergic contact dermatitis on the hands and quantitative patch test dose-response data lie many variables, most of which have only been addressed in a limited manner. These variables include interindividual and skin site variations, occluded versus open application, single versus repeated contact, and the existence (or not) of eczema or other impairment at the exposed skin site. Vehicles, duration of skin contact, weather conditions, and other factors also play their part in determining skin reactivity to allergen. Our studies with metal allergens have addressed some of what we believe are the key issues. Because the data are the most complete (or perhaps the least incomplete), the results with nickel will be taken as the example.

Nickel is a widespread and common contact allergen. Dose response studies using standard patch test techniques in allergic subjects suggest elicitation thresholds of from 1 ppm to at least 112 ppm.[18] In other words, there is a wide interindividual susceptibility. Subsequent studies in a panel of 20 subjects suggested there was little difference in reactivity between patch test reactions on the back and on the forearm, although the trend was toward greater reactions on the arms.[26] However, in these same subjects repeated treatment of the forearm with anionic surfactant to produce a moderate irritant reaction reduced the threshold for elicitation of allergic nickel reactions to 0.5 ppm. One half the panel reacted to 5 ppm nickel on this damaged skin. However, the experiment avoided the hand, the true target site, and was still based on a single 48-h occluded patch. So in a subsequent study, repeated surfactant treatment was retained but was combined with open treatment of a part of the hand with low levels of nickel, up to 1 ppm. The rationale for the selection of this level was as follows. Dose-response studies showed that sensitive nickel-allergic subjects were likely to react to 1 ppm nickel under patch test conditions on surfactant damaged,[25] or occasionally on normal skin.[18] Furthermore, 1 ppm nickel was being recommended by a European industry association as a suitable target level for consumer products, such as household cleaners and personal products.[38] The protocol that we developed incorporated repeated surfactant and nickel treatment, twice daily for a 23-day period (weekdays only). The repetition was important to allow for accumulated surfactant damage, additive subclinical effects, and for the buildup of nickel in the skin; it is well known that nickel binds avidly to skin where it is then persistent.[39] Nevertheless, in this experiment, despite the induction of an irritant response on both test and control hands, no nickel allergic reaction occurred in any of four subjects, three of whom had been previously shown to react to either 1 ppm or 10 ppm of nickel. It should be mentioned, however, that none of the four were, or had been, significant sufferers of hand eczema.

Although it must be stressed that these experiments have been conducted on only small numbers of subjects and did not progress to the point of eliciting a nickel allergic reaction, they do indicate certain conclusions. It is evident that individuals with an apparently high sensitivity to nickel do not respond on the hand to repeated, open contact, even when a concomitant inflammation is induced. Thus, it seems unlikely that persistent nickel hand eczema arises simply through an exquisite sensitivity to nickel at that site, nor perhaps does it arise through an enhanced ability to bind nickel over a period of time.

Ultimately, it will prove difficult to conduct definitive studies in this area. Except in special circumstances, the subjection of allergic individuals to allergen challenge on the hands will be judged unethical because of the risk of development of a chronic hand eczema. As a result, inferences from related studies are likely to be the best that can be achieved. In this context it is relevant to consider the position with chromium.[2] The available evidence suggests that prolonged (i.e., years of) contact with levels of no more than tens of parts per million can sensitize and then finally elicit a dermatitis. Cessation of exposure often fails to resolve the dermatitis. Experimental investigations that try to model this situation will clearly be difficult.

To summarize, although (allergic) hand eczema appears to be a particularly recalcitrant clinical problem that is often apparently associated with nickel allergy, our experimental studies with nickel-allergy subjects have failed to demonstrate an unexpectedly high sensitivity at this skin site. Consequently, it is reasonable to conclude, so far, that the cause of hand eczema requires more than an abnormally high allergic sensitivity.

REFERENCES

1. Friedman, P. S. and Moss, C., Quantification of contact hypersensivity in man, in *Models in Dermatology,* Vol. 2, Maibach, H. I. and Lowe, N., Eds., Karger, Basel, 1985, 275.
2. Burrows, D., Adverse chromate reactions on the skin, in *Chromium: Metabolism and Toxicity,* CRC Press, Boca Raton, FL, 1983, 137.
3. Fisher, A. A., *Contact Dermatitis,* Lea & Febiger, New York, 1986.
4. Landsteiner, K. and Chase, M. W., Studies on the sensitization of animals with simple chemical compounds, *J. Exp. Med.,* 69, 767, 1939.
5. Moss, C., Friedmann, P. S., and Shuster, S., DNCB reactivity in patients with multiple contact sensitivities, *Br. J. Dermatol.,* 107, 511, 1982.
6. Mosmann, T. R. and Coffman, R. L., Heterogeneity of cytokine secretion patterns and function of helper T cells, *Adv. Immunol.,* 46, 111, 1989.
7. Emmet, A. E., Risby, T. H., Jiang, L., Ng, S. K., and Feinman, S., Allergic contact dermatitis to nickel: bioavailability from consumer products and provocation threshold, *J. Am. Acad. Dermatol.,* 19, 314, 1988.
8. Eun, H. C. and Marks, R., Dose-response relationships for topically applied antigens, *Br. J. Dermatol.,* 122, 491, 1990.
9. Kim, H. O., Wester, R. C., McMaster, J. A., Bucks, D. A. W., and Maibach, H. I., Skin absorption from patch test systems, *Contact Dermatitis,* 17, 178, 1987.
10. Marzulli, F. N. and Maibach, H. I., Further studies of the effects of vehicles and elicitation concentration in experimental contact sensitization testing in humans, *Contact Dermatitis,* 6, 131, 1980.
11. Magnusson, B. and Hersle, K., Patch test methods. II. Regional variations of patch test responses, *Acta Derm. Venereol.,* 45, 275, 1965.
12. Wilkinson, D. S. and Wilkinson, J. D., Nickel allergy and hand eczema, in *Nickel and the Skin: Immunology and Toxicology,* CRC Press, Boca Raton, FL, 1989, 133.
13. Nater, J. P., Possible causes of chromate eczema, *Dermatologica,* 126, 160, 1963.

14. Malten, K. E. and Spruit, D., The relative importance of various environmental exposures to nickel in causing contact hypersensitivity, *Acta Derm. Venereol.*, 49, 14, 1969.

15. Nava, C., Campiglio, R., Caravelli, G., Galli, D. A., Cambini, M. A., Serboni, R., and Beretta, E., I sali di cromo e nickel come causa di dermatite allergica da contatto con detergenti, *Med. Lav.*, 78, 405, 1987.

16. Vilaplana, J., Grimalt, F., Romaguera, C., and Mascaro, J. M., Cobalt content of household cleaning products, *Contact Dermatitis*, 16, 139, 1987.

17. Kokelj, F., Nedoclan, G., Daris, F., and Crevatin, E., Nickel e cromo nei detergenti da toilette, *Boll. Dermatol. Allergol. Prof.*, 4, 31, 1989.

18. Allenby, C. F. and Goodwin, B. F. J., Influence of detergent washing powders on minimal eliciting patch test concentrations of nickel and chromium, *Contact Dermatitis*, 9, 491, 1983.

19. Allenby, C. F. and Basketter, D. A., Minimum eliciting patch test concentrations of cobalt, *Contact Dermatitis*, 20, 185, 1989.

20. Meneghini, C. L. and Angelini, G., Intradermal test in contact allergy to metals, *Acta Derm. Venereol.*, 59 (Suppl.), 89, 1979.

21. Goh, C. L., Ng, S. K., and Kwok, S. F., Allergic contact dermatitis from nickel in eyeshadow, *Contact Dermatitis*, 20, 380, 1989.

22. Kasahara, N. and Nakayama, H., Cosmetic dermatitis and metal sensitisation, *Hifubyo-Shinryo*, 12, 247, 1990.

23. Karlberg, A.-T., Lidén, C., and Ehrin, E., Colophony in mascara as a cause of eyelid dermatitis, *Acta Derm. Venereol.*, 71, 445, 1991.

24. Allenby, C. F., Basketter, D. A., Dickens, A., Barnes, E. G., and Brough, H. C., An arm immersion model for this study of compromised skin, *Contact Dermatitis*, 28, 84, 1993.

25. Allenby, C. F. and Basketter, D. A., An arm immersion model of compromised skin. II. Influence on minimal eliciting patch test concentrations of nickel, *Contact Dermatitis*, 28, 129, 1993.

26. Basketter, D. A., Barnes, E. G., and Allenby, C. F., Do transition metals in household and personal products play a role in allergic contact dermatitis?, *The Environmental Threat to the Skin*, Martin Dunitz, London, 1992, 215.

27. Basketter, D. A. and Allenby, C. F., Repeated immersion of the thumbs of nickel allergic subjects in surfactant solutions containing nickel, 1st Congress of the European Society of Contact Dermatitis, Brussels, 1992.

28. Weaver, J. E., Cardin, C. W., and Maibach, H. I., Dose-response assessments of Kathon biocide. I. Diagnostic use and diagnostic threshold patch testing with sensitized humans, *Contact Dermatitis*, 12, 141, 1985.

29. Cardin, C. W., Weaver, J. E., and Bailey, P. T., Dose-response assessments of Kathon biocide. II. Threshold prophetic patch testing, *Contact Dermatitis*, 15, 10, 1986.

30. Pasche, F. and Hunziker, N., Sensitization to Kathon CG in Geneva and Switzerland, *Contact Dermatitis*, 20, 115, 1989.

31. Cosmetic Ingredient Review, Final report of the Cosmetic Ingredient Review on methyl isothiazolinone and methylchloro isothiazolinone, *J. Am. Coll. Toxicol.*, 11, 75, 1992.

32. Kraus, A. L., Stotts, J., Altringer, L. A., and Allgood, G. S., Allergic contact dermatitis from propyl gallate: dose response comparison using various application methods, *Contact Dermatitis*, 22, 132, 1990.

33. Karlberg, A.-T. and Lidén, C., Comparison of colophony patch test preparations, *Contact Dermatitis*, 18, 158, 1988.

34. Jordan, W. P., Sherman, W. T., and King, S. E., Threshold responses in formaldehyde sensitive subjects, *J. Am. Acad. Dermatol.*, 1, 44, 1979.

35. Marzulli, F. N. and Maibach, H. I., Antimicrobials: experimental contact sensitization in man, *J. Soc. Cosmetic Chem.*, 24, 399, 1973.

36. Hannuksela, M. and Salo, H., The repeated open application test (ROAT), *Contact Dermatitis*, 14, 221, 1986.

37. Epstein, W. L., The use test for contact hypersensitivity, *Arch. Dermatol. Res.,* 272, 279, 1982.

38. Basketter, D. A., Briatico-Vangosa, G., Kästner, W., Lally, C., and Bontinck, W. J., Nickel, cobalt and chromium in consumer products: a role in allergic contact dermatitis?, *Contact Dermatitis,* 28, 15, 1993.

39. Fullerton, A. and Hoelgaard, A., Binding of nickel to human epidermis *in vitro, Br. J. Dermatol.,* 119, 675, 1988.

11

Hyperkeratotic Dermatitis of the Palms

Torkil Menné

CONTENTS

I. INTRODUCTION

Hersle and Mobacken[1] established hyperkeratotic dermatitis of the palms as an entity of its own, independent of psoriasis. Hyperkeratotic dermatitis of the palms occurs in otherwise healthy individuals with symmetrically hyperkeratotic plaques located centrally or proximally in the palms (Figure 1). Painful fissures may be a prominent feature. The margins of the lesions are less defined compared with psoriasis. Only rarely is simultaneous involvement of the sole present. The entity was originally described by Sutton and Ayres in 1953[2] as "hyperkeratotic dermatitis" of the palms and has later been discussed as "tylotic eczema".[3] Because of its distinct clinical features, this hand dermatosis deserves to be recognized as an entity of its own.

II. EPIDEMIOLOGY

Allergic and irritant contact dermatitis of the hands is more frequent in women than in men. The age of onset for these two skin diseases is in the 1920s and 1930s. In contrast, hyperkeratotic dermatitis of the palms mainly occurs in 40- to 60-year-old men.

Two Swedish population studies provided the relative frequency of hyperkeratotic dermatitis of the palms compared with other inflammatory hand dermatosis. Agrup,[4] in a 1968 field study, identified 1551 inflammatory hand dermatoses, among which 33 (2%) were classified as hyperkeratotic dermatitis of the palms. Agrup used the term "circumscribed palmar keratoderma". The median age in this study was 50 to 59 years with a female-to-male ratio of 0.6. In a more recent population study in Gothenberg, Meding and Swanbeck[5] identified 29 (2%) with hyperkeratotic eczema of the palms among 1457 individuals with eczematous skin lesions on the hands. The ratio between females and males was 0.8. It is reassuring that two independently organized studies within the same geographical area performed with a 20-year interval attain identical results.

In a study evaluating permanent disability from skin diseases, covering a 6-year period, 14 of 564 cases were caused by hyperkeratotic eczema of the palms. In comparison, 17 cases of persistent palmo-plantar pustulosis were identified in the same study.[6] The sex distribution follows the pattern seen in population studies with a female-to-male ratio of 0.8. Not unexpectedly, the female-to-male ratio for pustulosis palmo-plantaris was 16.

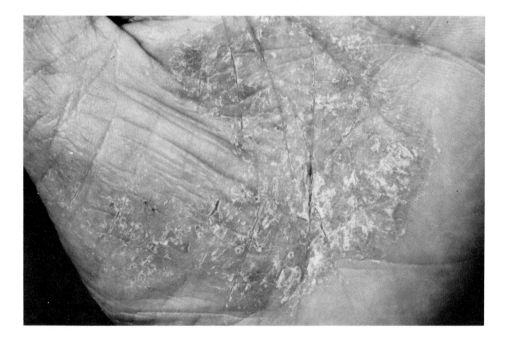

FIGURE 1. Hyperkeratotic dermatitis of the palms.

III. PATHOGENESIS

Hersle and Mobachen[1] performed a pivotal study on 32 cases of hyperkeratotic dermatitis of the palms. The inclusion criteria were as follows: presence of palmar, circumscribed, infiltrated scaling plaques, and an absence of psoriasis on the rest of the body at the initial visit. The study included 21 men and 11 women. The mean age of onset was 46 years. Dermatomycosis and contact allergy were excluded by the relevant investigations. No association to either former or present atopy or psoriasis was established. At the clinical investigation lesions were found in the palms and on the volar site of the fingers. Palmar and digital vesicular and pustular lesions, as well as nail changes, were absent. Only one third of the patients were engaged in hard manual labor at the onset of the symptoms. Histopathological investigations in nine of the patients revealed an identical picture of a spongiotic dermatitis with hyperkeratosis and slight focal parakeratosis. Neutrophils and microabscesses were not seen in epidermis. Investigations of human leukocyte antigen (HLA) types, known at that time, in 32 patients compared with 500 controls found identical HLA frequencies in the two groups. No clue by HLA types was given in that hyperkeratotic dermatitis of the palms might be genetically associated with psoriasis.

The only possible pathogenetic factor identified in the study was hard manual labor in one-third. It seems more significant that two thirds of the patients were not exposed to mechanical palmar trauma. Most cases tended to run a stable chronic course and only few patients experienced spontaneous clearing of the disease. No studies have indicated that hyperkeratotic dermatitis of the palms is associated with internal malignancy.

IV. DIFFFERENTIAL DIAGNOSES

Differentiation between hyperkeratotic dermatitis of the palms and palmar psoriasis is not of academic interest only. Why palmar psoriasis often is associated with nail changes, arthritis, pulpar involvement, and propensity to more disseminated psoriasis, skin lesions classified as the hyperkeratotic dermatitis of the palms are a localized inflammatory reaction and have no tendency to generalization.

In the study of Hersle and Mobachen,[1] only 1 of 32 patients developed psoriasis in an average observation period of 10 years. Mycosis, allergic contact dermatitis, and irritant contact dermatitis need to be excluded. Frictional contact dermatitis of the palms (Chapter XX), which might have similarities with hyperkeratotic dermatitis of the palms, is a distinct entity of its own because it is always possible to identify a mechanical trauma and the disease activity is closely related to the frictional trauma. If it is possible for the patient to avoid the trauma, the skin disease tends to disappear. Hyperkeratotic lesions in the palms mimic the initial symptoms of mycosis fungoides[7,8] and crusted scabies. Arsenical palmar hyperkeratoses are now rare.

IV. TREATMENT OF HYPERKERATOTIC DERMATITIS OF THE PALMS

Lesions are often dry and the patients often use greasy petroleum-based ointment particularly at night. Topically applied steroids only work under occlusion. Appropriate control is necessary to prevent skin atrophy. Palmar atrophy after use of potent steroids for prolonged periods is not as uncommon as generally thought. Treatment with crude coal tar or coal tar in petrolatum works in some cases. Treatment periods for 6 to 8 weeks need to be expected. Oral psoralen photochemotherapy (PUVA)[9] as well as Grenz rays are possible treatment modalities. Relapses are to be expected even after complete remissions have been induced. For some patients long-term treatment with retinoids is indicated and acceptable.[10]

REFERENCES

1. Hersle, K. and Mobachen, H., Hyperkeratotic dermatitis of the palms, *Br. J. Dermatol.*, 107, 195, 1982.
2. Sutton, R. L. and Ayres, S., Jr., Dermatitis of the hands, *Arch. Dermatol. Syphilol.*, 68, 266, 1953.

3. Bohnstedt, R. M., Hautkrankheiten der Handteller und Fuss-sohlen, in *Dermatologie und Venerologie,* Gottron, H. A. and Schönfeld, W., Eds., George Thieme Verlag, Stuttgart, 1960, 704.

4. Agrup, G., Hand eczema and other hand dermatosis in South Sweden, *Acta Derm. Venereol.,* 49 (Suppl. 61), 13, 1969.

5. Meding, B. and Swanbech, G., Epidemiology of different types of hand eczema in an industrial city, *Acta Derm. Venereol.,* 69, 227, 1989.

6. Menné, T. and Bachmann, E., Permanent disability from skin diseases, *Dermatosen,* 27, 37, 1979.

7. Major, T. S., Ploeg, E. E. V., and De Villez, R. L., Hyperkeratotic mycosis fungoides restricted to the palms, *J. Am. Acad. Dermatol.,* 7, 792, 1982.

8. Aram, H. and Zendenbaum, M., Palmoplantar hyperkeratosis in mycosis fungoides, *J. Am. Acad. Dermatol.,* 13, 897, 1985.

9. Mobachen, H., Rosén, K., and Swanbech, G., Oral psoralen photochemotherapy of hyperkeratotic dermatitis of the palms, *Br. J. Dermatol.,* 109, 205, 1983.

10. Reymann, F., Two years experience with tigason treatment of pustulosis palmo-plantaris and eczema keratoticum manuum, *Dermatologica,* 164, 209, 1982.

12

Risk Factors for Hand Dermatitis in Wet Work

Kaija Lammintausta

CONTENTS

0-8493-7355-7/94/$0.00 + $.50
© 1994 by CRC Press, Inc.

I. INTRODUCTION

Wet work is a major external risk factor for hand dermatitis. This fact has been verified in several studies.[1-4] Water, as such, decreases the protective capacity of the skin and occlusion further increases the irritant effect.[5-8] In many wet work occupations, lipid-soluble chemicals are added to water to achieve the cleaning effect. In the skin this effect is unfavorable because intercellular lipids are washed away. Those lipids are an important factor in the cutaneous protective capacity.[9-11] The removal of lipids induces structural and physiochemical alterations in the skin,[12-16] which apparently facilitates the process of cutaneous irritation. The cascade of cutaneous alterations leading to skin irritation is, however, dependent on many external and internal factors.

II. EXTERNAL FACTORS

Although the individual characteristics of the detergent itself are crucial concerning its irritation capacity, no reliable *in vivo* method exists to determine irritant potentials of chemicals. Simultaneously, a multitude of contributing external factors are important. For each individual chemical and for each individual worker, a different outcome can be seen after occupational exposure situations.

A. Irritant Exposure

1. Physicochemical Characteristics of the Chemical

Although the characteristics of the chemical are most important in irritation,[17] the concentration and the diluent of the chemical also determine the degree of the reaction. Even the reaction time may be different due to the alteration of the concentration.[18] Skin reaction is, for some part, dependent on the temperature of the irritant because the cutaneous blood flow alters with external temperature.[19] An increase of cutaneous temperature leads to an increase in the speed to react. When the normal pH of the skin is disrupted, the probability of the irritation increases. Both low and high pH extremes are poorly tolerated in the human skin.

2. Exposure Time

The duration and frequency of irritant contacts are influencing the development of skin reactions. Each exposure has its recovery time.[20] Even unexpected types of skin reactivity during that recovery time have been described.[21] The degree of irritation is correlated with the duration of the exposure and with the rest time after the previous exposure. The cumulation of irritant exposures seems to be contributing.[22]

3. Simultaneous Exposure Factors

Repeated physical trauma irritates. Friction, contact with rough materials, and repeated accidental exposure to minor cutaneous trauma eliciting factors are common in many wet work positions. Mechanical irritants, such as dusts from variable materials, may sometimes stay in occlusion below protective gloves.

B. Allergen Exposure

Contact allergens are not infrequently encountered in wet work. When the protective capacity of the epidermis is disrupted by wet work exposure, the penetration of the allergen is facilitated; thus, the probability of sensitization is increased. The need for protection is one important risk due to occlusion and allergen contact. Rubber sensitivity is not infrequent among these subjects.[1,2] When the sensitization develops slowly, the patient and the doctor often interpret the situation as an increasing need for protection. Immediate allergy to latex is a more poorly recognized etiologic factor leading to chronic dermatitis.

The sensitivities to nickel and perfumes are also common among these workers.[1,2] The specific importance of the allergy has to be evaluated for each patient individually. Sometimes it is difficult to determine whether the sensitization has already developed before the employee has become hired in the present work. The clinical appearance as well as the histology and the immunohistology of allergic and irritant contact dermatitis are indistinguishable.[23] The development of the clinical dermatitis, the anamnestic data, and the skin tests are diagnostic tools used in these cases of contact dermatitis.

C. Climate

Skin chapping is more frequent in winter. Dry cold wind induces chapping. Low humidity manifests symptoms, especially in subjects with a constitutional susceptibility.

III. INTERNAL FACTORS

A. Location

The face and the eyelids, in particular, are most susceptible to irritants because of skin-related reasons. Hands are most heavily exposed in wet work; thus, the probability for the development of hand dermatitis is great. The thick palmar epidermis reacts less than the back of the hand. The skin is thinnest between the fingers, where the reactions generally first appear.

B. Constitutional Factors

The interindividual variation in the susceptibility is extensive. Some individual groups of subjects have been characterized who have skin structure with a particular susceptibility to develop irritant contact dermatitis. The development of this skin disease is, however, multifactorial. We do not have any diagnostic tool to predict the susceptibility of one particular person to contact dermatitis.

1. Sweating

Palmar sweating may facilitate penetration of irritants and allergens. Sweating also makes it more difficult to protect the skin. Associations between the dyshidrotic type of hand dermatitis and palmar sweating have been questioned.

2. Age, Race, and Sex

Age seems to decrease the actual reactivity of the skin while the healing of the damage in the epidermal barrier is delayed.[24] The contribution of age-associated alteration of attitudes and behavior in skin protection may simultaneously change the risk.

Race-related differences in the structure of the skin exist. Those characteristics may influence the risk one has to develop contact dermatitis.[25-27] Results from studies on this topic are somewhat controversial. It appears that subjects with white and even poorly tanning skin may most easily develop dermatitis in wet work.[28]

Irritant contact dermatitis is more common among females compared with males.[1-3] This is probably due to more extensive household work performed by females in Western cultures. The importance of hormonal factors has not been verified.

3. "Sensitive" Skin

"Sensitive" skin is a poorly defined entity used to characterize the cutaneous structure of those subjects who easily develop skin irritation. The importance of this entity is most important in wet work occupations, although the usefulness is poor for practical purposes. Only anamnestic data can be used to diagnose individuals with sensitive skin. A history of previous hand dermatitis, however, can be regarded as a significant risk factor for developing irritant contact dermatitis.[29,30]

4. Atopy

Atopic subjects can be found as an important subgroup among subjects with sensitive skin. The importance of atopy in the etiopathogenesis of irritant contact dermatitis in wet work has been proven in several studies.[31-34] The wide spectrum of atopic symptoms makes this problem more complicated. Atopy without cutaneous symptoms does not increase one's risk to develop hand dermatitis.[32] The degree of divergence from "normal" skin structure and/or physiology may be just minimal in these subjects. No suspicion exists that a person who has a history of manifest atopic dermatitis has an increased risk for hand dermatitis if working in a wet work occupation.[31-34] If the atopic dermatitis symptoms have occurred in adulthood, the risk is even greater.

5. Other Skin Diseases

Dermatitis in any site of the skin increases the risk for simultaneous hand dermatitis when the threshold for cutaneous irritation is decreased.[35,36] Psoriatic skin reacts more to certain skin irritants because of increased penetration.[37]

6. Previous Contact Sensitivities

The subjects who have developed nickel allergy seem to develop irritant contact dermatitis in hands most easily.[38,39] This phenomenon seems to be a nonspecific factor without apparent relationship with nickel allergy. Because nickel is an unavoidable allergen in our environments and in wet work, allergen exposure may have some importance. Simultaneous exposure to wet conditions and nickel is not infrequent in occupational circumstances. Any other known contact sensitivity may be an apparent restriction in certain occupational environments. The knowledge about individual factors influencing the development of contact sensitization does not yet have useful applications for practical purposes.

IV. CONCLUSIONS

The stepwise evaluation of the risks in the work environments and the individual investigation of the work entering person are necessary to avoid cutaneous problems in wet work. In the susceptibility of an individual for hand dermatitis and in the secondary prevention as well, one of the most important factors is the worker's motivation to work because protective maneuvers and rationalization of the working processes need to be developed. Those factors are often crucial in wet work occupations.

REFERENCES

1. Agrup, G., Hand eczema and other hand dermatoses in South Sweden, *Acta Derm. Venereol.*, 49 (Suppl.), 61, 1969.
2. Fregert, S., Occupational dermatitis in a 10-year material, *Contact Dermatitis*, 1, 96, 1975.
3. Coenraads, P. J., Nater, J. P., and van der Lande, R., The prevalence of eczema and other dermatoses of the hands and arms in the Netherlands. Association with age and occupation, *Clin. Exp. Dermatol.*, 8, 495, 1983.
4. Lammintausta, K., Hand dermatitis in different hospital workers who perform wet work, *Dermatosen*, 31, 14, 1983.
5. van der Valk, P. G. M. and Maibach, H. I., Post-application occlusion substantially increases the irritant response of the skin to repeated short-term sodium lauryl sulfate (SLS) exposure, *Contact Dermatitis*, 21, 335, 1989.
6. Berardesca, E., Fideli, D., Gabba, P., Cespa, M., Rabbionic, G., and Maibach, H. I., Ranking of surfactant skin irritancy *in vivo* in man using the plastic occlusion stress test, *Contact Dermatitis*, 23, 1, 1990.

7. Mikulowska, A., Pronounced reactive changes in human skin produced by sodium lauryl sulfate and simple water occlusion, *Contact Dermatitis,* 23, 236, 1990.

8. Nieboer, C., Bruynzeel, D. P., and Boorsma, D. M., The effect of occlusion of the skin with transdermal therapeutic system on Langerhans' cells and the induction of skin irritation, *Arch. Dermatol.,* 123, 1299, 1987.

9. Elias, P. M., Lipids and the epidermal permeability barriers, *Arch. Dermatol. Res.,* 270, 95, 1981.

10. Hadby, N. F., Lipid water barriers in biological systems, *Prog. Lipid Res.,* 23, 1, 1989.

11. Potts, R. O. and Francolur, M. L., Lipid biophysics of water loss of the skin, *Proc. Natl. Acad. Sci. U.S.A.,* 87, 3871, 1990.

12. Willis, C. M., Stephens, C. J. M., and Wilkinson, J. D., Epidermal damage induced by irritants in man: a light and electron microscopic study, *J. Invest. Dermatol.,* 93, 695, 1989.

13. Grubauer, G. and Elias, P. M., Transepidermal water loss: the signal for recovery of barrier structure and function, *J. Lipid Res.,* 30, 323, 1989.

14. Elias, P. M., Menon, G. K., Grayson, S., and Brown, B. E., Membrane structural alterations in murine stratum corneum. Relationship to the localization of polar lipids and phospholipases, *J. Invest. Dermatol.,* 91, 3, 1988.

15. Menon, G. K., Feingold, K. R., and Elias, P. M., Lamellar body secretory response to barrier disruption, *J. Invest. Dermatol.,* 98, 279, 1992.

16. Menon, G. K., Feingold, K. R., Mao-Qiang, M., Schaude, M., and Elias, P. M., Structural basis for the barrier abnormality following inhibition of HMG CoA reductase in murine epidermis, *J. Invest. Dermatol.,* 98, 209, 1992.

17. Prottey, C. and Ferguson, T., Factors which determine the skin irritation potential of soaps and detergents, *J. Soc. Cosmetic Chem.,* 26, 29, 1975.

18. Anderson, C., The spectrum of non-allergic contact reactions. An experimental view, *Contact Dermatitis,* 23, 695, 1990.

19. Halkier-Sörensen, L., and Thestrup-Pedersen, K., The relationship between skin surface temperature, transepidermal water loss and electrical capacitance among workers in the fish processing industry: comparison with other occupations, *Contact Dermatitis,* 24, 345, 1991.

20. van der Valk, P. G. M. and Maibach, H. I., Post-application occlusion substantially increases the irritant response of the skin to repeated short-term sodium lauryl sulfate (SLS) exposure, *Contact Dermatitis,* 21, 335, 1989.

21. Lammintausta, K., Maibach, H. I., and Wilson, D., Human cutaneous irritation: induced hyporeactivity, *Contact Dermatitis,* 17, 193, 1987.

22. Malten, K. E., Thoughts on irritant contact dermatitis, *Contact Dermatitis,* 7, 238, 1981.

23. Brasch, J., Burgaard, J., and Sterry, W., Common pathogenetic pathways in allergic and irritant contact dermatitis, *J. Invest. Dermatol.,* 98, 166, 1992.

24. Elsner, P., Wilhelm, D., and Maibach, H. I., Irritant contact dermatitis and aging, *Contact Dermatitis,* 23, 275, 1990.

25. Berardesca, E. and Maibach, H. I., Racial differences in sodium lauryl sulphate induced cutaneous irritation, *Contact Dermatitis,* 18, 65, 1988.

26. Berardesca, E. and Maibach, H. I., Cutaneous reactive hyperemia: racial differences induced by corticoid application, *Br. J. Dermatol.,* 120, 787, 1989.

27. Weigand, D. A. and Gaylo, J. R., Irritant reactions in negro and caucasian skin, *South Med. J.,* 67, 548, 1974.

28. Frosch, P. J., Hautirritation und empfindliche Haut, Ph.D., thesis, Grosse Scripta 7, Grosse Verlag, Berlin, 1985.

29. Nilsson, E. and Beck, O., The importance of anamnestic information of atopy, metal dermatitis and earlier hand eczema for the development of hand dermatitis in women in wet hospital work, *Acta Derm. Venereol.,* 66, 45, 1986.

30. Lammintausta, K., Maibach, H. I., and Wilson, D., Susceptibility to cumulative and acute irritant dermatitis. An experimental approach in human volunteers, *Contact Dermatitis,* 19, 84, 1988.

31. Rystedt, I., Hand eczema in patients with history of atopic dermatitis in childhood, *Acta Derm. Venereol.,* 65, 305, 1985.

32. Lammintausta, K. and Kalimo, K., Atopy and hand dermatitis in hospital wet work, *Contact Dermatitis,* 7, 301, 1981.
33. Nilsson, E., Mikaelsson, B., and Andersson, S., Atopy, occupation and domestic work as risk factors for hand eczema in hospital workers, *Contact Dermatitis,* 13, 216, 1985.
34. Meding, B. and Swanbeck, G., Predictive factors for hand eczema, *Contact Dermatitis,* 23, 154, 1990.
35. Björnberg, A., Skin reactions to primary irritants in patients with hand eczema, Ph.D. thesis, Oscar Isacssons Tryckeri AB, Goethenburg, Sweden, 1968.
36. Bruynzeel, D. P. and Maibach, H. I., Excited skin syndrome (angry back), *Arch. Dermatol.,* 122, 323, 1986.
37. MacDonalds, K. J. S. and Marks, J., Short contact anthralin in the treatment of psoriasis: a study of different contact times, *Br. J. Dermatol.,* 114, 435, 1986.
38. Peltonen, L., Nickel sensitivity in the general population, *Contact Dermatitis,* 5, 27, 1979.
39. Menné, T., Borgan, Ö, and Green, A., Nickel allergy and hand dermatitis in a stratified sample of Danish female population: an epidemiological study including a statistics appendix, *Acta Derm. Venereol.,* 62, 35, 1982.

13

Hand Eczema and Long-Term Prognosis in Atopic Dermatitis*

Ingela Rystedt

CONTENTS

---

* This article is largely based on the author's thesis, "Hand Eczema and Long-Term Prognosis in Atopic Dermatitis",[1] with subtitles.[2-7]

I. BACKGROUND

Atopic dermatitis is one of the most common dermatoses of infancy and childhood. It is also regarded by many dermatologists as fairly common in adult life, even though opinions differ concerning the frequency of the disease. Data for incidence and prevalence vary widely, especially in earlier investigations,[8-12] partly because of variations between different groups studied and partly because of different opinions about the diagnostic criteria. To create homogeneity in the diagnosis and to facilitate communication between different investigations, Hanifin and Rajka in 1980 drew up guidelines for atopic dermatitis in which they proposed special diagnostic criteria (Table 1).[13] According to these guidelines, which have been followed in most recent investigations, the major characteristics of atopic dermatitis are pruritus, typical appearance and localization, chronic or relapsing course, and family history of atopy and/or personal respiratory allergy. Minor criteria include (among others) xerosis, facial pallor, and orbital darkening. Three of 4 major characteristics and 3 of 23 minor criteria must be met for the diagnosis to be accepted.

Most recent incidence and prevalence data of atopic dermatitis refer to groups of schoolchildren and adolescents. Taylor et al. found, in large cohort studies published in 1984, an increase in overall rates of childhood eczema from 5.1% in children born in 1946 to 7.3% and 12.2% in those born in 1958 and 1970, respectively.[14] The cumulative incidence of atopic dermatitis had increased from 3 to 10% during 10 years in a population of twins investigated by Schultz Larsen in Denmark in 1986.[15] In three Scandinavian articles, published in 1979, 1980, and 1989, 10 to 15% of investigated schoolchildren had past or present atopic dermatitis.[16-18] Meding and Swanbeck[19] reported in a recent investigation of 20,000 people in the age range of 20 to 65 years a childhood history of atopic dermatitis of 10.4% A reasonable conclusion seems to be that the rates of atopic dermatitis are increasing.

Data concerning persistent atopic dermatitis in adult life range from as much as 8% in earlier studies to 83% in different follow-up studies.[20-25] The investigations have varied greatly with respect to number of patients, patient material, diagnostic criteria, observation period, method of investigation, and response rate to follow-up studies, which partly explains the differences regarding the prognostic data.

Many authors have suggested that the hands are the most common site of atopic dermatitis in adulthood.[26-28] During the last few decades a lot of interest has been focused on the relationship between atopic dermatitis and hand eczema, with emphasis on work-related hand eczema in atopics.[29-32] These issues also have a central position in the author's thesis.[1,3-4,6-7]

II. THE AUTHOR'S INVESTIGATION

The thesis[1] shows the results of a study that was carried out during 1979 to 1982 at the Department of Occupational Dermatology, Karolinska Hospital, Stockholm. The aims of the investigation were as follows:

- To make a long term follow-up study of patients with a childhood history of atopic dermatitis, with emphasis on unfavorable prognostic factors.
- To study the occurrence of hand eczema and factors influencing the development of hand eczema in adults who have had atopic manifestations in childhood.
- To study work-related skin problems in atopics to distinguish risk individuals and risk occupations.

Five groups of people were studied. Group I comprised 549 individuals with a childhood history of atopic dermatitis who had received inpatient treatment for their dermatitis at the Department of Dermatology, Karolinska Hospital. Group 2 included 406 individuals also with a childhood history of atopic dermatitis, but having received outpatient treatment at the same department. Group 3 comprised 222 individuals treated at the Department of Paediatrics in the same hospital and having a childhood history of bronchial asthma and/or allergic rhinitis, but no history of atopic dermatitis. Group 4, 199 people with no history or current symptoms or signs of atopic disease and no familial

TABLE 1   Guidelines for the Diagnosis of Atopic Dermatitis

Must have three or more basic features
   Pruritus
   Typical morphology and distribution
      Flexural lichenification or linearity in adults
      Facial and extensor involvement in infants and children
   Chronic or chronically relapsing dermatitis
   Personal or family history of atopy (asthma, allergic rhinitis, atopic dermatitis)
Plus three or more minor features
   Xerosis
   Ichthyosis/palmar hyperlinearity/keratosis pilaris
   Immediate (type I) skin test reactivity
   Elevated serum immunoglobulin E
   Early age of onset
   Tendency toward cutaneous infections (especially *Staphylococcus aureus* and herpes simplex)/
      impaired cell-mediated immunity
   Tendency toward nonspecific hand or foot dermatitis
   Nipple eczema
   Cheilitis
   Recurrent conjunctivitis
   Dennie-Morgan infraorbital fold
   Keratoconus
   Anterior subcapsular cataracts
   Orbital darkening
   Facial pallor/facial erythema
   Pityriasis alba
   Anterior neck folds
   Itch when sweating
   Intolerance to wool and lipid solvents
   Perifollicular accentuation
   Food intolerance
   Course influenced by environmental/emotional factors
   White dermographism/delayed blanch

From Hanifin, J. M. and Rajka, G., *Acta Derm. Venereol.*, 92, 44, 1980. With permission.

history of atopy, was selected at random and served as a control group. Group 5 comprised 445 patients, treated at the aforementioned Department of Occupational Dermatology.

The studies were based on comprehensive questionnaires, previous medical records, telephone interviews, and clinical examinations with patch test of 345 people in groups 1 and 2, chosen at random. The follow-up period was a minimum of 24 years. The response rate in the various groups was 97 to 99%.

A.   Prognosis of Atopic Dermatitis

At the time of investigation 67% in group 1 and 40% in group 2 had eczematous lesions on hands and/or other parts of the body.[1,2] The hands were the most common sites of the dermatitis. After being free from lesions during long periods in childhood, about 25% of the atopic dermatitis patients had suffered from recurrence of the dermatitis in adult life, most often localized to the hands. Hand eczema was always recorded as recurrent atopic dermatitis in all patients in whom the adult eczema could be connected with atopic dermatitis in childhood. The degree of severity of dermatitis was in general low. In group 1 45% had mild, 6% moderate, and 9% severe dermatitis. The corresponding totals for group 2 were 60, 35, and 5%, respectively.[1,2]

The data for persistent or recurrent dermatitis were high compared with the results of most earlier investigations. It should be stressed, however, that contrary to most of the earlier investigations, the study was based on a large well-defined group of individuals with a history of atopic dermatitis in childhood (excluding all with doubtful diagnoses according to the criteria of Hanifin and Rajka[13]), with a long follow-up period (minimum 24 years) and with a high rate of response to follow up.

The follow-up showed that, in order of importance, dry/itchy skin, widespread dermatitis in childhood, associated bronchial asthma and/or allergic rhinitis, early age at onset, and female sex were prognostically unfavorable factors for the healing of atopic dermatitis. The same factors were also associated, in the same order, with increased severity of persistent or recurrent dermatitis. Even though the study was based on a selected material of patients with severe to moderate atopic eczema in childhood, it seems reasonable to attempt a generalization as to all patients with atopic dermatitis in childhood: the fewer and the less important the unfavorable factors involved, the better the prognosis.

B.   Prevalence of Hand Eczema in Atopics

The frequency of hand eczema was found to be significantly higher in people with a history of atopic dermatitis than in nonatopics.[25,28] At the time of investigation the prevalence of hand eczema was 41% in group 1, 25% in group 2, 5% in group 3, and 4% in group 4 (Figure 1). The significant difference in prevalence of hand eczema between people with a history of severe (group 1) and people with a history of mild to moderate (group 2) atopic dermatitis in childhood indicates that individuals with milder forms of atopic dermatitis develop hand eczema to a lesser extent than individuals with more severe forms of atopic dermatitis.[1,3]

An interesting observation was that the difference in frequency of hand eczema between people with past or present atopic dermatitis and nonatopics was much greater at the actual time of the investigation than when measured over a longer period; the frequency was from 4 to as much as ten times higher in the atopic dermatitis groups (Figure 1).[1] The most likely explanation for these discrepancies is that hand eczema is more protracted and occurs in lengthier episodes and/or shows more frequent recurrences in people with a history of atopic dermatitis than in nonatopics.

People with a history of respiratory allergy (atopic mucosal symptoms) (group 3) without concomitant atopic dermatitis showed a lower incidence of hand eczema than those who had had childhood atopic dermatitis, and were in general not significantly more prone to develop hand eczema than nonatopics (group 4).[1,3] In people with respiratory allergy and in nonatopics, however,

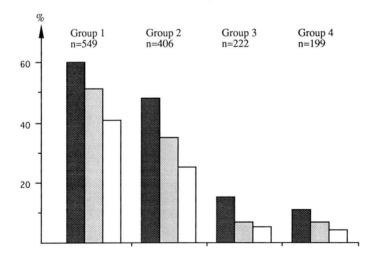

FIGURE 1.   Occurrence of sporadic or continuous hand eczema (HE) on some occasion after 15 years of age, during 12 months before investigation. Columns denote percentage of atopic and nonatopic individuals with HE. (▓) HE on some occasion after 15 years of age; (▒) HE during the 12 months before the investigation; (□) HE at the time of the investigation. (From Hanifin, J. M. and Rajka, G., *Acta Derm. Venereol.*, 92, 44, 1980. With permission.)

the simultaneous presence of dry/itchy skin,[1] in Lammintausta's study[29] in combination with white dermographism and facial pallor (atopic skin diathesis),[29] had markedly increased the incidence of hand eczema.

C. Severity of Hand Eczema

Severe hand eczema was found to be unusual in both atopics (groups 1 to 3) and nonatopics (group 4) (defined by a special severity index),[3] even though the hand eczema was found to be more intense and, as previously mentioned, more protracted in atopics. Higher figures for medical consultations and periods of sick leave among the atopics corroborate these findings.[1,3]

D. Localization and Morphology

No essential difference between atopics and nonatopics with regard to the localization of hand eczema was found in the study, the main site in both categories being the fingers.[1,3] In more than 85% of the people in the atopic dermatitis groups the fingers were involved, in the majority in combination with eczema on the backs or the palms of the hands. Eczema solely on the palms occurred in only 2%. No specific pattern of atopic hand eczema emerged. Consequently, it was not possible to tell simply by looking at the hands whether the hand eczema was of exogenous or endogenous origin. These observations have later been confirmed by Cronin.[33]

E. Etiology

The etiology of hand eczema is always multifactorial[34-36] and is influenced by both environmental and various constitutional factors. The relative importance of exogenous and endogenous factors is difficult to distinguish in the individual case. There is much evidence to indicate that in patients with atopic dermatitis there is an early defect in the skin barrier function as demonstrated by an increased transepidermal water loss and a decreased ability of the stratum corneum to bind water.[37,38] Probably as a consequence, atopic skin seems to have a reduced resistance to irritants, which varies from individual to individual.[39-42] There is overwhelming clinical evidence that irritants above all tensides aggravate any type of hand dermatitis.[43] Consequently, exogenous predictors for hand eczema should not be underestimated. However, the author's investigation gave no indication that exposure to irritants was the main cause of hand eczema in the majority of people with a history of atopic dermatitis.[4,6]

Several factors that might serve as indicators for a constitutional skin vulnerability include eczematous hand involvement of atopic dermatitis before 15 years of age, persistent eczema on parts of the body other than the hands, and persistent dry/itchy skin, all of which were found to be strong predictors for hand eczema.[1,6] Of these strong predictors hand involvement before 15 years of age was the predominant one. In individuals without such involvement, severe (widespread) dermatitis in childhood was a dominant factor. Female sex, family history of atopic dermatitis, and associated respiratory allergy were found to be weaker predictors.

Contact sensitivity was not found to be an important predictor for hand eczema;[1,5] 17% of the people with a childhood history of severe and 23% of those with mild to moderate dermatitis in childhood (groups 1 and 2) were sensitized to one or several of the contact allergens in a standard tray used in the investigation,[5] which is in agreement with other similar studies.[30,44,45] Neither the frequency nor the severity of hand eczema among the atopics was shown to be greater in sensitized rather than nonsensitized persons. Most atopics were unable to correlate current episodes of hand eczema with any obvious exposure to allergens to which they reacted. The allergic contact dermatitis that develops in atopics in association with contact with a known allergen may boost an existing dermatitis but seems as a rule to have nothing (or only little) to do with persistent or recurrent atopic hand eczema.

In summary, the predominant cause of hand eczema in atopics seems in most cases to be a skin vulnerability that varies from individual to individual. Many atopics therefore develop hand eczema independently of excessive exposure to irritants, but such exposure probably brings about additional irritant contact dermatitis. Atopics with hand eczema can also have a contributory allergic dermatitis, although contact sensitivity seldom seems to be the original cause of hand eczema in atopics.[5,30]

F.   Work-Related Hand Eczema in Atopics

Even though it is impossible to distinguish between irritant contact dermatitis on an atopic base in which the clinical picture is the result caused by exogenous factors and atopic hand eczema mainly caused by endogenous factors,[1,33] it is important for medicolegal reasons to emphasize the work-related implications of hand eczema in atopics. Only a few investigations concerning hand eczema among atopics in various occupations and trades have been reported.[4,29,32,46] Lammintausta and Kalimo[29] and Nilsson et al.[32] investigated atopics engaged in hospital work. Both groups found a high frequency of hand eczema among kitchen workers and cleaners and among assistant nurses. Hand eczema was, in the author's investigation, found to be significantly more common in atopics (groups 1 and 2) exposed to irritants, above all tensides, than in atopics not thus exposed.[1,4] The highest rate of hand eczema occurred among food handlers and wet workers, e.g., hairdressers, assistant nurses, other nursing staff, and domestic workers, in whom the occurrence of hand eczema after 15 years of age in people with a history of atopic dermatitis was between 81% and 68%; the corresponding value for office workers never exposed to irritants was 52%[1,4] (Table 2). The high frequency of hand eczema among food handlers may partly be due to the fact that hand eczema in such jobs is often caused by type I reactions giving rise to contact urticaria followed by protein contact dermatitis.[47]

It is important to point out that apart from occupational domestic exposure to irritants, domestic factors at home proved to be of significant importance for the development of hand eczema.[1,4] One of the dominating risk occupations is that of "housewife". A highly significant difference in prevalence of hand eczema was found between women exposed and women not exposed to irritants in their home environment[1,4] irrespective of occupational exposure. Further, the incidence of hand eczema increased with an increasing number of children and was also more common in women with children younger than 3 years of age (groups 1 and 2).

TABLE 2   Occurrence of Hand Eczema after
15 Years of Age among Atopics in
Various Occupations with and
without Exposure to Irritants (Groups
1 and 2)

Occupation	Occurrence of hand eczema (%)
Food handling	81[a]
Hairdressing	76[b]
Assistant nursing	75[b]
Other nursing occupations	71[c]
Laboratory work	43
Domestic work	68[a]
Cleaning	60
Building (concrete) work	57
Metalwork (wet)	57
Hotel and restaurant work	53
Garage work	49
Printing	48
Farming and forestry	56
Office work	52

Note: Only occupations with 15 individuals or more have
been included in the table; n = 955.

[a]   Significance versus office work: $p < 0.05$.
[b]   Significance versus office work: $p < 0.001$.
[c]   Significance versus office work: $p < 0.01$.

From Hanifin, J. M. and Rajka, G., *Acta Derm. Venereol.*,
92, 44, 1980. With permission.

In most studies of hand eczema there is a female predominance,[13,48-51] which in the author's study was significant only in groups exposed to irritants[1] (groups 1 to 5). It is unclear whether this is because women are more exposed to irritants than men, especially because they often both have a job and do housework, or because female skin withstands trauma less well than male skin.[52] A hormonal factor might also be involved. In considering the effect of irritants of the skin, it should be noted that ~25% of high-risk workers with a history of atopic eczema had never developed hand eczema.[1,4] (groups 1 and 2). This confirms the importance of constitutional factors in the etiology of atopic hand eczema.

G. Change of Occupation

Hand dermatitis can limit the choice of career because job factors sometimes elicit or exacerbate the eczema. People with a history of atopic dermatitis had changed occupations because of hand eczema to a somewhat higher extent than had nonatopics (9% in the atopic groups 1 and 2 and 3% in the nonatopic group 4), which, however, mainly parallels the higher incidence of hand eczema in atopics.[1,4]

Aggravation of the hand eczema by wet and dirty work seemed to be the main reason for change of job (groups 1 to 5), even though in most cases social, economic, and labor market factors also had contributed to the change. In many of these people the hand eczema was not particularly severe. Objectively, this was confirmed by a low sick-listing rate, few medical consultations, and a minor use of corticosteroids. The most common jobs people had not been able to keep up with were as follows: hairdressing, food handling, cleaning, printing, wet metalwork, assistant nursing, garage work, and hotel and restaurant work. It should be emphasized, however, that many atopics with and without hand eczema had been able to stand up to excessive exposure to irritants, often with the help of a good skin care program.

Opinions are divided concerning the value of change of job for patients who have contracted hand eczema at work. Some authors consider a change to be of value,[53] whereas others express doubt.[54] After perusal of 10 years of patient material at the Department of Occupational Dermatology[36] in Southern Sweden, it appeared that no difference in prognosis existed between patients who had changed jobs and those who continued in their original jobs. The beneficial effect of a change was, in the author's study, found to be more marked in nonatopics than in atopics (groups 1 to 5), which might be explained by the pronounced influence of constitutional factors on the development of hand eczema in atopics.[4,7] Even though the healing rate after change of work in people with a childhood history of atopic dermatitis was not more than about 20%, a change to clean, dry work had improved the cause of the hand lesions in most of them (groups 1 to 5).

H. Risk Individuals and Risk Occupations

For young atopic persons about to choose their first occupation it is important to emphasize the risk of developing hand eczema. It is possible to distinguish high- and low-risk individuals by assessing the appropriate strong predictors found in the investigation (eczematous hand involvement in childhood, persistent "body" eczema in adult life, and persistent dry/itching skin[1,6]). In the group of atopic people with all the strong predictors about 80% of those in "dry" jobs and 90% of those in "wet" jobs had had hand eczema in adult life. The corresponding value for those without any of the strong predictors was about 10%.[1] Previous hand eczema always puts an individual at high risk, especially if the predictor is combined with one or several of the other strong predictors. However, people without any or with only a few of the weak risk factors do not seem to run a much higher risk of developing hand eczema than nonatopics, even though the borderline between the categories must be regarded as diffuse.

In all likelihood, for a pronounced high-risk individual the choice of occupation is often of limited importance, insofar as hand eczema has already developed or will develop later independently of the occupation chosen. Even so, it is important to point out that contact with irritants (e.g., detergents) often causes a deterioration of an existing hand eczema, thus constituting a worsening factor that can make the patient incapable of working. Atopics who are constitutionally more moderately burdened, that is, with lesser indicators of a skin fragility, will probably manage with their hands in dry work, whereas work involving excessive contact with irritants may be the eliciting cause of hand eczema.

People with childhood respiratory allergy without simultaneous atopic dermatitis do not seem to be at risk more than nonatopics unless they have dry/itching skin. This is in accordance with the finding that dry/itchy skin was found to be a strong predictor, which also may make nonatopics risk individuals, although not to the same extent as high-risk atopics. A person with a history of atopic dermatitis must consider risk levels of different occupations. Jobs involving exposure to various irritants, above all tensides, belong to the very high-risk occupations as do jobs involving food handling. Domestic wet work can be an additional aggravating factor for hand eczema but can also, when intense, be looked upon as a risk occupation in itself.

Even though contact sensitivity does not seem to be more common in atopics than in nonatopics and even though the frequency of hand eczema in atopics does not seem to be higher in sensitized than in nonsensitized atopics, jobs in which potent allergens are present can sometimes be risk occupations for atopics. The traumatized skin barrier in atopics with an already existing atopic hand eczema may in some cases be a prerequisite for the development of a contact sensitivity, which may aggravate the dermatitis and cause occupational hindrance.

REFERENCES

1. Rystedt, I., Hand eczema and long-term prognosis in atopic dermatitis, *Acta Derm. Venereol.*, 117, 1, 1985.
2. Rystedt, I., Prognostic factors in atopic dermatitis, *Acta Derm. Venereol.*, 65, 206, 1985.
3. Rystedt, I., Hand eczema in patients with history of atopic manifestations in childhood, *Acta Derm. Venereol.*, 65, 305, 1985.
4. Rystedt, I., Work-related hand eczema in atopics, *Contact Dermatitis*, 12, 164, 1985.
5. Rystedt, I., Contact sensitivity in adults with atopic dermatitis in childhood, *Contact Dermatitis*, 13, 1, 1985.
6. Rystedt, I., Factors influencing the occurrence of hand eczema in adults with a history of atopic dermatitis in childhood, *Contact Dermatitis*, 12, 185, 1985.
7. Rystedt, I., Atopic background in patients with occupational hand eczema, *Contact Dermatitis*, 12, 247, 1985.
8. Hill, L. W. and Sulzberger, M. B., Evolution of atopic dermatitis, *Acta Dermatol. Syphilol.*, 32, 451, 1935.
9. Norrlind, R. and Prurigo, B., Atopic dermatitis: a clinical-experimental study of its pathogenesis with special reference to acute infections of the respiratory tract, *Acta Derm. Venereol.*, 13 (Suppl.), 1, 1946.
10. Rajka, G., *Atopic Dermatitis*, W. B. Saunders, Philadelphia, 1975.
11. Hecht, R., Infantile eczema, *J. Allergy*, 11, 195, 1940.
12. Grosfeld, I. C. M., Voorhorst, R., de Vries, J., and Kuiper, I. P., A study of the relation of some allergological factors with some clinical aspects of atopic dermatitis, Fifth European Congress of Allergy, Basel, 1982, 386.
13. Hanifin, J. M. and Rajka, G., Diagnostic features of atopic dermatitis, *Acta Derm. Venereol.*, 92 (Suppl.), 44, 1980.
14. Taylor, B., Wadsworth, J., Wadsworth, M., and Peckham, C., Changes in the reported prevalence of childhood eczema since the 1939-45 war, *Lancet*, 2, 1255, 1984.
15. Schultz Larsen, F., Holm, N. V., and Henningsen, K., Atopic dermatitis. A genetic-epidemiologic study in a population-based twin sample, *J. Am. Acad. Dermatol.*, 15, 487, 1986.
16. Haahtela, T. M. K., The prevalence of allergic conditions and immediate skin test reactions among Finnish adolescents, *Clin. Allergy*, 9, 53, 1979.
17. Haahtela, T., Heiskala, M., and Suoniemi, I., Allergic disorders and immediate skin test reactivity in Finnish adolescents, *Allergy*, 35, 433, 1980.
18. Åberg, N., Engström, I., and Lindberg, U., Allergic diseases in Swedish school children. *Acta Paediatr. Scand.*, 78, 246, 1989.

19. Meding, B. and Swanbeck, G., Predictive factors for hand eczema, *Contact Dermatitis*, 23, 154, 1990.
20. Berlinghoff, W., Die Prognose des Säulingsekzems, *Dtsch. Gesundheitswes.*, 16, 110, 1961.
21. Burrows, D. and Penman, R. W. B., Prognosis of the eczema-asthma syndrome, *Br. Med. J.*, 2, 825, 1960.
22. Roth, H. L. and Kierland, R. R., The natural history of atopic dermatitis, *Arch. Dermatol.*, 89, 209, 1964.
23. Musgrove, K. and Morgan, J. K., Infantile eczema. A long-term follow-up study, *Br. J. Dermatol.*, 95, 365, 1976.
24. van Hecke, E. and Leys, G., Evolusion of atopic dermatitis, *Dermatologica*, 163, 370, 1981.
25. Vickers, C. F. H., The natural history of atopic eczema, *Acta Derm. Venereol.*, 92 (Suppl.), 113, 1980.
26. Breit, R., Leutgeb, C., and Bandman, H.-J., Zum neurodermitischen Handekzem, *Arch. Dermatol. Forsch.*, 244, 353, 1972.
27. Bandmann, H.-J., and Agathos, M., Die atopische Handdermatitis, *Dermatosen*, 28, 110, 1980.
28. Cronin, E., Bandmann, H.-J., Calnan, C. D., Fregert, S., Hjorth, N., Magnusson, B., Maibach, H. I., Malten, K., Meneghini, C. L., Pirilä, V., and Wilkinson, D. S., Contact dermatitis in the atopic, *Acta Derm. Venereol.*, 50, 183, 1970.
29. Lammintausta, K. and Kalimo, K., Atopy and hand dermatitis in hospital wet work, *Contact Dermatitis*, 7, 301, 1981.
30. Forsbeck, M., Skog, E., and Åsbrink, E., Atopic hand dermatitis: comparison with atopic dermatitis without hand involvement especially with respect to influence of work and development of contact sensitization, *Acta Derm. Venereol.*, 63, 9, 1983.
31. Shmunes, E. and Keil, J. E., The role of atopy in occupational dermatoses, *Contact Dermatitis*, 11, 174, 1984.
32. Nilsson, E., Mikaelsson, B., and Andersson, S., Atopy, occupation and domestic work as risk factors for hand eczema in hospital workers, *Contact Dermatitis*, 13, 216, 1985.
33. Cronin, E., Clinical patterns of hand eczema in women, *Contact Dermatitis*, 13, 153, 1985.
34. Epstein, E., Hand dermatitis: practical management and current concepts, *J. Am. Acad. Dermatol.*, 10, 395, 1984.
35. Wilkinson, D. S., Contact dermatitis of the hands, *Trans. St. Johns Hosp. Dermatol. Soc.*, 58, 163, 1971.
36. Fregert, S., Occupational dermatitis in a 10-year material, *Contact Dermatitis*, 1, 96, 1975.
37. Werner, Y. and Lindberg, M., Transepidermal water loss in dry and clinically normal skin in patients with atopic dermatitis, *Acta Derm. Venereol.*, 65, 182, 1985.
38. Werner, Y., The water content of the stratum corneum in patients with atopic dermatitis, *Acta Derm. Venereol.*, 66, 281, 1986.
39. Blaylock, W. K., Atopic dermatitis: diagnosis and pathobiology, *J. Allergy Clin. Immunol.*, 57, 62, 1976.
40. Hanifin, J. M. and Lobitz, W. C., Newer concepts of atopic dermatitis, *Arch. Dermatol.*, 113, 663, 1977.
41. Hjorth, N. and Fregert, S., Contact dermatitis, in *Textbook of Dermatology*, 3rd ed., Rook, R., Wilkinson, D. S. and Ebling, F. S. G., Eds., Blackwell Scientific, Oxford, 1979.
42. Hanifin, J. M., Atopic dermatitis, *J. Allergy Clin. Immunol.*, 73, 211, 1984.
43. Frosch, P. J. and Kligman, M. M., The soap chamber test: a new method for assessing irritancy of soaps, *J. Am. Acad. Dermatol.*, 1, 35, 1979.
44. Bandman, H.-J., Breit, R., and Leutgeb, C., Kontaktallergie und Dermatitis atopica, *Arch. Invest. Dermatol.*, 244, 332, 1972.
45. Lammintausta, K., Kalimo, K., and Havu, V. K., Contact allergy in atopics, who perform wet work in hospital, *Dermatosen*, 30, 184, 1982.
46. Cronin, E. and Kullavanijaya, P., Hand dermatitis in hairdressers, *Acta Derm. Venereol.*, 59, (Suppl. 85), 47, 1979.

47. Hjort, N. and Roed-Petersen, J., Occupational protein contact dermatitis in food handlers, *Contact Dermatitis,* 2, 28, 1976.
48. Meding, B., Epidemiology of hand eczema in an industrial city, *Acta Derm. Venereol.,* 153 (Suppl.), 1, 1990.
49. Kavli, G. and Förde, O. H., Hand dermatoses in Tromsö, *Contact Dermatitis,* 10, 174, 1984.
50. Coenraads, P. J., Nater, J. P., and van der Lende, R., Prevalence of eczema and other dermatoses of the hands and arms in the Netherlands. Association with age and occupation, *Clin. Exp. Dermatol.,* 8, 495, 1983.
51. Lantinga, H., Nater, J. P., and Coenraades, P. J., Prevalence, incidence and course of eczema on the hands and fore-arms in a sample of the general population, *Contact Dermatitis,* 10, 135, 1984.
52. Mathias, C. G. T. and Maibach, H. I., Dermatoxicology monographs. I. Cutaneous irritation: factors influencing the response to irritants, *Clin. Toxicol.,* 13, 333, 1978.
53. Rajka, G., Katamnestische untersuchungen Beruflicher chemishallergische Kontaktekzeme, *Acta Allergol.,* 136, 236, 1966.
54. Neumann, Y. B., Rehabilitation problems in occupational skin diseases, *Proc. Intern. Congr. Occup. Health,* 7, 1966.

14

Individual and Environmental Risk Factors for Hand Eczema in Hospital Workers

Eskil Nilsson

CONTENTS

I. INTRODUCTION

Hand eczema is a multifactorial disease. Individual and environmental factors interact in a complex manner in this common disorder. The knowledge of the relative importance of various endogenous and exogenous factors is very limited. Extending this knowledge is important to understand the nature of hand eczema. This chapter is a summary of a study on hospital workers entitled, "Individual and environmental risk factors for hand eczema in hospital workers".[1] The study consists of three parts: (1) epidemiological, designed to investigate the relative importance of some individual and environmental factors in the etiology of current hand eczema in newly employed hospital workers;[2,3] (2) clinical, consisting of patients from the total cohort who consulted a dermatologist because of current hand eczema;[4] these patients being studied especially with regards to the importance of irritants, allergens, and contact urticants in the etiology of the current hand eczema; and (3) bacteriological, in which the microflora in hand eczema and the effects of a potent topical steroid on the microflora were studied.[5]

II. MATERIALS AND METHODS

A. Epidemiological Study

This part of the investigation was performed as a prospective cohort study, which makes it possible to quantitate and compare the relative importance of various factors. The study design is illustrated schematically in Figure 1. A history of atopy was taken at the preemployment examination. If the employee had a history of both atopic dermatitis (AD) and atopic mucosal symptoms (AMS), he/she was classified as AD. A history of metal dermatitis (HMD) and a history of hand eczema (HHE) were derived from a questionnaire as were information on occupational and domestic exposure. The following six domestic parameters were recorded: (1) the nursing of children younger than 4 years of age; (2) members of the household; (3) hours of housekeeping per week; (4) hours per week spent working with hands on a hobby; (5) use of washing machine; and (6) use of dishwasher. The occurrence of hand eczema during follow-up was identified by questionnaire. The employee was asked to characterize the hand eczema with one or more of the following five alternatives: (1) dry and chapped skin with rashes and small cracks; (2) itching red macular and papular skin lesion; (3) small vesicles; (4) ruptured vesicles or excoriated skin; and (5) rough skin with cracks and scaling. The consequence of the hand eczema with regard to medical consultation, sick leave, and change of work due to current hand eczema were recorded.

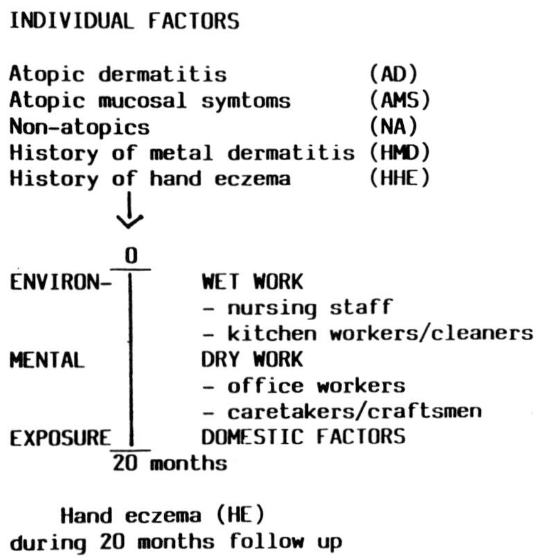

```
INDIVIDUAL FACTORS

Atopic dermatitis           (AD)
Atopic mucosal symtoms      (AMS)
Non-atopics                 (NA)
History of metal dermatitis (HMD)
History of hand eczema      (HHE)
                 ↓
               0
ENVIRON-          WET WORK
                  - nursing staff
                  - kitchen workers/cleaners
MENTAL            DRY WORK
                  - office workers
                  - caretakers/craftsmen
EXPOSURE          DOMESTIC FACTORS
              20 months

     Hand eczema (HE)
during 20 months follow up
```

FIGURE 1. Schematic illustration of the study design.

TABLE 1 Number of Employees, Sex, and Median Age in the Occupational Groups

	Number	Female (%)	Median age
Nursing staff	1613	87.7	25.0
Kitchen workers/cleaners	457	93.4	23.0
Office workers	269	91.8	22.5
Caretakers/craftsmen	113	16.8	29.0

From Nilsson, E., Mikaelsson, B., and Andersson, S., *Contact Dermatitis*, 13, 217, 1985. With permission.

The studied cohort consisted of 2651 newly employed hospital workers. The follow-up questionnaire was received from 2452 (92.5%) employees after a median observation time of 20 months. Table 1 shows the number, sex, and median age in the four occupational groups.

B. Statistics

The risk of developing hand eczema during follow-up was calculated as predicted relative odds ratios (OR) using a multivariate logistic regression technique.[2] The risk in percentage of developing hand eczema is expressed as predicted probability (PP). Student's *t* test was used to compare relative frequencies. The geometric means of groups of bacteria were compared with paired *t* tests. A significance level of 5% was chosen.

Three multivariate regression analyses of the relative importance of individual and environmental risk factors for hand eczema will be presented. The following factors were studied in the three analyses: first analysis: AD, AMS, nonatopic (NA) and occupation; second analysis: AD, AMS, NA, domestic factors, and the three occupations dominated by women; and third analysis: AD, AMS, NA, HMD, and HHE in women in wet hospital work.

C. Clinical Study

In this study 142 patients with current hand eczema were investigated, 91% of whom were women. These patients were questioned about factors they thought elicited the current hand eczema. The state of the current hand eczema and diagnosis of ongoing eczema at sites other than the hands were noted. A total of 120 of 142 patients were patch tested with a modified European standard series and 55 of 120 were tested with an additional hospital series. This series consisted of disinfectants, preservatives, emollients, perfumes, and colorings present in products in common use in the hospitals. Prick tests were performed on 41 of 49 patients with a history of immediate reactions. As a supplement to substances suspected from case histories, the same patients were tested with a hospital screening series.

D. Bacteriological Study

In 20 patients with hand eczema the density of the microflora was studied with a modification of the Williamson and Kligman scrub technique. Before treatment, samples were taken from three sites: (1) the most pronounced eczematous lesions; (2) skin affected only with erythema, and (3) clinically normal skin of the hands. The patients were treated with a potent topical corticosteroid, clobetasol propionate 0.05% cream (Dermovat®, Glaxo) in an intermittent schedule for 14 days. After treatment, new samples for a bacteriological culture were taken from the same sites as before treatment.

III. RESULTS

A. Prevalence of Individual Risk Factors

The following values for atopy were found in the total cohort: AD 10.2% (including 4.1% with AMS), pure AMS 12.4%, and NA 77.4%. In 1857 women employed in wet hospital work (nursing

TABLE 2   Hand Eczema and Its Consequences in Occupational Groups

	Hand eczema (%)	Medical consultation (%)	Sick leave (%)	Changed work (%)
Nursing staff	41	9.8	1.9	2.0
Kitchen workers/cleaners	37	14.0	3.6	2.4
Office workers	25	7.6	1.5	0.4
Caretakers/craftsmen	17	7.3	0	0

From Nilsson, E., Mikaelsson, B., and Andersson, S., *Contact Dermatitis*, 13, 218, 1985. With permission.

staff, kitchen workers, and cleaners) HHE was reported by 22.4%. The values for HHE in atopics and nonatopics were AD 48%, AMS 24%, NA 18%. The value for HMD was 26.3%. HMD was more common in atopics: AD 36.5% ($p < 0.01$) and AMS 31.4% ($p < 0.05$) compared with NA 24.1%. HMD was more common in subjects with HHE (atopics 46.9%, nonatopics 40.0%) than in subjects without HHE (atopics 26.7%, nonatopics 20.5%) ($p < 0.01$).

B.   Frequency of Current Hand Eczema

Before presenting the predicted relative risk of hand eczema, the frequency of current hand eczema for the various individual and environmental factors will be given. The predicted relative risk of developing hand eczema was calculated by the multivariate logistic regression technique applied on these absolute frequency values.

Table 2 shows the frequency of hand eczema, medical consultation, sick leave, and change of work due to current hand eczema in the four occupations during follow-up.

Table 3 shows the occurrence of hand eczema, medical consultation, sick leave, and change of work due to current hand eczema in atopics and nonatopics in the four occupations. During follow-up hand eczema was more common in subjects with atopic dermatitis than in subjects with atopic mucosal symptoms and nonatopics. The difference between atopics and nonatopics increased in the more severe forms of hand eczema (medical consultation, sick leave, and change of work). Sick leave was uncommon in most occupations. From subjects on sick leave, 75% had been absent from work less than 1 month. Most employees with hand eczema do not consult a doctor. The

TABLE 3   Hand Eczema and Its Consequences in Atopics and Nonatopics in Occupational Groups

	Hand eczema (%)	Medical consultation (%)	Sick leave (%)	Changed work (%)
Atopic dermatitis with or without atopic mucosal symptoms				
Nursing staff	61	31.0	7.3	5.5
Kitchen workers/cleaners	63	35.0	8.2	11.0
Office workers	45	31.0	3.4	0
Caretakers/craftsmen	20	20.0	0	0
Atopic mucosal symptoms				
Nursing staff	46	14.0	1.5	2.0
Kitchen workers/cleaners	35	13.0	1.9	3.7
Office workers	25	3.1	0	3.1
Caretakers/craftsmen	11	5.3	0	0
Nonatopics				
Nursing staff	37	6.2	1.3	1.5
Kitchen workers/cleaners	33	11.0	3.2	1.2
Office workers	22	4.9	1.5	0
Caretakers/craftsman	19	7.0	0	0

From Nilsson, E., Mikaelsson, B., and Andersson, S., *Contact Dermatitis*, 13, 219, 1985. With permission.

following reasons for not consulting a doctor were given by 677 employees: the hand eczema was mild (69.0%), the employee treated himself with various topical formulations (43.9%), the eczema healed fast spontaneously (36.5%), and other reasons (17.4%).

Table 4 provides data for hand eczema, medical consultations, sick leave, and change of work due to hand eczema in women in wet hospital work with AD, AMS, NA, HMD, and HHE.

C. Predicted Risk of Current Hand Eczema

Predicted relative ORs and PPs for hand eczema in atopics and nonatopics in the four occupations are presented in Table 5. The relative OR for subjects with atopic dermatitis was 2.8 times higher than nonatopics in both wet and dry work. Nursing staff showed ORs approximately three times higher than caretakers/craftsmen and twice as high as office workers. Figure 2 shows a schematic description of the predicted relative ORs presented in Table 5.

In the second analysis the interplay among atopy, occupation, and the domestic factors was studied. In this analysis the following factors significantly increased the risk of developing hand eczema during follow-up: atopic dermatitis ($p < 0.001$), occupation ($p < 0.001$), children younger than 4 years old ($p < 0.001$), and lack of a dishwasher ($p < 0.05$). From the population in this analysis 16.4% had children younger than 4 years old and 70.4% had no dishwasher.

Table 6 shows the predicted ORs and the PPs for hand eczema. Values for atopics, nonatopics, and three occupations dominated by women, and the most favorable and unfavorable combinations of the two significant domestic factors are given. Figure 3 shows a schematic description of the OR data in Table 6.

As shown in Table 6 and Figure 3, the relative ORs for hand eczema in an occupation are twice as high for subjects with an unfavorable combination of the two significant domestic factors (children younger than 4 years and no dishwasher) than for subjects with a favorable combination of the two factors. Office workers nursing children younger than 4 years and having no dishwasher showed as great a risk of developing hand eczema as wet workers without children younger than 4 years and having a dishwasher. Wet work in combination with the two significant domestic factors increased the odds by 4 times compared with dry work and a favorable combination of the two significant domestic factors (no children younger than 4 years and having a dishwasher).

The third analysis was performed on women in wet hospital work (nursing staff, kitchen workers, and cleaners). Atopy, HMD, and HHE were analyzed as risk factors for current hand eczema and its consequences regarding medical consultation, sick leave, and change of work. Table 7 shows the results of this analysis. Data for medical consultation, sick leave and change of work are given as a percentage of the PP of hand eczema in the various groups. In this analysis HHE increased the predicted relative OR by 12.9 times and created a subdivision of the population into two groups, which differ considerably regarding the risk of developing hand eczema during follow-up. HMD further increased the odds by 1.8 times and atopy (AD, AMS) by another 1.3 times.

The PP of hand eczema in this analysis ranged from 24% in subjects with no HHE, no HMD, and no atopy to 91% in subjects with HHE, HMD, and atopy. Figure 4 shows a schematic description of the predicted relative ORs presented in Table 7. Figure 5 shows the frequency of previous hand eczema, metal dermatitis, and atopy in the total cohort of women in wet hospital work. By comparing Figure 5 with Table 7 and Figure 4, it is possible to get information about how great a part of the total cohort belongs to the various groups in this analysis.

D. Severity of Current Hand Eczema

From the results presented in Table 7, it is clear that subjects with a history of atopic dermatitis get a more severe eczema. Thus, subjects with AD show higher values for medical consultation ($p < 0.01$), sick leave ($p < 0.01$), and change of work ($p < 0.01$). Table 8 shows additional evidence for a more severe hand eczema in subjects with a history of atopic dermatitis. Thus, vesicular lesions, permanent symptoms, and early debut were more common in subjects with AD. A mild eczema noted only as ''dry and chapped skin with rashes and small cracks'' was more common in subjects with AMS and NA.

TABLE 4 Current Hand Eczema and its Consequences in 1857 Women in Wet Hospital Work

Hand eczema (20 months)	Total	AD[a]	AMS[b]	NA[c]	HMD[d]	No HMD	HHE[e]	No HHE
Number	1857	194	227	1436	487	1342	410	1423
Current hand eczema (%)								
By questionnaire	41.0	61.0	45.0	37.0	56.0	35.0	84.0	28.0
Medical consultations	11.0	31.0	15.0	7.6	17.0	8.8	28.0	6.1
Sick leave	2.4	7.3	1.8	1.9	5.3	1.4	4.3	1.8
Changed work	2.2	6.7	3.1	1.5	3.9	1.6	5.1	1.4

[a] Atopic dermatitis with or without atopic mucosal symptoms.
[b] Atopic mucosal symptoms.
[c] Nonatopics.
[d] History of metal dermatitis.
[e] History of hand eczema.

From Nilsson, E. and Bäck, O., *Acta Derm. Venereol.*, 66, 46, 1986. With permission.

TABLE 5   Predicted Relative Odds Ratios (OR) and Predicted Probability (PP) for Hand Eczema in the Occupational Groups

	NA[a]		AMS[b]		AD[c]	
	OR	PP (%)	OR	PP (%)	OR	PP (%)
Nursing staff	3.2	37	4.1	44	8.8	62
Kitchen workers/cleaners	2.7	33	3.5	39	7.5	58
Office workers	1.5	22	2.0	27	4.2	44
Caretakers/craftsmen	1.0	16	1.3	20	2.8	34

[a]   Nonatopics.
[b]   Atopic mucosal symptoms.
[c]   Atopic dermatitis with or without atopic mucosal symptoms.

E.   Clinical Study

In the patients investigated because of current hand eczema risk individuals were overrepresented. The following values were found: HHE 67%, HMD 41%, atopy 58% (AD ± AMS 46%, pure AMS 12%). Corresponding values for the total cohort were HHE 22%, HMD 26%, and atopy 23%. From 65 patients with current hand eczema and a history of AD, 23 (35%) had ongoing atopic eczema on other locations. From the clinically investigated patients, 131 of 142 (92.3%) considered that the current hand eczema was elicited by external contacts. It was stated that the following agents had provoked the hand eczema in these 131 patients.

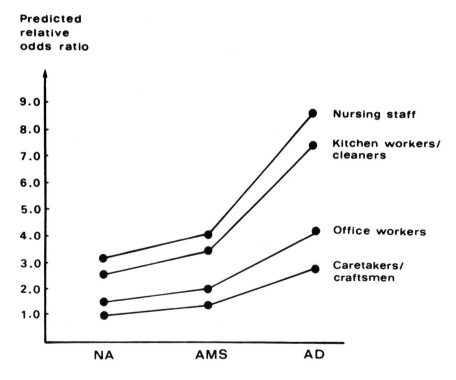

FIGURE 2.   Predicted relative odds ratios for hand eczema in atopics and nonatopics in the occupational groups. NA = nonatopics; AMS = atopic mucosal symptoms; AD = atopic dermatitis with or without atopic mucosal symptoms. (From Nilsson, E., Mikaelsson, B., and Andersson, S., *Contact Dermatitis,* 13, 220, 1985. With permission.)

TABLE 6 Predicted Odds Ratios (OR) and Predicted Probability (PP) for Hand Eczema in Atopics and Nonatopics with the Most Favorable and Unfavorable Combinations of Significant Domestic Factors

	Children <4 yr	Dishwasher	NA[a]		AMS[b]		AD[c]	
			OR	PP (%)	OR	PP (%)	OR	PP (%)
Nursing staff	Yes	No	4.1	48	5.5	55	11.4	72
Kitchen/cleaning	Yes	No	3.5	44	4.6	50	9.5	68
Nursing staff	No	Yes	2.1	32	2.7	38	5.6	56
Office workers	Yes	No	2.0	31	2.6	37	5.5	55
Kitchen/cleaning	No	Yes	1.7	28	2.3	34	4.7	51
Office workers	No	Yes	1.0	18	1.3	23	2.7	38

[a] Nonatopics.
[b] Atopic mucosal symptoms.
[c] Atopic dermatitis with or without mucosal symptoms.

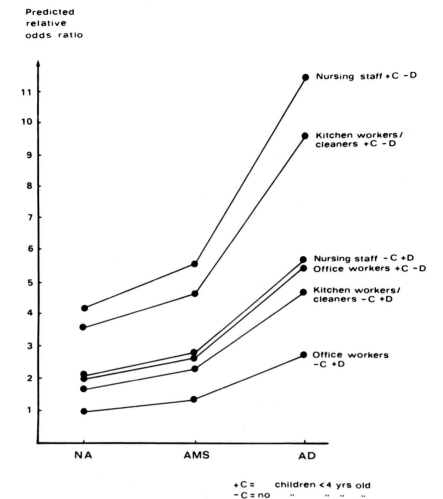

Predicted
relative
odds ratio

FIGURE 3. Predicted relative odds ratios for hand eczema in atopics with the most favorable and unfavorable combinations of domestic work. NA = nonatopics; AMS = atopic mucosal symptoms; AD = atopic dermatitis with or without atopic mucosal symptoms. (From Nilsson, E., Mikaelsson, B., and Andersson, S., *Contact Dermatitis,* 13, 220, 1985. With permission.)

Agents	Number of patients
Water and cleaning agents	111
Disinfectants	26
Physical factors	24
Various foods	23
Rubber gloves	17
Oils, solvents	11
Paper towels	9
Dirt and dust	8

From *Occupational Hazards in the Health Professions,* Brune, D. K. and Edling, C., Eds., CRC Press, Boca Raton, FL, 1989. With permission.

TABLE 7   Predicted Relative Odds Ratios (OR) and Predicted Probability (PP) for Hand Eczema and its Consequences in Women in Wet Work

			Hand eczema		Medical consultation PP[a]	Sick leave PP[a] (%)	Changed work PP[a] (%)
			OR	PP (%)			
	HHE[b]	HMD[c]	AD[d]	31	91	57	14.0	14.0
	HHE	HMD	AMS[e]	31	91	42	5.6	9.1
	HHE	HMD	NA[f]	23.1	88	28	5.6	5.5
	HHE	No HMD	AD	17.3	84	53	6.6	10.0
	HHE	No HMD	AMS	17.3	84	37	2.6	6.5
	HHE	No HMD	NA	12.9	80	25	2.6	3.9
No	HHE	HMD	AD	2.4	43	48	22.0	14.0
No	HHE	HMD	AMS	2.4	43	34	9.5	9.1
No	HHE	HMD	NA	1.8	36	22	9.5	5.5
No	HHE	No HMD	AD	1.3	30	44	11.0	10.0
No	HHE	No HMD	AMS	1.3	30	30	4.3	6.5
No	HHE	No HMD	NA	1.0	24	19	4.3	3.9

Note: Medical consultation: AD $p < 0.001$, HHE $p < 0.01$; sick leave: AD $p < 0.01$, HMD $p < 0.05$; changed work: AD $p < 0.01$.

[a]   Values are expressed as percentage of PP for hand eczema.
[b]   History of hand eczema.
[c]   History of metal dermatitis.
[d]   Atopic dermatitis with or without atopic mucosal symptoms.
[e]   Atopic mucosal symptoms.
[f]   Nonatopics.

From *Occupational Hazards in the Health Professions,* Brune, D K., and Edling, C., Eds., CRC Press, Boca Raton, FL, 1989, 284. With permission.

Contact with eliciting factors was considered to take place mostly at work by 57.2%, equally at work and at home by 21%, and mostly at home or in leisure time by 13.8% of the patients. Contact allergy was found in 45 of the 120 patients tested. The allergens are listed in Table 9. It is noteworthy that no positive test was found to the substances in the hospital epicutaneous series. Many patients suspected that they had contact allergy prior to patch testing and they had tried to avoid the allergens. Although minor exposure of the hands to different allergens was common, few patients thought that contact allergy played any significant role as a cause of the current episode of hand eczema. In only 2 of 10 patients allergic to rubber chemicals was there a clear correlation between occupational exposure to rubber gloves and the current hand eczema. Of 51 patients with a history of metal dermatitis, a positive patch test to nickel and/or cobalt was obtained in only 37.3%. The corresponding value for atopics was 36.4% and for nonatopics 38.9%. In subjects with no history of metal dermatitis in a positive test to nickel and/or cobalt was found in 11.4% of the atopics and 5.9% of the nonatopics.

A history suspect for contact urticaria was reported by 49 of the 142 patients (34.5%) and was more common after exposure to substances in the home. Various kinds of food, cleaning agents, and animals were more commonly considered to provoke contact urticaria at home and in leisure time.

Cleaning agents, vegetables, and rubber gloves were most commonly reported to elicit contact urticaria at work. One or more positive prick test reactions were seen in 32 of 41 patients tested. The total number of positives were 68, and 32 of 68 were considered relevant for contact urticaria on normal or dermatitic skin. In 24 atopics 46 positive prick tests were seen and in 17 nonatopics 22 were positive. Although the value in the atopics was higher, the difference is not significant. Most patients with contact urticaria were aware of it before testing and, if possible, they avoided the substances. In a small number of patients, predominantly those reacting to rubber and disinfectants, urticarial reactions caused real problems because of the difficulty of avoidance. In two patients prick tests were positive to both benzalconium chloride and the emollient Helosan which contains it.

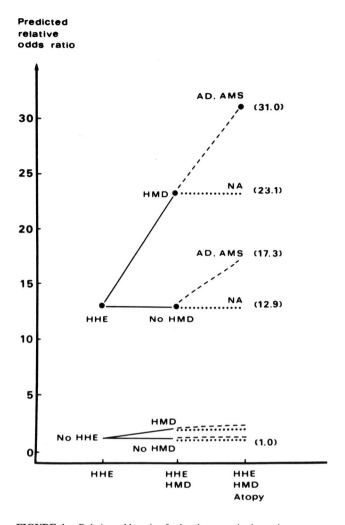

FIGURE 4.   Relative odds ratios for hand eczema in the various groups during 20 months of wet hospital work. HHE = history of hand eczema; AD = atopic dermatitis with or without atopic mucosal symptoms; AMS = atopic mucosal symptoms; NA = nonatopics; HMD = history of metal dermatitis. (From Nilsson, E. and Bäck, O., *Acta Derm. Venereol.*, 66, 47, 1986. With permission.)

F.   Bacteriological Study

The incidence of *Staphylococcus aureus* in eczema was 18 of 20, in erythema 13 of 16, and in normal skin 8 of 20. Treatment with clobetasol propionate reduced the incidence of *S. aureus* in the three sampling sites to 6 of 20, 4 of 16, and 2 of 20, respectively. Before treatment the mean density of *S. aureus* in eczema was 56,000 colony-forming units (cfu)/cm², in erythema 2,600 cfu/cm², and in normal skin 45 cfu/cm².

The mean counts of *S. aureus* in the three sampling sites differ significantly ($p < 0.01$). Treatment reduced the counts of *S. aureus* significantly: in earlier eczema to 22 cfu/cm² ($p < 0.001$), in previous erythema to 21 cfu/cm² ($p < 0.001$), and in normal skin to 13 cfu/cm² ($p < 0.05$). Before treatment *S. aureus* was found in densities exceeding 10^5 cfu/cm² in the eczematous lesions of 15 patients. Only one patient had more than 10^6 cfu/cm². The two patients who did not carry *S. aureus* in their eczematous lesions were nonatopics. The mean counts for *S. aureus* did not differ significantly between atopics and nonatopics. The density of other aerobes and anaerobes

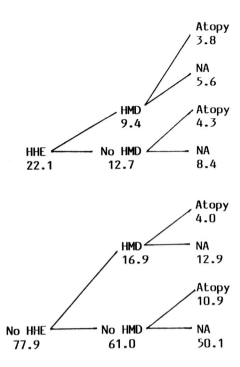

FIGURE 5. Frequency of HHE, HMD, and atopy in the total cohort of women in wet hospital work. Values are the percent in the total cohort. HHE = history of hand eczema; HMD = history of metal dermatitis; NA = nonatopics.

did not differ significantly in the three sampling sites before treatment. No significant reduction was seen in these bacterial groups after treatment. At follow-up after 14 days of intermittent treatment, the eczema was healed in 18 of 20 patients, and in 2 of 20 the eczema was much improved.

IV. COMMENTS

A. Individual Factors

A history of atopic dermatitis increased the odds of developing hand eczema only 2.8 times. As many as 40% of the women with a history of atopic dermatitis managed to work in wet work without hand eczema during the observation time. Thus, information about previous atopic dermatitis was of limited value as a predictor of hand eczema.

A history of hand eczema increased the odds of getting hand eczema during the observation time by 12.9 times. This increase is great and creates a subdivision of atopics and nonatopics in high-risk individuals and normal-risk individuals. Approximately one half of the subjects with atopic dermatitis, one fourth of the subjects with atopic mucosal symptoms, and one fifth of the nonatopics belong to the high-risk group. Thus, there are two subgroups among atopics and nonatopics that differ considerably with regard to the risk of developing hand eczema. A possible explanation for the great importance of earlier hand eczema is that the hands of most adult women have been exposed to some degree of irritant domestic or occupational work. This exposition, the usage irritancy test of womens hands, has caused hand eczema in some individuals. A history of hand eczema may be considered a positive usage irritancy test and indicate a skin vulnerability factor, a skin barrier with lowered resistance to irritants, which predispose to irritant hand dermatitis. This defective barrier may occur in atopics and nonatopics, in nonatopics probably especially in individuals with a family history of atopy. The vulnerability factor predisposing to irritant hand

TABLE 8   Severity of Hand Eczema

	AD[a]	AMS[b]	NA[c]
Number of employees with hand eczema	145	119	634
Vesicular lesions (%)	44	22[d]	22[e]
Permanent symptoms (%)	20	10[f]	6.1[e]
Onset of hand eczema within the first 4 months of occupation (%)	76	59[d]	54[e]
"Dry and chapped skin with rashes and small cracks" as the only symptoms of hand eczema (%)	24	43[d]	46[d]

[a]   Atopic dermatitis with or without atopic mucosal symptoms.
[b]   Atopic mucosal symptoms.
[c]   Nonatopics.
[d] $p < 0.01$ versus AD.
[e] $p < 0.001$ versus AD.
[f] $p < 0.05$ versus AD.

From Nilsson, E., Mikaelsson, B., and Andersson, S., *Contact Dermatitis*, 13, 219, 1985. With permission.

eczema is probably due to a defect in the skin barrier, which may be clinically manifested as various features of atopic skin, which is sometimes named atopic skin diathesis (ASD). ASD, as defined by Lammintausta and Kalimo,[6] was shown to increase the risk of hand eczema considerably in subjects with atopic mucosal symptoms and nonatopics.

Various signs of atopic skin (wool intolerance, xerosis, white dermografism, itch when sweating, keratosis pilaris, hyperlinear palms, perlèche) were predictors for hand eczema of various importance according to results reported by Diepgen and Fartasch.[7]

Although a history of atopic dermatitis as a single factor was of limited value as a predictor for hand eczema, it is important to observe that individuals with a history of atopic dermatitis will suffer from a more severe hand eczema. The reason for this may be that the current hand eczema in these patients has developed as a combination of "pure" atopic dermatitis located on the hands

TABLE 9   Positive Patch-Test Reactions in 120 Patients

Nickel	18.2
Cobalt	7.4
Balsam of Peru	5.8
Carba mix	4.1
Formaldehyde	4.1
Benzalkonium chloride	4.1
PPD mix	3.3
Wood tars	3.3
Thiuram mix	2.5
Caine mix	1.8[a]
Fragrance mix	1.8[a]
Colophony	1.7
Chromium	1.7
p-Phenylenediamine	0.8

Note: Values are percentages.

[a]   N = 55 patients.
From Nilsson, E., *Contact Dermatitis*, 13, 323, 1985. With permission.

and the vulnerable effect of irritants. This suggestion is supported by the finding that from the clinically investigated patients with a history of atopic dermatitis and current hand eczema, 35% had ongoing atopic dermatitis on locations other than the hands.

A history of metal dermatitis increased the odds of developing hand eczema by a factor of 1.8. This increase was seen on a high-risk level in patients with a history of hand eczema and on a normal-risk level in others. Metal dermatitis may develop as a cause of contact allergy and certainly even through irritant effects of metals, especially in subjects with vulnerable skin.

Thus, it was found in this study that a history of metal dermatitis was more common in subjects with previous hand eczema. From clinically investigated patients dominated by risk individuals with vulnerable skin, less than 40% with a history of metal dermatitis had a positive patch test to nickel and/or cobalt. Similar findings were made in a later study by Möller and Svensson in which they stated that metal sensitivity with a negative test indicates atopy.[8] Regarding the importance of individual factors, it is noteworthy that simple anamnestic information about earlier hand eczema, metal dermatitis, and atopic disease gives valuable prognostic information about the risk of developing hand eczema and its consequences in women in wet hospital work.

B. Environmental Factors

In the epidemiological part of this study, it was found that if you compare the various occupations without considering individual factors, wet work only doubled the odds of developing hand eczema compared with dry office work. This difference between what is considered a high-risk and a low-risk occupation is unexpectedly small, and individual factors are obviously much more important than occupational exposure. However, in the clinically investigated patients, which were dominated by risk individuals with vulnerable skin, trivial irritants were considered important causes of the current hand eczema.

Contact allergy and contact urticaria were rather common, but most employees could not correlate the current hand eczema to any obvious exposure to contact allergens or contact urticants. Contact allergens, such as nickel and fragrances, and some contact urticants are, however, common in the environment and some exposure of the hands is inevitable. Therefore, the relevance for positive tests to common allergens may be hard to assess.

C. Colonization of *S. aureus* in Hand Eczema

The frequent colonization of hand eczema by *S. aureus* in high counts is an important observation. Exposure to *S. aureus* may involve a threat to various groups of patients. The reduction of *S. aureus* by successful topical treatment of the eczema with a potent corticosteroid underlines the importance of efficient topical treatment of hand eczema. In a recent study on atopic dermatitis, it was found that the reduction of *S. aureus* increased with the potency of the corticosteroid and *S. aureus* was eliminated after 2 weeks of successful treatment with a potent corticosteroid.[9]

V. CONCLUSIONS

The predicted relative ORs of hand eczema for the individual and environmental factors found in the three analyses are given.

Atopy (analyses 1 and 2)	Increased OR for hand eczema
AD	2.8
AMS	1.3
compared with	
NA	

Occupation (analyses 1 and 2)	Increased OR for hand eczema
Wet work dominated by women compared with Dry work dominated by women	~2.0
Wet work dominated by women compared with Dry work dominated by men	~3.0

Domestic factors in occupations dominated by women (analysis 2)	
Children <4 years, no dishwasher compared with No children <4 years, having dishwasher	~2.0

Atopy, HMD, and HHE in women in wet work (analysis 3)	
HHE	12.9
HMD	1.8
AD, AMS compared with No HHE, no HMD, and NA	1.3

The following semiquantitative importance of risk factors for hand eczema in women in hospital work is suggested based on the findings in this study.

"Pure" atopic dermatitis located on the hands	+ + + + +
Vulnerable skin with lowered resistance to irritants (in atopics and non-atopics)	+ + + +
Wet work (without considering individual factors)	+
Contact allergy	+ ? (0-≫ + + + + +)
Contact urticaria	+ ? (0-≫ + + + + +)

REFERENCES

1. Nilsson, E., Individual and environmental risk factors for hand eczema in hospital workers, *Acta Derm. Venereol.* (Suppl.), 128, 1986.
2. Nilsson, E., Mikaelsson, B., and Andersson, S., Atopy, occupation and domestic work as risk factors for hand eczema in hospital workers, *Contact Dermatitis*, 13, 216, 1985.
3. Nilsson, E. and Bäck, O., The importance of anamnestic information of atopy, metal dermatitis and earlier hand eczema for the development of hand dermatitis in women in wet hospital work, *Acta Derm. Venereol.*, 66, 45, 1986.
4. Nilsson, E., Contact sensitivity and urticaria in "wet" work, *Contact Dermatitis*, 13, 321, 1985.
5. Nilsson, E., Henning, C., and Hjörleifsson, M.-L., Density of the microflora in hand eczema before and after topical treatment with a potent corticosteroid, *J. Am. Acad. Dermatol.*, 15, 192, 1986.

6. Lammintausta, K. and Kalimo, K. Atopy and hand dermatitis in hospital wet work, *Contact Dermatitis,* 7, 301, 1981.

7. Diepgen, T. L. and Fartasch, M., The role of atopic skin diathesis in hand eczema, Free Communication, FC7, Abstracts 155, EADV 2nd Congress Athens, Greece, 1991.

8. Möller, H. and Svensson, Å., Metal sensitivity: positive history but negative test indicates atopy, *Contact Dermatitis,* 14, 57, 1986.

9. Nilsson, E., Henning, C., and Magnusson, J., Topical corticosteroids and *Staphylococcus aureus* in atopic dermatitis, *J. Am. Acad. Dermatol.,* 27, 29, 1992.

15

Prediction of Skin Irritation by Noninvasive Bioengineering Methods

Tove Agner

CONTENTS

I.   INTRODUCTION

Irritant contact dermatitis is a common disease, and was reported to constitute 35% of all hand eczema cases.[1] Prevention is advantageous because severe cases may turn into chronic and disabling disease.[2] It is essential to diminish environmental hazards to the skin, in the home, as well as in the workplace. However, epidemiological[3] and experimental[4] studies indicate that individual-related factors are also important and should be considered for development of irritant contact dermatitis. All subjects exposed to strong acid and alkali develop an irritant reaction, although only some individuals will develop an eczematous reaction when exposed to low-grade irritation, and the skin of other individuals will remain normal. This expresses a physiological difference in skin susceptibility to irritants in healthy subjects.

It has been debated whether a group of individuals with generally sensitive skin actually exists. Due to varying bioavailability and different mechanisms of irritancy, the skin response to one particular irritant does not necessarily predict the response to irritants in general.[5,6] However, Frosch and Wissing were able to identify individuals with sensitive skin by assessment of the susceptibility to seven different irritants and the susceptibility to ultraviolet (UV) light.[7] It was concluded that ''hyperreactors'' exist and can be identified.[8] This conclusion was recently indirectly supported by Tupker et al.[9] who tested 33 healthy volunteers with 11 different detergents and found the same ranking order in almost all subjects.

Identification of high-risk subjects before development of more severe irritant contact dermatitis reactions, followed by information and counseling, may limit or even prevent the development of this disease.

II.   SKIN SUSCEPTIBILITY

The skin susceptibility to irritants depends partly on the environment-related (exogenous) factors and partly on individual-related (endogenous) factors (Figure 1).

A.   Exogenous Factors

Repetitive exposure to a low-grade irritant stimulus is an important external factor that may gradually influence the skin, as classically described by Malten.[10] Skin susceptibility varies with climatic factors. Increased susceptibility has been found during wintertime in Denmark.[11] Low ambient relative humidity is associated with decreased resistance to irritants.[12] Some external factors, such as the use of harsh soaps, may simply be changed whereas other external factors, such as climate, cannot easily be influenced.

B.   Endogenous Factors

Endogenous factors that determine skin susceptibility are inherent and constitutional of nature, but some individual-related risk factors vary over time. Thus, the skin susceptibility for an individual cannot generally be settled once and for all but may change over a lifetime, although some individual risk factors are essentially permanent. A difference in skin resistance to irritants in relation to body region is well documented.[13,14] Changes in skin resistance with age, with increased skin reactivity in childhood,[15] and decreased skin reactivity in older age[16] has been demonstrated. Although irritant contact dermatitis appears more frequently in women than in men,[1] increased skin susceptibility to irritants in women has never been experimentally confirmed.[4,17-19] Recently, variation in skin susceptibility to an irritant stimulus with menstrual cycle was demonstrated.[20] The significance of a history of atopic dermatitis for development of irritant skin reactions has been thoroughly demonstrated.[1,3,21-24] It is a clinically and scientifically supported observation that an active eczema somewhere on the body leads to a generally increased skin susceptibility to irritants.[5,25]

Lately biophysical properties of the skin also have been demonstrated to be of importance for the development of an irritant skin response. For the investigation of these properties a number of noninvasive measuring methods have been used. When the skin is exposed to an irritant stimulus, the skin response is initially determined by the skin barrier function and the current inflammatory

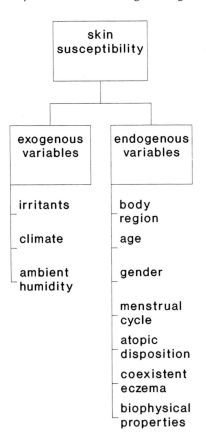

FIGURE 1. Skin susceptibility depends on exogenous (environment-related) and endogenous (individual-related) variables, all of which interact with each other.

reactivity of the skin. The noninvasive measuring methods reviewed herein reflect these parameters by examination of the biophysical properties of the skin.

III. TRANSEPIDERMAL WATER LOSS (TEWL) FOR PREDICTION OF SKIN IRRITATION

A. Technical Part

TEWL is the passive diffusion of water through the stratum corneum. TEWL can be measured by the Evaporimeter® EP-1, which records the total water loss from the skin. It is implied that eccrine sweating should be suppressed or kept to a minimum during measurements. When measurements are performed after a period of 30-min rest, this criterion is usually fulfilled. In the probe of the Evaporimeter two sensors are mounted in an open chamber. These sensors determine the water vapor pressure gradient between the skin surface and the ambient air to quantify the diffusion of water through the skin, i.e., the TEWL. Guidelines for measurement of TEWL have been established.[26]

TEWL depends on the relative ambient humidity and the ambient temperature. When relative humidity, temperature, and eccrine sweating are controlled, TEWL will reflect the integrity of stratum corneum. Basal TEWL studied in 30 healthy volunteers over a period of 10 days was found to be a stable individual characteristic.[27]

B. TEWL in Pathophysiological Conditions

A number of studies have demonstrated that TEWL values are significantly increased after sodium lauryl sulfate (SLS) exposure to the skin and that the TEWL response depends on the concentration and dose of SLS used.[28-30] TEWL is also increased in both involved and uninvolved skin in patients with atopic dermatitis,[24,31] in scaly hand eczema,[32] and in psoriasis,[33] whereas TEWL on noninvolved skin in patients with hand eczema was normal.[25]

C. Prediction of Skin Susceptibility

It is thus well documented that TEWL is increased in a number of pathophysiological conditions. The interesting question is, however, whether clinically normal skin with slightly increased TEWL values has a clinically relevant increased susceptibility to skin irritants. Are subjects with high basal TEWL values at risk and may the individual susceptibility to develop irritant contact dermatitis be reliably characterized by measuring basal TEWL values? A number of studies support this hypothesis.

In 1986 Murahata et al.[34] found a correlation between increased basal TEWL and increased visual reaction to an irritant stimulus in healthy subjects. Tupker et al.[19] studied the role of basal TEWL in susceptibility to weak irritants in 37 healthy subjects. Volunteers were exposed to low molarity SLS two times daily for 4 days, and the skin response was evaluated by measurement of TEWL and a visual scoring system. The degree of barrier damage, as evaluated by TEWL, and the degree of inflammation, as evaluated by visual scoring, were strongly related to barrier function before exposure (i.e., basal TEWL). In a study including 27 healthy volunteers exposed to SLS for 1 and 4 days, respectively, the same group found basal TEWL to be a good indicator of an individual's susceptibility to an irritant stimulus.[35] In a group of 70 healthy volunteers challenged with SLS, baseline TEWL was found to contribute significantly to a multiple regression analysis model using TEWL after SLS exposure as the dependent variable,[4] and in the same study subjects with high visual scores after SLS exposure had increased basal TEWL compared with those with low visual scores.[4] The relationship between high basal TEWL and increased susceptibility to SLS was supported in a study of 39 hand eczema patients and controls.[25] Only few studies have until now utilized individual basal TEWL values for prediction of risk of irritant contact dermatitis in epidemiological studies. Repetitive measurements of basal TEWL in workers in the metal industry in Singapore indicated that high TEWL values obtained from the back of the hands may predict later development of irritant contact dermatitis.[36] However, due to poorly standardized measuring conditions and a low number of participants, these results can only be accepted as preliminary. Currently, a prospective study on TEWL and hand dermatitis in apprentice nurses and apprentice hairdressers in being performed, but data from this study are still not available.[37]

Although the presented results are encouraging for utilizing basal TEWL as an indicator for susceptibility to irritant contact dermatitis, data have not generally been confirmed by all groups.[38-41] Differences in the experimental irritant trauma used, differences in experimental designs, and lack of standardization of the measuring method until recently may partly explain the conflicting results. It can be concluded that, although the method is difficult to handle, measurement of basal TEWL is a promising tool for identification of subjects with increased susceptibility to chemical irritants, and possibly increased risk for development of irritant contact dermatitis. However, future epidemiological studies are necessary to confirm the usefulness of TEWL measurement as a clinically relevant predictor of irritant contact dermatitis.

IV. ELECTRICAL CONDUCTANCE AND CAPACITANCE

A. Technical Part

Different electrical methods can be used for registration of skin hydration,[42] and new methods are still being developed. Skin conductance can be measured by the Skicon 100®.[43] The resistance to a high frequency current between two concentrically arranged electrodes separated by an insulator is measured and reported in $1/\mu$ohm. The electrical capacitance of the skin can be measured by a

Corneometer CM 420®.[44] The probe of the instrument functions as one electrode, and the skin functions as the other. Generally, the Skicon instrument is more sensitive for measurement of increased hydration and the Corneometer for decreased hydration.[45]

B. Electrical Parameters in Pathophysiological Conditions

The hydration state of normal skin, as measured by the Skicon 100, was decreased during the winter.[11] Increased response to irritants was found in the same season. Clinically normal skin in patients with atopic dermatitis did not differ significantly from that in healthy volunteers with respect to skin hydration, as measured by electrical capacitance[44] or electrical conductance.[46] Generally, low molarity SLS causes decreased hydration of the stratum corneum, which may last for several days.[47] However, information on dose-response relation to SLS irritation is not available.

C. Prediction of Skin Susceptibility

Increased susceptibility to SLS was reported in clinically dry skin compared with clinically normal skin in patients with eczema and in healthy volunteers,[23] but measurement of skin hydration by the Corneometer in the same study was found to have no predictive value for development of irritant skin reactions. A negative correlation between TEWL and skin hydration, as measured by electrical conductance or capacitance, has been reported in normal skin and various skin diseases.[44,48,49] A decreased hydration state of the stratum corneum is undoubtedly important for skin susceptibility to irritants. However, the measuring methods are sensitive and the intraindividual variation in the obtained results is high, which complicates the use of these methods for prediction of an irritant skin response. Careful arrangement of measuring conditions, including controlled skin temperature and ambient relatively humidity, may improve the predictive value of the electrical methods for measurement of skin hydration.

V. SKIN COLOR FOR PREDICTION OF SKIN IRRITATION

A. Technical Part

The skin surface color can be quantified by use of the standard tristimulus system proposed by the Commission Internationale de l'Eclairage.[50] The color is expressed as a value in a three-dimensional coordinate system[51] (Figure 2). Another method for determination of erythema and melanin index

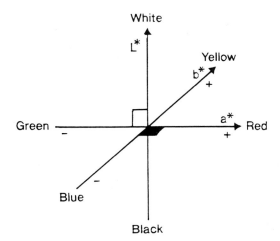

FIGURE 2. A schematic drawing of the L*a*b* three-dimensional color system. The a* axis represents the color range from red (+) to green (−); the b* axis represents the color range from yellow (+) to blue (−). L* expresses reflection of light from the skin ranging from black (low values) to white (high values).

is based on the amount of reflected green and red light from the skin.[52] The methods have been found to correlate well (Takiwaki and Serup, unpublished data) and to reflect the volume of blood under a given area of skin.

B. Skin Color in Pathophysiological Conditions

Changes in erythema (a*) correlate well with visually scored skin damage in a dose-dependent manner after testing with SLS.[29,30,51,53] Light reflection from the skin (L) was found increased (fair complexion) in patients with hand eczema compared with controls,[25] whereas no significant difference in light reflection was found between uninvolved skin of patients with atopic dermatitis and controls.[24]

C. Prediction of Skin Susceptibility

Clinically assessed fair skin and blue eyes were reported to correlate well with skin susceptibility to a mechanical trauma.[54] Frosch and Wissing[7] reported a positive correlation between sensitivity to UV light and to seven different chemical irritants in healthy volunteers. In a study on 70 healthy volunteers a statistically significant association between increased light reflection from the skin surface (fair skin), as measured by a tristimulus colorimeter, and increased susceptibility to SLS was demonstrated.[4] Tanning is well known to influence the skin response to irritants,[15,55] and measurements of skin color for determination of the individual skin sensitivity should therefore be obtained from areas not normally exposed to UV light.

In conclusion, experimental data support that the skin complexion is associated with skin susceptibility to irritants. The association is until now unexplained, but structural differences other than the melanin content of the skin should be considered. Measurement of skin color may be useful for determination of the individual skin susceptibility. The method is easy to use and highly reproducible, but the results may be complicated by changes due to UV exposure, which by itself will influence skin susceptibility to irritants.

VI. SKIN pH FOR PREDICTION OF SKIN IRRITATION

Skin surface pH can be measured by a surface electrode for pH measurements, connected to a pH meter.[38] The pH of normal skin is acidic, i.e., pH 3 to 6. Skin pH is increased after SLS exposure, and high skin pH has been demonstrated to correlate with increased TEWL values.[56] In a study including 10 healthy volunteers, a significant positive correlation between skin surface pH and the severity of SLS-induced irritancy was found.[38] In the same study skin pH after five tape strippings of the stratum corneum correlated even stronger to TEWL after SLS exposure. Apart from the aforementioned studies, other investigations of pH as a predictor for sensitive skin are to the author's knowledge not available. The observation on pH is interesting but needs confirmation.

VII. SKIN SURFACE LIPIDS FOR PREDICTION OF SKIN IRRITATION

The skin surface lipids can be measured by a Sebumeter®.[57] An opaque plastic film, on the probe of the instrument, is pressed against the skin surface with/under a standard load. The film becomes transparent by lipids, and the transmission is measured by photometry.

Sebum excretion, which accounts for most of the skin surface lipids, is normally regarded as being of questionable importance for the skin barrier function, although reduced skin surface lipid was reported to correlate with increased TEWL values.[56] In a recent study skin surface lipids were measured over the scapulae on 10 volunteers and compared with the magnitude of SLS-induced dermatitis in the same body region. No correlation was found, but the interindividual variation in sebum content of the skin was found to be considerable.[38,56] There is for the moment no clear indication that measurement of skin surface lipids can be utilized for prediction of skin irritation. However, this matter has not been sufficiently studied in the past.

VIII. ULTRASOUND FOR PREDICTION OF SKIN IRRITATION

A-mode ultrasound 20 MHz scanning is an accurate technique for the measurement of skin thickness.[58,59] The time lag between the echo from the skin surface and the echo from the interface between the dermis and the subcutaneous fat can be measured and the distance in millimeters calculated from the sound velocity in the tissue. Measurement of skin thickness includes the epidermis and the dermis together, the latter constituting the major part of the recorded distance, and minor changes in the thickness of the epidermis are thus beyond the detection limit of the method. B-scan for two-dimensional and C-scan for three-dimensional study of the skin are also now commercially available. Basal skin thickness, measured on the upper arm, has been reported to be decreased in patients with chronic hand eczema.[25] Although interesting, this observation needs to be explained. Basal skin thickness in patients with atopic dermatitis did not differ significantly from that in controls.[24] Skin thickness after SLS exposure is increased and dose-dependent,[29] as a result of edema formation. A more sophisticated evaluation of irritant skin reactions by B-scan and computerized image analysis was recently reported.[60]

In a study of 70 healthy volunteers basal skin thickness did not correlate with the irritant skin response to SLS.[4] Apart from the observation of decreased skin thickness in hand eczema patients, there is at present no clear indication that basal skin thickness can be used as an indicator for sensitive skin. Further studies are surely needed. However, the new advanced ultrasound examination techniques may provide detailed information about biophysical skin properties and may be utilized in the future.

IX. SKIN BLOOD FLOW FOR ASSESSMENT OF SKIN IRRITANCY

Noninvasive assessment of blood flow is possible by laser Doppler flowmetry, which is based on the Doppler phenomenon.[61] Assessment of the relationship between basal skin blood flow and skin susceptibility has not been the subject of much investigation. In one study on healthy volunteers basal blood flow, as measured by laser Doppler flowmetry, was not found to influence skin susceptibility to SLS exposure significantly.[4] There is until now no indication that basal skin blood flow can be used for prediction of skin irritancy.

X. CONCLUSIONS

Biophysical properties of the skin are important for the skin susceptibility to irritant trauma. These properties can be evaluated by a number of noninvasive bioengineering methods. For prediction of skin susceptibility, examination of the skin barrier is essential. Provisional data, mainly based on observations on SLS-induced skin irritation, indicate that measurement of basal TEWL may be critical for determination of skin susceptibility, whereas measurement of skin hydration due to great intraindividual variation and need of standardization of the measuring methods and conditions has not yet proved its utility. Light reflection from the skin (L*), as measured by a colorimeter, reflecting skin complexion, correlates well with skin susceptibility to irritancy as studied with SLS, but intermittent exposure to UV light might interfere with the accuracy. Measurement of skin pH has in one study proved to correlate significantly with skin sensitivity. The predictive value for skin irritation of basal skin thickness and skin surface lipids needs further evaluation.

Studies of the value of biophysical properties of the skin for predicting skin susceptibility are still in a preliminary phase. It is important to consider that almost all studies have used SLS-induced skin irritation as the experimental model. Although detergent-induced dermatitis is indeed highly relevant, this focus on SLS dermatitis may bias the results. Further studies using varying experimental designs are necessary, and final conclusions can only be obtained from large-scale epidemiological studies.

REFERENCES

1. Meding, B. and Swanbeck, G., Epidemiology of different types of hand eczema in an industrial city, *Acta Derm. Venereol.*, 69, 227, 1989.
2. Wall, L. M. and Gebauer, K. A., A follow-up study of occupational skin disease in Western Australia, *Contact Dermatitis*, 24, 241, 1991.
3. Nilsson, E. and Bök, O., The importance of anamnestic information of atopy, metal dermatitis and earlier hand eczema for the development of hand dermatitis in women in wet hospital work, *Acta Derm. Venereol.*, 66, 45, 1986.
4. Agner, T., Basal transepidermal water loss, skin thickness, skin blood flow and skin colour in relation to sodium-lauryl-sulphate-induced irritation in normal skin, *Contact Dermatitis*, 25, 108, 1991.
5. Björnberg, A., *Skin Reactions to Primary Irritants in Patients with Hand Eczema,* Isacson, Göteborg, 1968.
6. Coenraads, P. J., Bleumink, E., and Nater, J. P., Susceptibility to primary irritants, *Contact Dermatitis*, 1, 377, 1975.
7. Frosch, P. J. and Wissing, C., Cutaneous sensitivity to ultraviolet light and chemical irritants, *Arch. Dermatol. Res.*, 272, 269, 1982.
8. Frosch, P. J. and Kligman, A. M., Recognition of chemically vulnerable and delicate skin, in *Principles of Cosmetics for the Dermatologist*, Frost, P. and Horwitz, S., Eds., C. V. Mosby, St. Louis, 1982, 287.
9. Tupker, R. A., Pinnagoda, J., Coenraads, P. J., and Nater, J. P., The influence of repeated exposure to surfactants on the human skin as determined by transepidermal water loss and visual scoring, *Contact Dermatitis*, 20, 108, 1989.
10. Malten, K. E., Thoughts on irritant contact dermatitis, *Contact Dermatitis*, 7, 238, 1981.
11. Agner, T. and Serup, J., Seasonal variation of skin resistance to irritants, *Br. J. Dermatol.*, 121, 323, 1989.
12. Rycroft, R. J. G. and Smith, W. D. L., Low humidity occupational dermatoses, *Contact Dermatitis*, 6, 488, 1980.
13. Magnusson, B. and Hersle, K., Patch test methods. Regional variation of patch test responses, *Acta Derm. Venereol.*, 45, 257, 1965.
14. Frosch, P. J. and Kligman, A. M., Rapid blister formation in human skin with ammonium hydroxide, *Br. J. Dermatol.*, 96, 461, 1977.
15. Frosch, P. J., *Hautirritation und empfindliche Haut,* Grosse Verlag, Berlin, 1985.
16. Wilhelm, K. P., Cua, A. B., and Maibach, H. I., Skin aging, *Arch. Dermatol.*, 127, 1806, 1992.
17. Björnberg, A., Skin reactions to primary irritants in men and women, *Acta Derm. Venereol.*, 55, 191, 1975.
18. Lammintausta, K., Maibach, H. I., and Wilson, D., Irritant reactivity in males and females, *Contact Dermatitis*, 17, 276, 1987.
19. Tupker, R. A., Coenraads, P. J., Pinnagoda, J., and Nater, J. P., Baseline transepidermal water loss (TEWL) as a prediction of susceptibility to sodium lauryl sulphate, *Contact Dermatitis*, 20, 265, 1989.
20. Agner, T., Damm, P., and Skouby, S. O., Menstrual cycle and skin reactivity, *J. Am. Acad. Dermatol.*, 24, 566, 1991.
21. Rystedt, I., Work-related hand eczema in atopics, *Contact Dermatitis*, 12, 164, 1985.
22. Rystedt, I., Atopic background in patients with occupational hand eczema, *Contact Dermatitis*, 12, 247, 1985.
23. Tupker, R. A., Pinnagoda, J., Coenraads, P. J., and Nater, J. P., Susceptibility to irritants: role of barrier function, skin dryness and history of atopic dermatitis, *Br. J. Dermatol.*, 123, 199, 1990.
24. Agner, T., Susceptibility of atopic dermatitis patients to irritant dermatitis caused by sodium lauryl sulphate, *Acta Derm. Venereol.*, 71, 296, 1991.
25. Agner, T., Skin susceptibility in uninvolved skin of hand eczema patients and healthy controls, *Br. J. Dermatol.*, 125, 140, 1991.

26. Pinnagoda, J., Tupker, R. A., Agner, T., and Serup, J., Guidelines for transepidermal water loss (TEWL) measurement, *Contact Dermatitis,* 22, 164, 1990.

27. Pinnagoda, J., Tupker, R. A., Smit, J. A., Coenraads, P. J., and Nater, J. P., The intra- and interindividual variability and reliability of transepidermal water loss measurements, *Contact Dermatitis,* 21, 255, 1989.

28. van der Valk, P. G. M., Nater, J. P., and Bleumink, E., Skin irritancy of surfactants as assessed by water vapour loss measurements, *J. Invest. Dermatol.,* 82, 291, 1984.

29. Agner, T. and Serup, J., Sodium lauryl sulphate for irritant patch testing. A dose-response study using bioengineering methods for determination of skin irritation, *J. Invest. Dermatol.,* 95, 543, 1990.

30. Wilhelm, K. P., Surber, C., and Maibach, H. I., Quantification of sodium lauryl sulphate dermatitis in man: comparison of four techniques: skin color reflectance, transepidermal water loss, laser Doppler flow measurement and visual scores, *Arch. Dermatol. Res.,* 281, 293, 1989.

31. Werner, Y. and Lindberg, M., Transepidermal water loss in dry and clinically normal skin in patients with atopic dermatitis, *Acta Derm. Venereol.,* 65, 102, 1985.

32. Blichmann, C. and Serup, J., Hydration studies on scaly hand eczema, *Contact Dermatitis,* 16, 155, 1987.

33. Blichmann, C. and Serup, J., Epidermal hydration of psoriasis plaques and the relation to scaling, *Acta Derm. Venereol.,* 67, 357, 1987.

34. Murahata, R., Crove, D. M., and Roheim, J. R., The use of transepidermal water loss to measure and predict the irritation response to surfactancts, *Int. J. Cosmetic Sci.,* 8, 225, 1986.

35. Pinnagoda, J., Tupker, R. A., Coenraads, P. J., and Nater, J. P., Prediction of susceptibility to an irritant response by transepidermal water loss, *Contact Dermatitis,* 20, 341, 1989.

36. Coenraads, P. J., Lee, J., and Pinnagoda, J., Changes in water vapour loss from the skin of metal industry workers monitored during exposure to oils, *Scand. J. Work Environ. Health,* 12, 494, 1986.

37. van Rijssen, T., Coenraads, P. J., and Nater, J. P., A prospective study on TEWL and hand dermatitis in apprentice nurses and apprentice hairdressers, paper presented as a poster on Int. Symp. Irritant Contact Dermatitis, Groningen, Holland, October 1991.

38. Wilhelm, K. P. and Maibach, H. I., Susceptibility to irritant dermatitis induced by sodium lauryl sulfate, *J. Am. Acad. Dermatol.,* 23, 122, 1990.

39. Freeman, S. and Maibach, H. I., Study of irritant contact dermatitis produced by repeat patch testing with sodium lauryl sulphate and assessed by visual methods, transepidermal water loss and laser Doppler velocimetry, *J. Am. Acad. Dermatol.,* 19, 496, 1988.

40. Berardesca, E. and Maibach, H. I., Racial differences in sodium lauryl sulphate induced cutaneous irritation: black and white, *Contact Dermatitis,* 18, 65, 1988.

41. Berardesca, E. and Maibach, H. I., Sodium-lauryl-sulphate-induced cutaneous irritation. Comparison of white and hispanic subjects, *Contact Dermatitis,* 19, 136, 1988.

42. Leveque, J. L. and de Rigal, J., Impedance methods for studying skin moisturization, *J. Soc. Cosmetic Chem.,* 34, 419, 1983.

43. Tagami, H., Ohi, M., Iwatsuki, K., Kannamaru, Y., Yamada, M., and Ichijo, B., Evaluation of the skin surface hydration *in vivo* by electrical measurement, *J. Invest. Dermatol.,* 75, 500, 1980.

44. Werner, Y., The water content of the stratum corneum in patients with atopic dermatitis, *Acta Derm. Venereol.,* 66, 281, 1986.

45. Agner, T. and Serup, J., Comparison of two electrical methods for measurement of skin hydration. An experimental study on irritant patch test reactions, *Bioengineering Skin,* 4, 263, 1988.

46. Al-jaberi, H. and Marks, R., Studies of the clinically uninvolved skin in patients with dermatitis, *Br. J. Dermatol.,* 111, 437, 1984.

47. Agner, T. and Serup, J., Skin reactions to irritants assessed by non-invasive, bioengineering methods, *Contact Dermatitis,* 20, 352, 1989.

48. Blichmann, C. and Serup, J., Assessment of skin moisture, *Acta Derm. Venereol.*, 68, 284, 1988.

49. Tagami, H., Impedance measurement for evaluation of the hydration state of the skin surface, in *Cutaneous Investigation in Health and Disease*, Leveque, J., Ed., Marcel Dekker, New York, 1990, 79.

50. Robertson, A. R., The CIE 1976 color difference formulas, *Color Res. Appl.*, 2, 7, 1977.

51. Serup, J. and Agner, T., Colorimetric quantification of erythema — a comparison of two colorimeters (Lang Micro Color and Minolta Chroma Meter CR-200) with a clinical scoring scheme and laser Doppler flowmetry, *Clin. Exp. Dermatol.*, 15, 267, 1990.

52. Farr, P. M. and Diffey, B. L., Quantitative studies on cutaneous erythema induced by ultraviolet radiation, *Br. J. Dermatol.*, 111, 673, 1984.

53. Babulak, S. W., Rhein, L. D., Scala, D. D., and Simion, F. A., Quantitation of erythema in a soap chamber test using the Minolta Chroma (reflectance) Meter: comparison of instrumental results with visual assessment, *J. Soc. Cosmetic Chem.*, 37, 475, 1986.

54. Björnberg, A., Löwhagen, G., and Tengberg, J., Relationship between intensities of skin test reactions to glass-fibres and chemical irritants, *Contact Dermatitis*, 5, 171, 1979.

55. Larmi, E., Lahti, A., and Hannuksela, M., Effect of ultraviolet B on nonimmunologic contact reactions induced by dimethyl sulfoxide, phenol and sodium lauryl sulphate, *Photodermatology*, 6, 258, 1989.

56. Thune, P., Nilsen, T., and Hanstad, I. K., The water barrier function of the skin in relation to the water content of stratum corneum, pH and skin lipids. The effect of alkaline soap and syndet on dry skin in elderly, non-atopic patients, *Acta Derm. Venereol.*, 68, 277, 1968.

57. Serup, J., Formation of oiliness and sebum output — comparison of a lipid-absorbant and occlusive-tape method with photometry, *Clin. Exp. Dermatol.*, 16, 258, 1991.

58. Agner, T. and Serup, J., Individual and instrumental variations in irritant patch-test reactions: clinical evaluation and quantification by bioengineering methods, *Clin. Exp. Dermatol.*, 15, 29, 1990.

59. Serup, J., Ten years' experience with high-frequency ultrasound examination of the skin: development and refinement of technique and equipment, in *Ultrasound in Dermatology*, Altmeyer, P., el-Gammal, S., and Hoffmann, K., Eds., Springer-Verlag, Berlin, 1992.

60. Seidenary, S., Sonographic evaluation of skin reactions, paper presented at the Int. Symp. Irritant Contact Dermatitis, Gronigen, Holland, October 1991.

61. Shepherd, A. P., History on LDV flowmetry, in *Laser Doppler Blood Flowmetry*, Shepherd, and Öberg, T., Eds., Kluwer Acadmic, MA, 1990, 1.

16

General Aspects of Risk Factors in Hand Eczema

Thomas L. Diepgen and Manigé Fartasch

CONTENTS

0-8493-7355-7/94/$0.00 + $.50
© 1994 by CRC Press, Inc.

I. INTRODUCTION

Although eczema of the hand is one of the most common skin diseases, a clear and worldwide accepted definition of what is included as "hand eczema" (HE) does not exist, and even dermatologists differ in their interpretation. After having excluded disorders of known etiology (e.g., tinea manuum, scabies), well-defined noneczematous morphology (e.g., psoriasis, lichen planus, granuloma annulare, porphyria cutanea tarda, keratosis palmo-plantaris, fixed drug eruption), and neoplastic disorders from the category of HE, and if hands are not involved as part of an extensive skin disorder, the diagnosis of characteristic and established cases of HE usually presents little difficulty. Yet opinions differ on the validity of including mild and transient cases or those in which dryness, cracking, and superficial fissuring are the only features.[1] It is also difficult to subclassify HE according to morphologic, etiologic, or pathogenetic classifications used in dermatology.[2] He is a multifactorial disease in which both exogenous and endogenous factors play a role. General aspects of those risk factors in HE will be considered in this chapter. In addition to the fact that HE is not a single entity but an affliction with multiple causes,[2] an attempt to discuss the general role of risk factors by the literature poses additional problems: some studies are based on selected samples, as with patch test patients or special occupational groups (e.g., hairdressers, nurses), other population-based studies are based on questionnaires, and often control groups were not included. Finally, there is no clear agreement on the definition of endogenous risk factors, such as an atopic skin diathesis (ASD), which is believed to be often related to HE.[2-15] In this chapter some demographic characteristics of patients with HE will be introduced, and general aspects of exogenous and endogenous risk factors of HE will be reported according to several studies.

II. DEMOGRAPHIC CHARACTERISTICS OF HAND ECZEMA

The presented data are from our special occupational dermatoses clinic, established in 1984, in the Department of Dermatology of the Friedrich-Alexander University of Erlangen. Diagnoses and treatment of all the skin patients in which hands are predominantly affected are performed here. This sample is not population based and will be biased toward inpatients and outpatients. From 1469 patients with skin diseases of the hands in 83% (n = 1221) HE was diagnosed, and in 17% (n = 248) other skin conditions, including psoriasis, pustolosis palmaris et plantaris, tinea manuum, lichen planus, and others, were diagnosed. It is difficult to subclassify HE, and mostly several skin conditions are responsible. Table 1 lists some general clinical and morphological characteristics of different HE. According to that definition, the results of patch test, and the course of the HE, we distinguished the main diagnoses of HE as follows: atopic hand eczema was diagnosed in 36% (n = 443), allergic contact dermatitis of the hands in 23% (n = 279), irritant contact dermatitis of the hands in 21% (n = 258), and other HE, such as nummular HE, tylotic eczema of the palms, or pompholyx (if this was not an atopic HE), in 20% (n = 241). In the last group no known exogenous factors seemed to play an important role in the pathogenesis of the HE. If the same patient had more than one diagnosis of HE, the main diagnosis was documented. In atopic, allergic, or irritant HE females outnumbered males in contrast to nummular/tylotic HE (Table 2).

The age distributions of patients with HEs showed different patterns according to their diagnoses (Figure 1). Whereas patients with atopic, allergic, or irritant HE were mostly younger than 30 years, the distribution of the age in patients with nummular/tylotic HE showed no peak and was uniformly distributed. Most patients with nummular/tylotic HE were older than 30 years. In the group of patients with allergic HE there was also a second small peak of patients between 40 and 45 years of age. Further analyses showed that the peak was mainly caused by construction workers with type IV allergies against potassium dichromate.

III. EXOGENOUS RISK FACTORS

In all allergic HE it was possible to identify contact allergens that were relevant to the HE. That means that the person has come into contact with the allergen, and this contact is believed to play a causative role in his HE. Because we lack a test to determine whether an irritant is relevant to a patient's HE, it remains a clinical decision to judge the etiologic role of irritants in HE. Well-

TABLE 1   General Aspects of Different Kinds of Hand Eczema (HE)

Clinical characteristics of atopic HE

Morphologic presentation and localization
- 53% of all atopic HE show vesicular volar eruption, sometimes with extension from the distal part of the palm to proximal fingers (apron sign)
- Often nail involvement, in some cases fissuring and cracking of fingertips (pulpite séche)
- Involvement of the metacarpophalangeal joint of the thumb (tabatière)
- Involvement of other body regions (neck, flexural, dorsa of the feet)

Clinical characteristics of allergic HE

- Relationship between time of occurrence and occupational context
- Effects of weekends, vacations, and trips away from home, recurrence after return to work
- The regional pattern may give hints as to the cause
- Detection of relevant allergens by patch testing
- Spreading and dissemination possible

Characteristics of irritant HE

Etiopathology
- Frequency of mild irritant exposure is too high in relation to skin recovery time
- Predisposing individual factors, including atopic skin diathesis, sebostasis, hyperhidrosis

Region of eczema
- Dorsa and dorsal fingers and exposed distal parts of forearm, later spreading to palms
- Lesions sharply limited to the usual site of contact

Morphology
- First dry scaling and cracking
- Later erythema, infiltration, and fissures
- Itching is not so intense as in allergic HE but painful rhagades may appear

Clinical characteristics of nummulare (discoid) HE

- Characteristic feature, confluence of tiny papules and papulovesicles on erythematous ground into coin-shaped plaque
- Peripheral extension with central clearing
- Lesions are highly irritable, burning sensations in 21 to 33% initial patch at the dorsa of hands and dorsal fingers
- Onset as post-traumatic eczema within weeks of cutaneous injury

Characteristics of tylotic HE

- Mostly men affected, age >40 years
- Localization
  Proximal or middle part of palms and/or soles
  Additionally, fingertips or tip of the toes
- Without itching, without vesicular eruptions
- Persistence of sharply demarcated hyperkeratotic plaques of chronic course
- Histology
- Hyperkeratosis, focal parakeratosis, akanthosis, and spongioses

known irritants are water and wet work, detergents and cleansing agents, hand cleaners, unspecific chemicals, oils, and abrasives.

In 895 HE patients (73%) at least one of those exogenous risk factors was found to play an important role in the pathogenesis of HE. Figure 2 shows the frequencies of the different exogenous risk factors in those HE according to female and male patients. Water and wet work was found to be the most frequent exogenous risk factor in females and males. In females detergents and cleansing agents played an important role, too. In males hand cleaners, detergents and cleansing agents, oils, and unspecific chemicals were also important irritants. At least one of those irritants was always involved in irritant HE but also in 60% in atopic HE, in 84% in allergic HE, and in 63% in nummular/tylotic HE.

TABLE 2 Demographic Characteristics of Hand Eczema (HE)

Main diagnosis	Patients			Females			Males		
	No.	%	Age (years)	No.	%	Age (years)	No.	%	Age (years)
Atopic HE	443	36	25	288	65	23	155	35	28
Allergic HE	279	23	24	177	63	22	102	37	41
Irritant HE	258	21	28	174	67	27	84	33	35
Nummular/tylotic HE	241	20	41	101	42	36	140	58	43
Total	1221	100	28	740	61	24	481	39	35

Note: Values for age are medians.

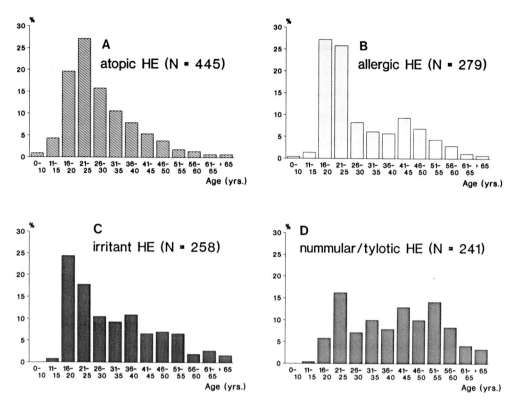

FIGURE 1. Age distribution of patients with different hand eczema: (A) atopic HE, (B) allergic HE, (C) irritant HE, and (D) nummular/tylotic HE.

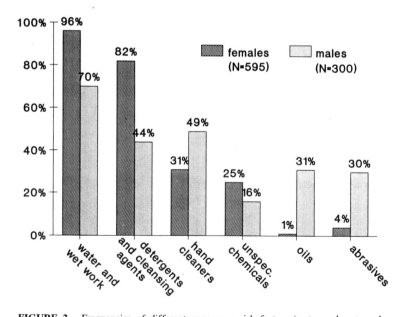

FIGURE 2. Frequencies of different exogenous risk factors (water and wet work, detergents and cleansing agents, hand cleaners, unspecific chemicals, oils, abrasives) in female and male patients with hand eczema, in which at least one exogenous risk factor was found to play an important role in the pathogenesis of HE (n = 895).

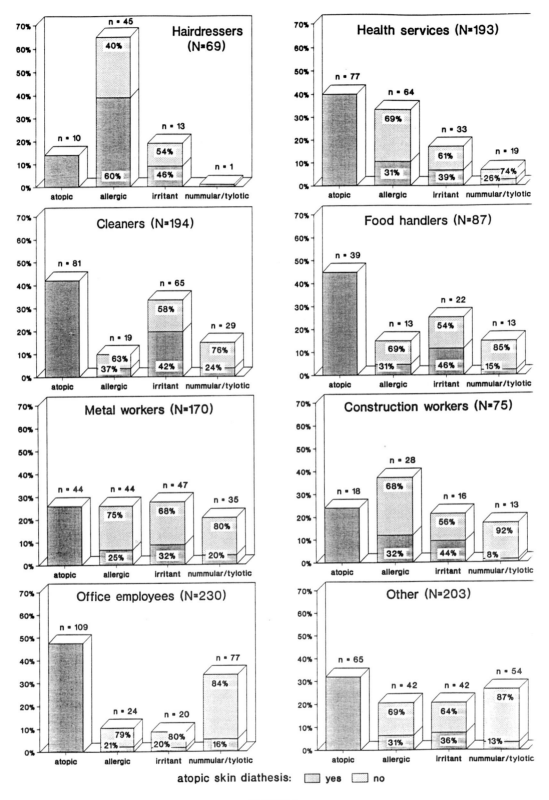

FIGURE 3.

A complex interplay of exogenous risk factors, such as several irritants and/or multiple well-known and unknown allergens, and of the endogenous disposition (atopy) is believed to be responsible for the occurrence and the course of HE in humans. The exposure to irritants and allergens by work and hobbies determines whether the main causative factor of the HE is more irritant or allergic. Another important factor is the individual susceptibility to HE, which is influenced by the atopic disposition. Water and wet work were found to play a major role in atopic HE in 54%, detergents and cleansing agents in 44%, hand cleaners in 21%, but oils only in 6%. In Figure 3 the pattern of different HE (atopic, allergic, irritant, and nummular/tylotic) is shown according to several occupational groups, i.e., hairdressers, food handlers, cleaners, health services, construction workers, metalworkers, office employees, and others. The diagnoses were established according to defined criteria and course of the disease (Table 1). Additionally, the percentage of patients with an atopic disposition is presented in each HE group. In this context an atopic disposition was defined as the presence of at least two of the following variables: personal or family history of atopy, dry skin, white dermographism, hyperlinear palms, retroauricular rhagades, pityriasis alba, and elevated immunoglobulin E (IgE) (>100 U/ml).

In some occupational groups, e.g., hairdressers, health services, and construction workers, allergic HE was more frequently diagnosed compared with irritant HE. In other groups, e.g., food industry or cleaners, irritant HE outnumbered allergic HE. Atopic HE was often diagnosed in all professions and an atopic disposition was found to be an important cofactor in allergic and irritant HE. Nummular/tylotic HE was found to be normally not work related. Looking to the pattern of HEs in several professions shown in Figure 3, it must be taken into consideration that this was not a population-based study on occupational HE but a sample of patients in an HE clinic.

IV. ENDOGENOUS RISK FACTORS

A. The Relationship between Hand Eczema and Atopy

Atopy and especially atopic eczema (AE) are well-known factors influencing the course and prognosis of HE,[2-15] but the role of atopic features in the developing of HE is still unclear. There are two ways of looking at the relationship between atopy and HE: the frequency of HE in atopics and the frequency of atopy in patients with HE (Table 3). In comparing the findings in the literature, one is faced with the same difficulties of selection and interpretation that have been mentioned before. Additionally, the definition of atopy itself differs considerably. Some authors include a family history as well as a personal history of atopy, others divide their subjects into those with AE and those with respiratory allergy, and some would accept only positive prick tests as evidence for the atopic diathesis. Finally, only few studies have included a matched control group. Considering these objections it must be mentioned that the frequencies of atopy in patients with HE are increased over the that expected in the general population according to most studies[19,23] (Table 3).

Atopic disease and especially AE in childhood are risk factors for HE in adults.[3,4,8,9] However, these studies also found that a considerable number of subjects with a personal history of AE managed to work in risk occupations without developing HE. Therefore, a reduced resistance to irritants does not occur in all subjects with AE and may occur in subjects with respiratory atopy and in nonatopics.

B. Atopic Skin Diathesis and Hand Eczema

Lammintausta[4] introduced the term ''atopic skin diathesis'' as a prognostically useful definition of the skin condition that might be involved in the development of HE. This condition was defined

FIGURE 3.   Frequencies of atopic, allergic, irritant, and nummular/tylotic HE in different occupational groups: hairdressers (n = 69), health services (n = 193), cleaners (n = 194), food handlers (n = 87), metal workers (n = 170), construction workers (n = 75), office employees (n = 230), and others (n = 203). Additionally, the percentage of patients with an atopic disposition is given in the different HE groups.

TABLE 3   The Relationship Between Hand Eczema (HE) and Atopy

Study	Year	Subjects (atopics)		Frequencies of HE
		HE among Atopics (Selection)		
Cronin[16]	1970	AE	N = 233	68%
Breit[17]	1974	AE	N = 130	69%
Rystedt[9]	1985	Severe AE	N = 549	60%
		Moderate AE	N = 406	48%
		Respiratory	N = 222	14%
		Nonatopics	N = 199	11%
Diepgen[18]	1991	AE	N = 428	72% Often or sometimes HE
		Atopics among HE (Selection)		
Lammintausta[3]	1981	HE in hospital wet work	N = 259	54% Atopics
Cronin[19]	1985	HE in women	N = 263	34% Personal history of atopy
				67% Personal or family History of atopy
Meding[20]	1990	HE in a population-based sample	N = 1,238	27% Childhood eczema
				28% Asthma/hay fever
Lodi[21]	1992	Pompholyx	N = 104	50% Personal or family History of atopy
Diepgen[22]		HE	N = 458	19% Respiratory allergy
				34% Family history of atopy
				62% Personal or family History of atopy

as (1) dry skin, (2) a history of low pruritus threshold for two of three nonspecific irritants (sweat, dust, rough material), (3) white dermographism, and (4) facial pallor/infraorbital darkenings. This ASD was found in 35% of subjects with respiratory atopy and in 18% of the nonatopics and significantly increased the risk of HE among employees engaged in wet work.[3] Rystedt[8,9] found in her follow-up studies of atopic children that the frequency of HE was 4 to 10 times higher in people who had had AE in childhood than in those who had not. Patients with a history of respiratory allergy without associated AE (n = 222; 14% HE) showed no increased frequencies of HE than controls without personal or family atopy (n = 199; 11% HE). Therefore, it seems necessary to subclassify the atopic state of possible skin involvement for occupational risk assessment.

For the diagnosis of AE an array of clinical (basic and minor) features proposed by Hanifin and Rajka[24] are in common use because there are no laboratory or other objective markers for the diagnosis of the disease. However, many of the atopic features can be found in normal individuals who never previously had skin problems or eczema at the time of examination.[25,26]

1.   Study 1

To establish a diagnostic score of AE we evaluated basic and minor features of AE systematically in established cases of AE and in subjects randomly collected from the caucasian normal population (NP) of young adults in a prospective computerized study.[18,26-29] Anamnestic and clinical atopic (basic and minor) features were investigated in all test subjects by two investigators to obtain a good interobserver agreement. On the base of statistical modeling of those atopic features with the highest odds ratios (ORs) a diagnostic score system was constructed, which should be based on anamnestic and clinical features without laboratory investigations.[18,26] Atopic features that were seen to be less frequent than 20% in AE were not included. The presence of an itching flexural dermatitis was not included because this was the selection base. On the base of chi-square values every atopic feature obtained a value between 1 and 3 points according to its statistical significance (Table 4). By using the proposed score system both groups were separated fairly clearly with minimal overlapping (Figure 4). Based on this score system patients with more than 10 points should be considered to have an ASD and patients with more than 6 points are suspicious of ASD.

TABLE 4 Atopy Score Based on Chi-Square Values without Laboratory Investigations

Atopic feature	Points	Chi-square	OR	95% CI of OR
Xerosis	3	429	27.9	23.2–33.8
Itch when sweating	3	410	25.4	21.1–30.1
White dermographism	3	357	19.3	16.2–23.2
Wool intolerance	3	355	15.8	13.4–18.5
Pityriasis alba	2	304	60.1	41.6–87.0
Infraorbital fold	2	292	11.0	9.4–12.7
Hertoghe sign	2	282	44.8	32.1–62.6
Palmar hyperlinearity	2	242	11.7	9.8–13.9
Ear rhaghade	2	236	19.2	15.2–24.4
Perlèche	1	201	7.0	6.1–8.2
Cradle cap	1	184	10.6	8.7–12.9
Family history of atopy	1	69	2.9	2.6–3.3
Facial pallor/erythema	1	117	5.3	4.5–6.3
Keratosis pilaris	1	103	4.9	4.2–5.8
Food intolerance	1	85	4.7	4.0–5.7
Allergic rhinitis	1	65	3.1	2.7–3.6
Allergic asthma	1	55	4.8	3.4–6.0
Metal sensitivity	1	55	2.7	2.4–3.1
Photophobia	1	41	2.6	2.3–3.1

Note: Atopy score: chi-square >350, 3 points; 350 > chi-square >220, 2 points; chi-square <220, 1 point. The statistical analysis is based on 428 AE patients and 628 noneczematous controls.

Adapted from Diepgen.[18]

2. Study 2

In the second study we evaluated the role of these atopic features in the development of HE. Therefore, we prospectively investigated the occurrence of atopic symptoms and signs in a case-control study of 458 patients with HE and in a noneczematous control group (NP) of 458 individuals matched by sex and age. During a 2-year period, in all inpatients and outpatients with HE at our HE clinic, atopic features as described elsewhere[30] were investigated consecutively. The median age in both groups was 26 years, and females predominated males (60 to 40%). According to the proposed score system, the distribution of the summarized atopic points in HE patients are shown in Figure 4. Independently, in the final diagnosis of the HE (atopic, allergic, irritative, nummular/tylotic) in 52% of the consecutively investigated patients with HE 10 or more points were found, in 19% between 7 and 9 points, and in only 29% less than 7 points. This investigation clearly demonstrates that atopic symptoms and signs play a major role in the development of HE.

In a further statistical analysis of this case-control study the importance of the different atopic features for the development of HE was estimated. Table 5 shows the frequencies of some atopic features in patients with HE and in noneczematous control subjects. Additionally, the ORs including 95% confidence intervals (CI) and the *p* values (chi-square test) are given. Dry skin or xerosis as a sign of ASD was found in 59% in HE and differed significantly from that found in noneczematous controls. Signs of an abnormaly low threshold for pruritis for nonspecific irritants, such as the atopic features wool intolerance and itch when sweating, were found to be significantly increased in patients with HE. Constitutional atopic signs, such as hyperlinear palms, keratosis pilaris, and white dermographism, were also found to be significantly increased in HE patients. Minor clinical manifestations often seen in ASD, e.g., perlèche and retroauricular rhagades, were significantly more common in patients with HE. The ORs of these features range from 6.2 to 2.6.

Laboratory markers, such as elevated serum IgE and a positive Phadiatop® test (specific radioallergosorbent tests of the eight most important inhalant allergens), showed in comparison with

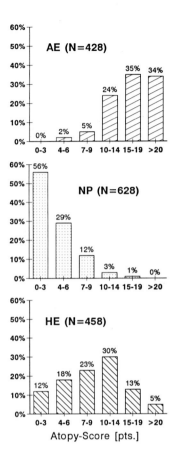

FIGURE 4. Distributions of evaluated points of an atopic skin diathesis[18] in patients with atopic eczema (AE, n = 428), noneczematous control subjects (NP, n = 628), and patients with hand eczema (HE, n = 458).

TABLE 5 **Frequencies of Some Atopic Features, Odds Ratios (OR), 95% Confidence Intervals, and *p*-Values (Chi-Square Test) of 458 Patients with HE and 458 Noneczematous Control Subjects (Matched Pairs According to Sex)**

Atopic feature	HE (%)	NP (%)	OR	95% CI	*p* value
High risk for developing HE					
Wool intolerance	46	15	4.6	3.4–6.4	>0.001
Palmar hyperlinearity	34	7	6.4	4.2–9.7	>0.001
Itch when sweating	30	8	5.3	3.5–7.9	>0.001
Keratosis pilaris	34	11	4.1	2.8–5.9	>0.001
Xerosis	59	28	3.7	2.8–4.9	>0.001
White dermographism	25	9	3.3	2.2–4.8	>0.001
Perlèche	35	16	2.7	2.0–3.8	>0.001
Low risk for developing HE					
Phadiatop positive	38	26	1.8	1.3–2.4	>0.001
Elevated IgE (>150 U/ml)	24	16	1.6	1.2–2.2	<0.01
Cradle cap	10	6	1.7	1.1–2.8	<0.05
Family history of atopy	34	33	—	—	NS
Allergic rhinitis	18	17	—	—	NS
Allergic asthma	5	5	—	—	NS

Note: $p < 0.001$.

TABLE 6 The Role of Sex and Endogenous Factors (Atopic Features) Related to HE According to a Multivariate Logistic Regression Analysis

Variable	β coefficient	Standard error	p value	Odds ratio	95% CI of OR
Intercept	−2.34	0.200	<0.0001		
Itch when sweating	1.62	0.238	<0.0001	5.07	3.18–8.09
Hyperlinear palms	1.45	0.249	<0.0001	4.25	2.61–6.93
Wool intolerance	1.35	0.207	<0.0001	3.87	2.57–5.81
Keratosis pilaris	0.95	0.229	<0.0001	2.59	1.65–4.07
Xerosis	0.87	0.187	<0.0001	2.38	1.65–3.44
White dermographism	0.86	0.262	<0.0001	2.37	1.42–3.96
Female sex	0.60	0.198	<0.001	1.82	1.23–2.68
Elevated IgE (>150 U/ml)	0.48	0.228	<0.05	1.61	1.03–2.53

our control group only low ORs. The family history of atopy and the personal history of respiratory (rhinitis and asthma) did not differ significantly. Additional endogenous factors hyperhidrosis and acrocyanosis (persistent dusky discoloration of the hands and feet) were found to be significantly more often seen in patients with HE than in control subjects (hyperhidrosis: HE 36%, NP 15%, OR 3.2, 95% CI 2.3 to 4.4; acrocyanosis: HE 27%, NP 8%, OR 4.0, 95% CI 2.8 to 5.9).

Previous studies have shown that HE is more common in women than in men.[31,32] The reason for this sex difference is not known, but one reason could be the greater exposure of women to wet work and surfactant.[2] Additionally, AE is also more common in females than in males.[33] By a multivariate logistic regression model the prognostic value of the investigated atopic features as risk factors for HE were analyzed under consideration of sex as an additional covariable (Table 6). According to stepwise (backward and forward) elimination technique the most important factors (OR >2.0) are itch when sweating, hyperlinear palms, wool intolerance, dry skin (xerosis), keratosis pilaris, and white dermographism. Female sex remains in the model as a significant covariable (OR 1.82) as well as elevated IgE (OR 1.61).

According to the study of Rystedt,[9] endogenous factors, such as eczematous involvement of the hands in childhood, persistent body eczema in childhood, and dry/itchy skin, were of predominant importance, whereas female sex, family history of atopy, and associated respiratory allergy were of lesser importance. In subjects with a respiratory allergy or family history of atopy, we propose the evaluation and validation of an array of atopic features to estimate the ASD, which seems to be an important endogenous risk factor for the development of HE. For vocational guidance this could also be helpful in noneczematous subjects and those with no history of childhood eczema.

In an epidemiological population-based study, Meding[34,35] investigated factors related to HE my mailed questionnaires in a random sample of the 20,000 individuals 20 to 65 years of age of the inhabitants of Gothenburg, Sweden. Of those individuals who reported having had childhood eczema, the reported period prevalence of HE (during the last 12 months) was 27.3% compared with 9.0% among the others. Excluding those who had had childhood eczema, the reported prevalence of HE decreased to 11.4% for individuals with asthma/hayfever compared with 8.5%. According to stepwise logistic regression analysis the five most important factors to HE were childhood eczema, female sex, occupational exposure (to solvents, oils, paints, glues, unspecific chemicals, cement, water and detergents, foodstuffs, plants and soil, dust and dry dirt, and coins), hayfever/asthma, and service occupation.

C. Metal Sensitivity, Atopy, and Hand Eczema

The incidence of nickel sensitivity appears to lie between 40 and 56% in patients with past or present HE.[1,36-39] In our 458 patients with HE a history of nickel allergy was found in 38%, which was significantly increased compared with the control group. Yet it must be taken into consideration that a number of other factors are known to be related to nickel sensitivity and play an important role in the development of HE in nickel-sensitive patients. The discussion of all the factors involved in the etiology of HE and nickel sensitivity is outside the scope of this chapter. One important aspect of the interrelationship between nickel sensitivity and HE could be the role of atopy, which

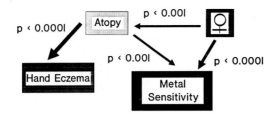

FIGURE 5.   Log-linear model of complex interrelationship among hand
eczema, history of metal sensitivity, and atopic skin diathesis.

is also discussed. In our study we also found a statistically significant increase of a history of metal
sensitivity (HMS) in subjects with a positive ASD (10 and more atopy points). Therefore, we
analyzed the complex interrelationship among HE, sex, ASD, and HMS by a multivariate model.[18]
According to this analysis (Figure 5), the strongest relationships were found between female sex
and HMS and between ASD and HE, and a less significant statistical association between ASD
and HMS. Using the multivariate analysis there was no longer a significant direct association
between HE and HMS. Atopy might trigger both the occurrence of HE and nickel sensitivity, but
these observations need further confirmation by additional studies.

V.   HAND ECZEMA AND OCCUPATIONAL SKIN DISEASES

More than 90% of work-related skin diseases are hand HE. However, most studies about endogenous
and exogenous factors of occupational dermatoses are based on inpatients or outpatients of hospitals
and are therefore not randomly selected. Thus, epidemiological conclusions without constraints are
not possible. There are only a few reports on systematic epidemiological investigations of occupational skin diseases.[40-46] The comparison of these studies is difficult because there is no uniform
definition of occupational skin diseases. Additionally, in most work-related HE there is rarely
anything about their location and appearance to differentiate clearly from dermatitis of nonoccupational origin.[47]

   According to the U.S. Department of Labor, skin disorders represented almost 50% of all
occupational illnesses in the U.S. in 1979.[5] Occupation-related skin problems are the most frequent
cause of workers' disability claims in Germany. In 1981 of 61,156 medical reports of an occupational
disease, 20,584 cases (34%) were related to occupational skin diseases. According to German law,
under No. 5101, i.e., occupational skin disorders without skin cancer (''severe or repeatedly
relapsing dermatoses which have clearly necessitated the cessation of all occupational activities
which were or could be responsible for causing the disease or its relapse or aggravation''). About
8% of all cases of workers' disability claims for dermatitis were reported in North Bavaria, in the
last years.

   In a population-based epidemiological study we prospectively investigated all closed cases of
occupational skin disease (OSD) that were registered between March 1990 and March 1992 in
North Bavaria according to possible involved risk factors. For these reasons, the data presented
are representative of the overall situation of occupational dermatoses in North Bavaria. The survey
of all these cases was performed prospectively and encompassed a record review of all case files
and medical records, a mailed questionnaire, and, if necessary, physical examination, patch test,
laboratory findings, and factory visiting.[46] Patch testing was performed in more than 92%. Of all
2582 cases, 1912 (74%) were diagnosed as having a pathological condition of the skin for which
occupational exposure can be shown to be a major causal, or contributory, factor. The aims of the
study were as follows: (1) to establish demographic characteristics, (2) to give frequencies of the
main diagnoses of OSD, and (3) to evaluate the roles of allergy and atopy. The basic data were
as follows: 1912 occupational dermatoses, 60% females (n = 1144), median of age 22 years; 40%
males (n = 768), median of age 32 years; 76% of all cases included hairdressers (26%), metalworkers (19%), health services (11%), food handlers (10%), construction workers (7%), and

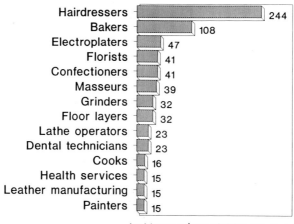

Incidences (per 10,000 employed)

FIGURE 6. Incidences of occupational skin diseases in North Bavaria (number of new cases of OSD per 10,000 employed in 1-year period).

cleaners (3%). The median age of onset was lowest in hairdressers (median 19 years) and highest in cleaners (median 39 years). Based on the number of employees in the different occupations in the same area of North Bavaria during that time, the incidences for work-related skin diseases in the different occupations could be calculated (Figure 6). The highest incidences were estimated for hairdressers and bakers. In South Carolina the average incidence for all industries was 10.8% per 10,000 employees.[5]

In our study the most common diagnoses were allergic contact eczema (females 55%; males 44%) and irritant contact eczema (females 52%; males 60%). In 92% of all OSD the hands were involved. Figure 7 details the main diagnoses of OSD. Isolated allergic contact eczema occurred in 33%, irritant contact eczema in 34%, the combination of allergic and irritant contact eczema in 9%, and in 18% an isolated or additional AE was diagnosed. The ratio of irritant to allergic contact eczema was found in hairdressers (68%) and construction workers (71%), mostly irritant contact eczema in food handlers (75%), metalworkers (66%), and cleaners (64%). OSDs in health services were in 53% of irritant and in 54% of allergic origin. The percentages of work-related allergies differed in the main professions as follows: according to patch test results at least one work-related allergy was found in hairdressers in 74%, in construction workers in 72%, in health services in 55%, in cleaners in 41%, in food handlers in 39%, and in metalworkers in 37%. The most frequent delayed-type sensitizations were diagnosed against nickel sulfate, cobalt chloride, glyceryl mon-

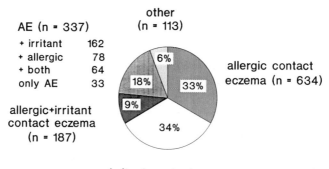

FIGURE 7. Main diagnoses of occupational skin diseases in North Bavaria.

othioglycolate, *p*-phenylenediamine, potassium dichromate, ammonium persulfate, toluylene diamine sulfate, isothiazolinone, and fragrance mixture.

According to our analysis, atopy seems to play an important role in OSD. Female subjects with OSD had in 45%, males in 39% an ASD. These observations correspond with other studies: Keil and Shmunes[5] estimated that atopics have a 13.5 times greater risk of developing an OSD than nonatopics. The prevalence of a personal or family history of atopy was found in 101 of the 134 respondents to a mailed questionnaire.[5] However, retrospective studies based on mailed questionnaire could be biased heavily. According to a study performed in Singapore,[41] 35% of cases with contact dermatitis were occupational eczema. In this epidemiological comparison between occupational and nonoccupational HE, in the occupational group a significantly larger proportion of males (65% versus 51%), a lower prevalence of a personal or family history of atopy (7% versus 15%), and a larger proportion of irritant contact dermatitis (76% versus 39%) were found.[41] In Australia, atopy was more prevalent in females with OSD (62%) than males (39%).[43] In an epidemiological study of dermatoses in construction workers[42] a history of atopy was present in 32 (24%) of 133 cases of eczema compared with only 35 (11%) of 327 noneczematous controls. The highest proportion of atopics (24%) was in irritant dermatitis. In our study, of 126 construction workers with OSD the percentage of atopics was found to be 27%.

REFERENCES

1. Wilkinson, D. S. and Wilkinson, J. D., Nickel allergy and hand eczema, in *Nickel and the Skin: Immunology and Toxicology,* Maibach, H. I. and Menné, T., Eds., CRC Press, Boca Raton, FL, 1989, 133.
2. Epstein, E., Hand dermatitis: practical management and current concepts, *J. Am. Acad. Dermatol.,* 10, 395, 1984.
3. Lammintausta, K. and Kalimo, K., Atopy and hand dermatitis in hospital wet work, *Contact Dermatitis,* 7, 301, 1981.
4. Lammintausta, K., Risk Factors for Hand Dermatitis in Wet Work, Ph.D. thesis, University of Turku, Finland, 1982.
5. Keil, J. E. and Shmunes, E., The epidemiology of work-related skin diseases in South Carolina, *Arch. Dermatol.,* 119, 650, 1983.
6. Forsbeck, M., Skog, E., and Asbrink, E., Atopic hand dermatitis: a comparison with atopic dermatitis without hand involvement, especially with respect to influence of work and development of contact sensitization, *Acta Derm. Venereol.,* 63, 9, 1983.
7. Shmunes, E. and Keil, J. E., The role of atopy in occupational dermatoses, *Contact Dermatitis,* 11, 174, 1984.
8. Rystedt, I., Factors influencing the occurrence of hand eczema in adults with a history of atopic dermatitis in childhood, *Contact Dermatitis,* 12, 185, 1985.
9. Rystedt, I., Hand eczema and long-term prognosis in atopic dermatitis, *Acta Derm. Venereol.,* 117, 1, 1985.
10. Bäurle, G., Hornstein, O. P., and Diepgen, T. L., Professionelle Handkzeme und Atopie. Eine klinische Prospektivstudie zur Frage des Zusammenhangs, *Dermatosen,* 33, 161, 1985.
11. Bäurle, G., Hornstein, O. P., and Diepgen, T. L., Atopic als Kausal- und Kofaktor bei der Entstehung und Unterhaltung beruflicher Ekzeme, *Arbeitsmed. Sozialmed. Praeventivmed.,* 20, 100, 1985.
12. Nilsson, G. E., Mikaelsson, B., and Andersson, S., Atopy, occupation and domestic work as risk factors for hand eczema in hospital workers, *Contact Dermatitis,* 13, 216, 1985.
13. Nilsson, E., Individual and environmental risk factors for hand eczema in hospital workers, *Acta Derm. Venereol.,* 128 (Suppl.), 1, 1986.
14. Fartasch, M., Diepgen, T. L., Meister, G., and Hornstein, O. P., Diagnostik der Handekzeme und Relevanz der atopischen Diathese als ätiologischer Kausalfaktor, in *Aktuelle Beiträge zu Umwelt und Berufskrankheiten der Haut,* Hornstein, O. P., Ed., BMV-Verlag, Berlin, 1991, 105.
15. Fartasch, M., Diepgen, T. L., and Hornstein, O. P., Evaluation of endogenous factors and metal sensitivity in hand eczema, *Contact Dermatitis,* 23 (Abstr.), 281, 1990.

16. Cronin, E., Bandmann, H.-J., Calnan, C. D., Fregert, S., Hjorth, N., Magnuson, B., Maibach, H. I., Malten, K., Meneghini, C. L., Pirilä, V., and Wilkinson, D. S., Contact dermatitis in the atopic, *Acta Derm. Venereol.*, 50, 183, 1970.
17. Breit, R., Leutgeb, Ch., and Bandmann, H. J., Zum neurodermitischen Handekzem, *Arch. Dermatol. Forsch.*, 244, 353, 1972.
18. Diepgen, T. L., *Die atopische Hautdiathese*, Gentner, Stuttgart, 1991, 51.
19. Cronin, E., Clinical patterns of hand eczema in women, *Contact Dermatitis*, 13, 153, 1985.
20. Meding, B. and Swanbeck, G., Predictive factors for hand eczema, *Contact Dermatitis*, 23, 154, 1990.
21. Lodi, A., Betti, R., Chiarelli, G., Urbani, C. E., and Crosti, C., Epidemiological, clinical and allergological observations on pompholyx, *Contact Dermatitis*, 26, 17, 1992.
22. Diepgen, T. L., unpublished data.
23. Glickman, F. S. and Silvers, S. H., Hand eczema and atopy in housewives, *Arch. Dermatol.*, 95, 487, 1967.
24. Hanifin, J. M. and Rajka, G., Diagnostic features of atopic dermatitis, *Acta Derm. Venereol.*, 92 (Suppl.), 44, 1980.
25. Diepgen, T. L., Fartasch, M., Bäurle, G., and Hornstein, O. P., Atopiekriterien in der Normalbevölkerung: berufliche Konsequenzen, *Dermatosen*, 37, 222, 1989.
26. Diepgen, T. L., Fartasch, M., and Hornstein, O. P., Evaluation and relevance of atopic basic and minor features in patients with atopic dermatitis and in the general population, *Acta Derm. Venereol.*, 144 (Suppl.), 50, 1989.
27. Diepgen, T. L. and Fartasch, M., Stigmata and signs of atopic eczema, in *New Trends in Allergy*, Vol. 3, Ring, J., and Przybilla, B., Eds., Springer-Verlag, Berlin, 1991, 222.
28. Diepgen, T. L. and Fartasch, M., Statistische Evaluierung klinisch-diagnostischer Kriterien beim atopischen Ekzem, *Allergologie*, 8, 301, 1991.
29. Diepgen, T. L. and Fartasch, M., Recent epidemiological and genetic studies in atopic dermatitis, *Acta Derm. Venereol.*, 176, 13, 1992.
30. Diepgen, T. L., Fartasch, M., and Hornstein, O. P., Kriterien zur Beurteilung der atopischen Hautdiathese, *Dermatosen*, 39, 79, 1991.
31. Agrup, G., Hand eczema and other dermatoses in South Sweden, *Acta Derm. Venereol.*, 61, 1, 1969.
32. Peltonen, L., Nickel sensitivity in the general population, *Contact Dermatitis*, 5, 27, 1979.
33. Rajka, G., *Essential Aspects of Atopic Dermatitis*, Springer, New York, 1989.
34. Meding, B. and Swanbeck, G., Prevalence of hand eczema in an industrial city, *Br. J. Dermatol.*, 116, 527, 1987.
35. Meding, B., Epidemiology of hand eczema in an industrial city, *Acta Derm. Venereol.*, 153, 1, 1989.
36. Christensen, O. B. and Möller, H., Nickel allergy and hand eczema, *Contact Dermatitis*, 1, 129, 1975.
37. Menné, T., Borgen, O., and Green, A., Nickel allergy and hand dermatitis in a stratified sample of the danish female population: an epidemiological study including a statistics appendix, *Acta Derm. Venereol.*, 62, 35, 1982.
38. Wahlberg, J. E. and Skog, E., Nickel allergy and atopy: threshold of nickel sensitivity and immunoglobulin E determinations, *Br. J. Dermatol.*, 85, 97, 1971.
39. Cronin, E., Nickel, in *Contact Dermatitis*, Cronin, E., Ed., Churchill Livingstone, Edinburgh, 1980, chap. 7.
40. Plotnick, H., Analysis of 250 consecutively evaluated cases of workers' disability claims for dermatitis, *Arch Dermatol.*, 126, 782, 1990.
41. Goh, C. L., An epidemiological comparison between occupational and non-occupational hand eczema, *Br. J. Dermatol.*, 120, 77, 1989.
42. Coenraads, P. J., Nater, J. P., Jansen, H. A., and Lantinga, H., Prevalence in construction workers in the Netherlands, *Clin. Exp. Dermatol.*, 9, 149, 1984.
43. Wall, L. M. and Gebauer, K. A., Occupational skin disease in Western Australia, *Contact Dermatitis*, 24, 101, 1991.
44. Wall, L. M. and Gebauer, K. A., A follow-up study of occupational skin disease in Western Australia, *Contact Dermatitis*, 24, 241, 1991.

45. Meding, B. and Swanbeck, G., Occupational hand eczema in an industrial city, *Contact Dermatitis*, 22, 13, 1990.
46. Diepgen, T. L., Schmidt, A., Schmidt, M., and Fartasch, M., Epidemiologie berufsbedinger Hautkrankheiten in Nordbayern, *Z. Hautkr.*, 66 935, 1991.
47. Adams, R., Medicolegal aspects of occupational skin diseases, in *Dermatologic Clinics: Occupational Dermatoses*, Taylor, J. S., Ed., W. B. Saunders, Philadelphia, 1988, 121.

17

Epidemiology of Hand Eczema

Birgitta Meding

CONTENTS

I. INTRODUCTION

Hand eczema is a common cause of medical consultation for skin disease. It is also the most important occupational skin disease. There are several reports on the prevalence of hand eczema, in particular from the Scandinavian countries. Agrup[1] reported the prevalence to be 2 to 3% in the general population of mainly rural parts of south Sweden in the mid-1960s. In a Finnish population selected for studying nickel allergy in 1976–77, Peltonen[2] found the prevalence of hand eczema to be 4%. Menné et al.[3] in 1982 reported a cumulative incidence of 22% in Danish women. In Tromsö, Norway, the 1-year period prevalence of allergic hand eczema was estimated to 8.9% by Kavli and Förde[4] in 1979. In the Netherlands, the 3-year period prevalence was reported to be 6 to 7% in two samples of the general population.[5,6]

To estimate with sufficient precision the distribution of a disease and its consequences, it is desirable to obtain information from the general population. This is also of value for allocating health care resources and planning preventive measures. To estimate the occurrence and importance of hand eczema in the general population of a large industrial city, Gothenburg, Sweden, an epidemiologic study was performed in 1983–84.[7-12]

II. STUDY DESIGN

In Sweden, population registers are kept by the County Administrations. From the 1982 register of Gothenburg a random sample of 20,000 individuals, aged 20 to 65 years, was drawn. These individuals received a mailed questionnaire asking about the occurrence of hand eczema on some occasion in the previous 12 months, atopy history, occupation, and occupational exposure. Answers were obtained from 83% (16,584 subjects). Those who reported hand eczema were invited to a dermatological examination including patch testing with a standard series and, when appropriate, with complementary test substances — 71% attended the examination. Nonresponse and nonattendance were investigated via telephone interviews.

The design of the study was thus cross-sectional, i.e., a prevalence study. Point prevalence (or simply, prevalence) is the proportion of diseased individuals at a certain point in time. For a relapsing disease such as hand eczema, period prevalence can also be a useful measure — meaning the proportion of individuals having the disease at any time during a defined period, e.g., 1 year. The term hand eczema covered allergic contact dermatitis, irritant dermatitis, atopic hand eczema, nummular eczema, hyperkeratotic dermatitis of the palms, and pompholyx.

III. PREVALENCE OF HAND ECZEMA

Of the 16,584 responders to the questionnaire, 11.8% reported having hand eczema on some occasion in the previous 12 months. Taking into account several possible sources of error, such as different response rate according to age, wrong self-diagnoses, actual symptoms at the time of dermatological examination, and the results of the dropout analysis, the 1-year period prevalence was estimated to be 10.6% and the point prevalence 5.4%. The error in these proportions was estimated to be not larger than ±0.1%. Hand eczema was almost twice as common in females as in males, with a ratio of 1.9, and particularly was more frequent in young females (Figure 1). Hand eczema being more common among women has also been observed in other prevalence studies.[1,4-6]

IV. TYPES OF HAND ECZEMA

The most common types of hand eczema were irritant dermatitis (35%), atopic hand eczema (22%), and allergic contact dermatitis (19%). The corresponding female/male ratios were 2.6, 1.9, and 5.4, respectively. The point prevalence in different age groups is illustrated in Figures 2 and 3. The figures are minimum figures, not corrected for dropouts.

The most frequent positive patch test results are shown in Table 1. Totally, 32% of the patients had one or more positive reactions to the standard series. The results resemble those of other publications on patch test results.[13,14] When comparing the different occupational groups the only

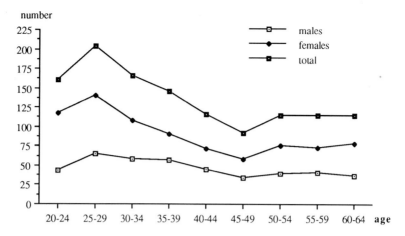

FIGURE 1.   Number of hand eczema patients in relation to age and sex.

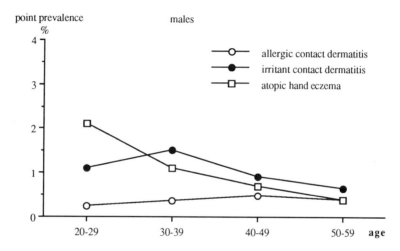

FIGURE 2.   Point prevalence of the three most common types of hand eczema in men in relation to age (minimum figures).

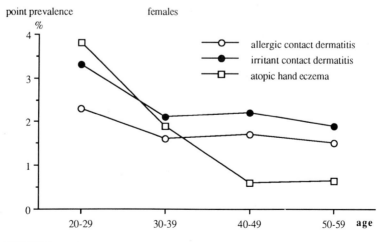

FIGURE 3.   Point prevalence of the three most common types of hand eczema in females in relation to age (minimum figures).

TABLE 1   The Most Frequent Positive Test
Reactions to the Standard Series in
1081 Patients (Females, 67%)

Test substance	Conc. (%)	Total (%)
Nickel sulfate	5	14.8
Cobalt chloride	1	6.7
Fragrance mix	16	5.8
Balsam of Peru	25	4.9
Colophony	20	3.2
Thiuram mix	1	1.8
Neomycin sulfate	20	1.8
Carba mix	3	1.7
Formaldehyde	2	1.6
Potassium dichromate	0.5	1.5

Note: The vehicle used was petrolatum, except for formaldehyde where water was used.

statistically significant increase in the prevalence of a contact allergy was noted among women in administrative work for colophony (p <0.01). Whether this is attributable to exposure to rosin in paper[15-17] is not known, but this is an hypothesis for further research.

Hand eczema was shown to be a long-lasting disease, with a mean duration of 12 years from the first appearance to the time of examination. A relapsing course was reported, with 77% having eczema-free intervals. This implies that the prognosis for a total cure is not very favorable. It might be improved by better treatment and more careful instructions to the patients about preventive measures.

V.   OCCUPATION AND HAND ECZEMA

Experience, clinical observations, and earlier studies indicate that some occupations involve a higher risk of hand eczema than others, e.g., hospital workers who perform wet work.[18,19]

The questionnaire included questions on occupation and occupational exposure. Not unexpect- edly, those who reported any of the exposures listed had a higher risk of hand eczema, 1.6, than those who had jobs that did not expose the hands. The most harmful exposures seemed to be to water and detergents, dust and dry dirt, and to unspecified chemicals.

Service occupations had a statistically significant higher period prevalence of hand eczema than other groups (15%). The occupation with the overall highest period prevalence was cleaning (21%). Otherwise, the differences between occupations were not very large when age and sex differences were taken into consideration. One of the main reasons for this is probably the cross-sectional design of the study, which does not afford information on changes over time. People with eczematous tendencies may avoid certain occupations, thus equalizing the prevalence of hand eczema in different occupations and masking its harmfulness — the "healthy worker effect". To compare the risk in different occupations, a different study design should be used.

One way of estimating the relationship between a particular occupation and hand eczema is to study job changes caused by the condition. All the hand eczema patients interviewed were asked this question. It showed that change of jobs also was most frequent in service occupations. The abandoned occupations, in relation to the number of individuals in each occupation, are shown in Table 2. That hairdressing tops the list is not surprising.[20-22]

VI.   CONSEQUENCES OF HAVING HAND ECZEMA

Having hand eczema is inconvenient. It causes disturbances in the patient's daily life, and social consequences in the form of loss of working days and costs for medical care.

TABLE 2   The Occupations Most
Frequently Abandoned
Because of Hand Eczema

Occupation	%[a]
Hairdresser	18
Baker	11
Dental nurse	5
Cleaner	4
Kitchen maid	4
Cook	4
Machine tool operator	3
Practical nurse	2

[a]   Proportion of total number of individuals in
each occupation.

Of the hand eczema patients, 69% had visited a doctor at least once and 21% had been on sick leave (minimum 7 days) on one occasion or more. A few persons had a very long total sick leave, with a high mean of 19 weeks, and a median of 8 weeks.

Some kind of disturbance attributable to hand eczema, at work or during leisure time, was reported by 81% of the hand eczema patients. Women seemed to be more concerned than men. Every third patient reported cosmetic problems influencing interpersonal relations. Frequent itching was reported by just over half the patients and occasional itching by another third.

Information of this kind, of course, is subjective and has to be interpreted cautiously. However, to be able to offer the patient optimal care it is important to consider the impact of the disease on the patient's total situation. There are only a few publications on the psychosocial influences of skin disease, mostly regarding psoriasis.[23-25] More documentation and research in this field is desirable.

VII.   SEVERITY OF HAND ECZEMA

The severity of hand eczema can be estimated from different parameters such as duration, continuity of symptoms, extent of involvement of the hands, need for medical consultations, treatment, sick leave, and whether the hand eczema causes a change of work. Taking all these parameters into account when comparing the three most common diagnoses, it is obvious that irritant dermatitis is the mildest form of hand eczema. An investigation performed on a sample of the general population includes mild cases of irritant contact dermatitis. Allergic contact dermatitis presents the most serious consequences, but atopic hand eczema is a more widespread and longstanding disease.

VIII.   HAND ECZEMA AND ATOPY

Atopics have an increased risk of hand eczema. This was clearly confirmed in studies by Rystedt,[26] Lammintausta and Kalimo,[27] and Nilsson et al.[28] In the Gothenburg study, 10% of the persons who answered the questionnaire reported childhood eczema, 6% bronchial asthma, and 17% hay fever on some occasion. Of the 1238 individuals with hand eczema, 27% reported childhood eczema. Among those with childhood eczema, a threefold increase in the risk of hand eczema was found. For persons with asthma/hay fever, the hand eczema risk was increased by 1.6 times.

The relevant question in the questionnaire concerned childhood eczema. Hence, the answers include not only atopic dermatitis, but also other types. From other studies of childhood eczema[29] one can estimate 70 to 80% as being atopic dermatitis. Young persons reported childhood eczema far more often than older people (Figure 4). This indicates that the prevalence of atopic dermatitis is increasing, as do other epidemiological studies of atopy.[30-33]

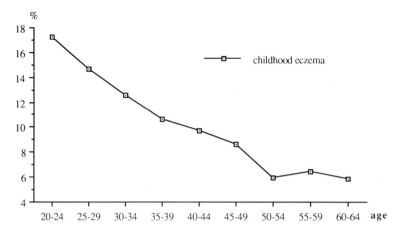

FIGURE 4. History of childhood eczema in relation to age (n = 16,584). (From Meding, B. and Swanbeck, G., *Contact Dermatitis*, 23, 154, 1990. With permission.)

IX. PREDICTIVE FACTORS FOR HAND ECZEMA

In the study, information was obtained on the following factors possibly related to hand eczema: age, sex, occupation, occupational exposure, childhood eczema, and asthma/hay fever. The relative importance of these factors was evaluated by using stepwise multiple logistic regression analysis. The most important predictive factor for hand eczema turned out to be a history of childhood eczema, followed by sex, occupational exposure, asthma/hay fever, service occupation, and age (negatively correlated). From this analysis it is possible to calculate the risk for an individual to develop hand eczema in a 12-month period. Examples are shown in Figure 5.

X. COMMENTS

Since the prevalence of atopic dermatitis is increasing, and as it is the most important predictive factor for hand eczema, a rising prevalence of hand eczema can be expected in the future. There

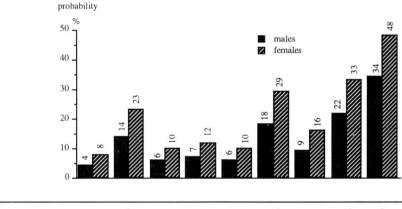

childhood eczema	-	+	-	-	-	+	-	+	+
hay fever/asthma	-	-	+	-	-	+	-	-	+
occupational exposure	-	-	-	+	-	-	+	+	+
service occupation	-	-	-	-	+	-	+	-	+

FIGURE 5. Example of the estimated probability of hand eczema on some occasion during a 12-month period in relation to sex, childhood eczema, hay fever/asthma, occupational exposure, and service occupation. (From Meding, B. and Swanbeck, G., *Contact Dermatitis*, 23, 154, 1990. With permission.)

are indications that an increase has in fact taken place in the last few decades. In Agrup's[1] study of hand dermatoses in the mid-1960s the prevalence of hand eczema was about half of that found in Gothenburg 20 years later. Comparing the different diagnoses it is obvious that the increase mostly concerns atopic hand eczema. The diagnostic criteria were mainly the same in the two studies.

This prediction very strongly suggests a need for further research and the improvement of treatment and preventive measures regarding hand eczema.

REFERENCES

1. Agrup, G., Hand eczema and other hand dermatoses in South Sweden, *Acta Derm. Venereol. Stockholm,* 49 (Suppl. 61), 1969.
2. Peltonen, L., Nickel sensitivity in the general population, *Contact Dermatitis,* 5, 27, 1979.
3. Menné, T., Borgan, Ö., and Green, A., Nickel allergy and hand dermatitis in a stratified sample of the Danish female population: an epidemiologic study including a statistic appendix, *Acta Derm. Venereol. Stockholm,* 62, 35, 1982.
4. Kavli, G. and Förde, O. H., Hand dermatoses in Tromsö, *Contact Dermatitis,* 10, 174, 1984.
5. Coenraads, P. J., Nater, J. P., and van der Lende, R., Prevalence of eczema and other dermatoses of the hands and arms in the Netherlands. Association with age and occupation, *Clin. Exp. Dermatol.,* 8, 495, 1983.
6. Lantinga, H., Nater, J. P., and Coenraads, P. J., Prevalence, incidence and course of eczema on the hands and forearms in a sample of the general population, *Contact Dermatitis,* 10, 135, 1984.
7. Meding, B., Epidemiology of hand eczema in an industrial city, *Acta Derm. Venereol. Stockholm,* Suppl. 153, 1990.
8. Meding, B. and Swanbeck, G., Prevalence of hand eczema in an industrial city, *Br. J. Dermatol.,* 116, 627, 1987.
9. Meding, B. and Swanbeck, G., Epidemiology of different types of hand eczema in an industrial city, *Acta Derm. Venereol. Stockholm,* 69, 227, 1989.
10. Meding, B. and Swanbeck, G., Occupational hand eczema in an industrial city, *Contact Dermatitis,* 22, 13, 1990.
11. Meding, B. and Swanbeck, G., Consequences of having hand eczema, *Contact Dermatitis,* 23, 6, 1990.
12. Meding, B. and Swanbeck, G., Predictive factors for hand eczema, *Contact Dermatitis,* 23, 154, 1990.
13. Lynde, C. W., Warshawski, L., and Mitchell, J. C., Screening patch tests in 4190 eczema patients 1972–81, *Contact Dermatitis,* 8, 417, 1982.
14. Enders, F., Przybilla, B., Ring, J., Burg, G., and Braun-Falco, O., Epikutantestung mit einer Standardreihe. Ergebnisse bei 12026 Patienten, *Hautartz,* 39, 779, 1988.
15. Wikström, K., Allergic contact dermatitis caused by paper, *Acta Derm. Venereol. Stockholm,* 49, 547, 1969.
16. Bergmark, G. and Meding, B., Allergic contact dermatitis from newsprint paper, *Contact Dermatitis,* 9, 330, 1983.
17. Karlberg, A.-T. and Lidén, C., Colophony (rosin) in newspapers may contribute to hand eczema, *Br. J. Dermatol.,* 126, 161, 1992.
18. Lammintausta, K., Hand dermatitis in different hospital workers, who perform wet work, *Dermatosen,* 31, 14, 1983.
19. Singgih, S. I. R., Lantinga, H., Nater, J. P., Woest, T. E., and Kruyt-Gaspersz, J. A., Occupational hand dermatoses in hospital cleaning personnel, *Contact Dermatitis,* 14, 14, 1986.
20. Marks, R. and Cronin, E., Hand eczema in hairdressers, *Aust. J. Dermatol.,* 18, 123, 1977.
21. Cronin, E. and Kullavanijaya, P., Hand dermatitis in hairdressers, *Acta Derm. Venereol. Stockholm,* 59 (Suppl. 85), 47, 1979.
22. Lindemayr, H., Das Friseurekzem, *Dermatosen,* 32, 5, 1984.

23. Jobling, R. G., Psoriasis — a preliminary questionnaire study of sufferers' subjective experience, *Clin. Exp. Dermatol.,* 1, 233, 1976.

24. Stankler, L., The effect of psoriasis on the sufferer, *Clin. Exp. Dermatol.,* 6, 303, 1981.

25. Jowett, S. and Ryan, T., Skin disease and handicap: an analysis of the impact of skin conditions, *Soc. Sci. Med.,* 20, 425, 1985.

26. Rystedt, I., Hand eczema in patients with history of atopic manifestations in childhood, *Acta Derm. Venereol. Stockholm,* 65, 305, 1985.

27. Lammintausta, K. and Kalimo, K., Atopy and hand dermatitis in hospital wet work, *Contact Dermatitis,* 7, 301, 1981.

28. Nilsson, E., Mikaelsson, B., and Andersson, S., Atopy, occupation and domestic work as risk factors for hand eczema in hospital workers, *Contact Dermatitis,* 13, 216, 1985.

29. Hambly, E. M. and Wilkinson, D. S., Sur quelques formes atypiques d'eczéma chez l'enfant, *Ann. Dermatol. Venereol. Paris,* 105, 369, 1978.

30. Taylor, B., Wadsworth, J., Wadsworth, M., and Peckham, C., Changes in the reported prevalence of childhood eczema since the 1939–45 war, *Lancet,* 2, 1255, 1984.

31. Schultz-Larsen, F., Holm, N. V., and Henningsen, K., Atopic dermatitis. A genetic-epidemiologic study in a population-based twin sample, *J. Am. Acad. Dermatol.,* 15, 487, 1986.

32. Åberg, N., Engström, I., and Lindberg, U., Allergic diseases in Swedish school children, *Acta Paediatr. Scand.,* 78, 246, 1989.

33. Haahtela, T., Heiskala, M., and Suoniemi, I., Allergic disorders and immediate skin test reactivity in Finnish adolescents, *Allergy,* 35, 433, 1980.

18

Principles of Occupational Hand Eczema

Magnus Bruze

CONTENTS

0-8493-7355-7/94/$0.00 + $.50
© 1994 by CRC Press, Inc.

I. INTRODUCTION

For dermatologists, and even for general practitioners, hand eczema is a common cause for consultation. Of course, this reflects the fact that hand eczema is common in the general population, but it probably also reflects the profound effects hand eczema may have occupationally and socioeconomically, both in terms of influence on beginning a job as well as the possibility of continuing a particular job, and causation of various disturbances of daily life activities.[1,2]

In an industrial city the 1-year period prevalence of hand eczema was estimated to be around 11% and the prevalence at a certain time 5.4%.[1] In a Finnish population of approximately 1000 persons, the hands were examined and eczema was found in 4%.[3] A cumulative hand eczema incidence of 22% was reported in a sample of Danish women.[4] In two samples of the general population in the Netherlands a 3-year period prevalence of hand eczema was found to be 6 to 7%.[5]

Occupational dermatitis was diagnosed in 30% of the men and 12% of the women in a joint European study of consecutive clinic patients with dermatitis.[6] In different countries dermatoses comprise 20 to 70% of all occupational diseases and 20 to 90% of the dermatoses are contact dermatitises.[6-13] Furthermore, the hands, either alone or together with other sites, are affected in 80 to 90% of the cases of occupational contact dermatitis.[6,14,15]

From the referred figures it is obvious that occupational hand eczema (OHE) is sufficiently common to expect a wide knowledge of the condition among dermatologists. Furthermore, it is a condition caused by exogenous factors, which means that correct diagnosis and characterization of the causative agent(s) are necessary prerequisites for successful preventive measures to lessen a possibly great impact on the subject's well-being and financial situation.[1,2,7,11,16-18]

II. DEFINITION

The three words comprising OHE often cause difficulties in defining them precisely. The last word, "eczema", is often used interchangeably with dermatitis by dermatologists. Some dermatologists use the term dermatitis for the acute stages and the term eczema for the subacute and chronic stages of the disease.[19] However, dermatitis simply means inflammation of the skin and encompasses a wide spectrum of disorders. Eczema is synonymous with eczematous dermatitis and refers to the generation of serous exudate in the epidermis (spongiosis, histologically) causing papules and vesicles.[20,21] These efflorescences are characteristic for the acute stages of eczemas while the subacute and chronic stages are characterized more by scaling and lichenification, making the differentiation from other types of dermatitis hard. However, histologically the subacute and chronic stages display the eczematous features with spongiosis accompanied by lymphocytosis,[20,21] and when the course of the skin disease is followed frequently in patients with subacute and chronic eczema, exacerbations with the typical morphological features of acute eczema will be seen now and then. In this chapter the word eczema refers to all stages of eczematous dermatitis.

Usually, eczemas are divided into two major groups: exogenous and endogenous eczemas (Table 1). The exogenous group in Table 1 includes some eczemas that are rarely discussed. However, both infective eczema (if existing) and dermatophytide present with eczematous features macroscopically and microscopically, and both are caused by microorganisms, which is why these two eczemas have been included in this chapter. On the other hand, phototoxic contact dermatitis is not included, although it is usually discussed together with irritant, allergic, and photoallergic contact dermatitis.

However, even if phototoxic contact dermatitis principally is caused by the same type of chemicals and ultraviolet radiation as the other major exogenous dermatitises listed in Table 1, it is not an eczematous dermatitis.[22]

The second word, "hand", in OHE does not need any additional elucidation. By definition, all exogenous eczemas can localize to the hand and this is also true for most endogenous eczemas (Table 1).

The first word, "occupational", is the hardest to define. A medical definition adopted by the Committee on Occupational Dermatoses of the American Medical Association (1939) was "An occupational dermatosis is a pathological condition of the skin for which occupational exposure can be shown to be a major causal or contributory factor."[7,23] Occupational dermatoses are also

TABLE 1   Examples of Exogenous and Endogenous Eczematous Dermatitis, Their Location, and Occupational Connection

Eczema type	Hand localization	Occupational connection Causation	Occupational connection Aggravation
Exogenous dermatitis			
Irritant contact dermatitis	x	x	x
Allergic contact dermatitis	x	x	x
Photoallergic contact dermatitis	x	x	x
Infective dermatitis	x	x	x
Dermatophytide	x	x	x
Post-traumatic eczema	x	x	x
Endogenous dermatitis			
Atopic dermatitis	x		x
Seborrhoic dermatitis			x
Asteatotic eczema	x		x
Nummular eczema	x		x
Neurodermatitis (lichen simplex)	x		x
Stasis dermatitis			x
Hyperkeratotic palmar dermatitis	x		x
Pompholyx (dyshidrotic eczema)	x		x

defined as cutaneous abnormalities primarily caused by components of the work environment,[24] or a skin disease which would not have occurred if the patient had not been doing the work or in that occupation.[25] These medical definitions include the various exogenous eczemas listed in Table 1 as possible occupational dermatoses. However, the medico-legal definitions of occupational dermatosis can differ from the medical definitions and can also vary from one country to another. For example, in Sweden and the U.S. a substantial aggravation of an endogenous hand eczema can be approved and compensated for as an occupational dermatosis (the aggravation), provided there is reasonable probability that the aggravation was caused by work exposures.[21] With this legislation, it is important to know which endogenous eczemas can present as hand eczema (Table 1).

III. DIAGNOSIS

Considering the difficulties in arriving at an indisputable definition of OHE it is obvious that there is no single and easy way to diagnose OHE. Making the diagnosis is the final step in a series of steps and evaluations founded on facts, but also includes assessments more or less influenced by the dermatologist's interest in, and knowledge of, occupational dermatology. Circumstances and conditions considered to be evidence in favor of an OHE are

1. Exposure to agents known to have caused hand eczema
2. Occurrence of hand eczema in fellow workers or within the same occupation
3. Correct time relationship between exposure and onset of hand eczema
4. Anatomical distribution of lesions consistent with exposure
5. Attacks of hand eczema after exposure and improvement or clearing after exposure ceases
6. Patch and provocation tests supporting history and examination [7,15,24,26-30]

Expressed slightly differently, a diagnosis of OHE requires (1) identification of an occupational hazardous factor, (2) exposure to this factor, and (3) demonstration of a relationship between this hazardous exposure and the dermatitis under investigation with regard to its type, localization, and course.

A. Hazardous Exposures

The first and necessary step in the development of OHE is occupational exposure to a hazardous factor. There are three major groups of hazardous factors: chemical compounds, physical factors, and microorganisms.

TABLE 2   The Induction of Various Exogenous Eczemas Caused by Various Hazardous Exposures

	Induction of eczema			
Exogenous eczema	Chemically	Physically	Chemically and physically	By microorganism
Irritant contact dermatitis	x	x		
Allergic contact dermatitis	x			
Photoallergic contact dermatitis			x	
Infective dermatitis				x
Dermatophytide				x
Post-traumatic eczema	x	x		

Table 2 shows the various exogenous eczemas that can be caused by the different hazardous factors. An irritant contact dermatitis can either be induced chemically or physically. Many substances are known irritants and they exert their irritancy in different ways which can give rise to different irritant reactions, including chemical burns.[31] Various physical factors such as radiation, heat, cold, high and low humidity, and mechanical irritation can damage/influence the skin in different ways.[32] Still, one of the intriguing issues concerning irritant contact dermatitis is the transformation from a pure irritant reaction type of dermatitis to an eczematous one.[33] Commonly, an allergic contact dermatitis is preceded by an irritant contact dermatitis. An allergic contact dermatitis is always caused by a chemical substance. However, in natural and synthetic compound products sometimes the nature of the sensitizer is not known. Presently, approximately 3000 compounds are known contact sensitizers[34] and this figure is constantly increasing as new compounds are established as sensitizers. These sensitizers are low molecular weight substances — most of them with a molecular weight under 600. Photoallergic contact dermatitis can be considered to be the result of the combined effect of exposure to a chemical and a physical factor. The physical factor, of course, is ultraviolet radiation (most often, long-wave ultraviolet radiation) and the chemical factor is similar to, and sometimes the same as, the substances which can cause an allergic contact dermatitis.

Both irritant, allergic, and photoallergic contact dermatitis can be caused by biologic organisms and materials due to their physical properties or content/secretion of irritating and/or sensitizing/photosensitizing substances. Microorganisms can cause skin infection, and when such an infection is superimposed on a preexisting exogenous or endogenous eczema an aggravation of the eczema can occur (Table 1). Whether microorganisms alone can cause an eczema is more controversial.[20] Infective dermatitis is considered by some dermatologists to be an eczema caused by microorganisms.[20] In case this is correct, of course the exposure to the microorganisms might be occupational. Less controversial is dermatophytide, which is an allergic eczematous reaction to a dermatophyte infection elsewhere in the skin.[20,35] A dermatophytide is more likely to develop with inflammatory dermatophytes[35] which can be acquired occupationally. Anyway, eczema due to infections by fungi or other microorganisms is rare, so they will not be further considered in this chapter.

Post-traumatic eczema is a poorly understood complication of skin injuries which can present as a discoid (nummular) eczema.[36,37] It can appear occupationally after physical or chemical skin injuries and is always unrelated to infection and topical treatment.

The recognition of exposure to an occupational hazardous factor in a patient with hand eczema is not sufficient to establish a diagnosis of OHE. It has to be shown that the type, localization, and course of the eczema is understandable and explainable with regard to the occupational hazardous exposure.

B.   Ways of Exposure

Principally, there are three ways of hazardous exposure to the skin. Direct contact between the skin and the hazardous factor, of course, is the most important and common route; the second route of exposure is via the airways and the lungs; and the third route is via the gastrointestinal canal.

It is obvious that any hazardous factor, i.e., chemicals, physical factors, and microorganisms, in direct contact with the skin can cause damage to it under certain circumstances. However, it is not as obvious that the absorption of a hazardous factor through the lungs or the gastrointestinal canal can cause an eczematous eruption in the skin. Sensitizers and photoallergens, after ingestion, can reach the skin and cause an eczematous dermatitis without or with the help of ultraviolet radiation.[38] On the other hand, irritant substances generally exert their irritancy to all types of cells, including the cells of the gastrointestinal canal, and it is therefore very unlikely that an irritant can be ingested during a sufficient period of time and to such a degree that an irritant eczema will be evoked in the skin. The same principal discussion used for ingestion is also applicable to the inhalation of sensitizers, irritant substances, and photoallergens. However, an eczematous eruption in the skin exclusively due to inhalation seems to be a rare event,[39-42] although it has been reported from inhalation of a few contact sensitizers; for example chromate, turpentine, and mercury.[39-41] Exanthem seems to be the most common clinical presentation of inhaled mercury in a hypersensitive person.[41] Before giving rise to a remote eczema most airborne agents are expected to cause a facial dermatitis unless the face is protected, for example, by a face mask. Face dermatitis caused by exposure to airborne sensitizers, irritants, and photosensitizers is well known,[43] and spreading of the dermatitis to remote parts of the skin due to simultaneous inhalation, excluding direct skin contact, is possible. Substances nonhazardous to the skin can be ingested and then metabolized to either sensitizers or photoallergens, which then can cause an eczematous dermatitis in the skin. Theoretically, this should also be possible for inhaled substances, but examples of this mechanism for the development of an eczema after inhalation do not seem to have been reported.

C. Determination of Hazardous Potential

From the experience of dermatologists and toxicologists, as well as from the results of scientific investigations, a lot of information has been gained and collected through the years about the hazardous potential of various physical factors and chemical compounds. Before new substances are introduced into the market and work sites, predictive tests should have been carried out to determine the substances' skin-irritating and sensitizing capacity.[44,45] Predictive tests concerning photosensitizing potential are available, but are not carried out as frequently as tests for allergenicity and irritancy. It is sometimes easy to predict the irritant capacity of a compound/product from its chemical properties, i.e., with regard to its alkalinity/acidity, solvent properties, oxidizing capacity, and so on.

Many substances are known sensitizers. However, in a particular patient with hand eczema it is not sufficient to know that a compound/product is a potential sensitizer to make a diagnosis of allergic contact dermatitis, but it has also to be shown that the patient is hypersensitive to the compound/product. When suspecting an allergic OHE, patch testing frequently has to be performed with materials from the work site. Though getting positive test reactions to work materials of the allergic type morphologically, still, the possibility of a false positive test reaction has to be substantially diminished by patch testing with serial dilutions of the incriminating agent and also by patch testing controls.[46,47] In the event that the sensitizer is a compound product, it is also important to patch test known ingredients separately. The corresponding photopatch testing can establish the substance/product as a photoallergen or photoirritant when a photosensitive OHE is suspected. When the patient is hypersensitive to a compound/test preparation present in a patch/photopatch test series, it has also to be shown that this sensitizer/photosensitizer is present in the patient's work environment.

D. Localization of Eczema

Sometimes, hand eczema is not the sole manifestation of an eczematous dermatitis. Localization on other parts of the body can give clues to the nature of the eczema with regard to endogenicity and exogenicity and, in the case of an exogenous eczema, also with regard to the route of hazardous exposure.[43] Of course, a person with an endogenous dermatitis that also can manifest as hand eczema (Table 1) can get a hand eczema entirely caused by exogenous factors.

Knowing that a patient with hand eczema is occupationally exposed to a hazardous factor (irritant, sensitizer, or photosensitizing compound) means that this exposure is a possible explanation for the eczema. If the entire hands are exposed in a similar way, for example exposure to a hazardous liquid or powder, the first sites on the hands to be affected are the finger webs, the sides of the fingers, and the dorsal parts. An eczema can also appear on the volar aspects of the hands, particularly concerning a sensitizer but also for an irritant, when there is frequent exposure to a potent hazardous factor. Sometimes the hazardous exposure, especially with regard to solid objects and occasionally liquids, is entirely or predominantly on the volar aspects of the hands, and a subsequent eczema can then be localized to this part exclusively. Such an eczema from a solid object can be sharply demarcated and confined to the area of contact, which can provide diagnostic clues. When the hands are exposed to a hazardous liquid the eczema can still show a patchy appearance on the dorsal aspects. However, such an eczema almost always consists of low-active lesions; i.e., red scaling lesions rather than a papular-vesicular eruption. Well-demarcated areas with vesicles on the central palms or eczematous lesions extending from the volar aspects of the proximal fingers to the contiguous distal part of the palms to form a half circle or "apron" pattern are suggestive of an endogenous dermatitis.[48]

E. Course of Eczema

The course of an OHE will follow, at least initially, exposure to the incriminating agent. When the worker is off work during sick leaves and vacations, the eczema will improve and eventually heal, and then reappear when back at work.

On daily exposure to an irritant the eczema will usually recur slowly, while the eczema will appear sooner on the corresponding exposure to a sensitizer. However, there might be iatrogenic confounding factors. For example, a severe OHE may require systemic corticosteroids, and if this treatment is terminated in close connection with a vacation period there might be a "spontaneous" flare during the vacation, although there is no hazardous exposure.

A hand eczema with a multifactorial background and where an occupational hazardous exposure is contributing to the eczema will improve during sick leave and vacation periods to a degree determined by the significance of the exogenous hazardous exposure for the initial eczema, provided that the exogenous hazardous exposure ceases during the time off from work. At a given time, the sole manifestation of an endogenous dermatitis may be hand eczema. Endogenous dermatitis may have a seasonal variation and, not infrequently, show improvement or healing during the summer. When following the course of a hand eczema under investigation in a worker, the hand eczema may heal during a period of sick leave in early summer. The hand eczema will then usually stay away during the summer vacation but can recur when going back to work after the vacation. Such a course is suggestive of an OHE, which, of course, is one possibility, but an endogenous dermatitis with summer healing has to be considered and ruled out by following the hand eczema course over an extended period of time.

F. Diagnostic Problems

Much of the time it is easy to diagnose an OHE. For patients with hand eczema and occupational exposure to a hazardous factor, and where the extension and intensity of the eczema follows the exposure to the exogenous factor, the diagnosis is easy. However, sometimes it is hard to arrive at a diagnosis of OHE due to various circumstances, some of which will be discussed in the following.

1. Concealed Hazardous Exposure

When investigating a person with OHE any occupational hazardous exposure is concealed unless considering an occupational origin as a possibility. For any adult and many young people with hand eczema, exogenous factors, including occupational ones, should be considered. However, there are situations when the occupational hazardous exposure remains concealed although a careful occupational history has been taken. Sometimes the worker is not aware of occupational exposures, independent of being hazardous or nonhazardous, and consequently can not disclose any information on a possible hazardous exposure. For example, a cleaner in a plastics industry may not clean within the manufacturing area, but in the workers' changing-rooms, where the cleaner has to take care of clothes and protective equipment which can be contaminated with hazardous plastics chemicals. Also, door handles, table surfaces, hand grips of tools, etc., may be contaminated with various substances. According to the author's experience, most cleaners know about the hazards of their cleansers, but almost nothing about any hazardous exposures related to the places and work sites they clean. In these situations the dermatologist has to inquire about the activities in the rooms cleaned and, if necessary, get additional information from the employer. Other examples of occupations with this type of possible concealed hazardous exposure are caretakers and repairmen. An irritant contact dermatitis is unlikely from this type of concealed exposure as it requires both a more frequent and exaggerated exposure (as opposed to an irritant reaction and chemical burn), which makes the exposure more obvious. However, for potential sensitizers a brief exposure may be sufficient for sensitization and elicitation of allergic contact dermatitis. The author, for example, has seen cleaners without any knowledge of occupational exposures apart from their cleansers, but with allergic OHE from resins based on phenol and formaldehyde and from grinding dust based on an epoxy resin system.

2. Infrequent Hazardous Exposure

Most jobs imply exposure to irritants and possible sensitizers and sometimes also photosensitizers on a regular and frequent basis, not infrequently on a daily basis. However, sometimes the exposure to a potential hazardous factor is both irregular and infrequent. Examples of occupations with such possible occasional exposures are craftsmen and certain industrial workers, e.g., assembly workers in the aircraft industry. In this industry hundreds of chemical compounds are used, many of them are potential sensitizers and irritants, and a few are photosensitizers. It is fairly unlikely that a brief isolated exposure to an irritant should be sufficient to cause an irritant contact dermatitis in a healthy individual, but rather an irritant reaction or a chemical burn. On the other hand, in a hypersensitive worker, temporary exposure to a sensitizer/photosensitizer can suffice to elicit an allergic/photoallergic contact dermatitis provided that the hypersensitivity is strong; i.e., only a few molecules of the sensitizer/photosensitizer are required in the skin to elicit a dermatitis.[49] For this type of transient but relapsing hand eczema the occupational origin is easily overlooked. The major clues to suspect OHE are the occupational history revealing a possible occasional hazardous exposure, and the course of the eczema with relapses of eczema only during working periods or closely after such periods (within a few days).

3. No Demonstrable Hazardous Factor

As mentioned before, establishing a diagnosis of OHE requires the identification of an occupational hazardous factor. Thus, without the identification of an exogenous factor, it is by definition impossible to make a diagnosis of OHE. However, occasionally no hazardous factor can be identified although the type of hand eczema, its localization, and course strongly suggest OHE. Repeatedly, the hand eczema may disappear when off work and recur when resuming work. In these situations, skill in taking occupational history[50] and having a good knowledge of hazardous factors and their presence in various occupations[51] is needed. Also, investigations with extended patch testing with work materials[52] and plant visits can be required.[53] On the whole, the importance of plant visits for the management of suspected occupational dermatosis can not be overemphasized. The hazardous factor may still remain unidentified, but since our knowledge of the environment will never be complete, a diagnosis of OHE may be justified in these situations as an expression of our ignorance as well as of the imperfectness of our investigative methods and diagnostic tools. However, this statement must never be used as an evasion or excuse for not making a serious attempt through extensive investigations to identify the occupational hazardous factor before making a diagnosis of OHE. Unless this is done, the diagnosis has to be confined to hand eczema.

4. Multifactorial Background

When a worker is occupationally exposed to a hazardous factor the assessment of the clinical relevance for this exposure is simple in two extreme occasions: (1) when the exposure does not explain the eczema at all, and (2) when the exposure explains the eczema entirely (Figure 1).

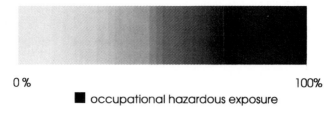

0 %   100%

■ occupational hazardous exposure

FIGURE 1.   The contribution of an occupational hazardous exposure for
a hand eczema.

However, many hand eczemas, particularly those with a chronic course, have a multifactorial
background, so factors other than occupational ones may contribute to the hand eczema. Theoretically, the contribution of occupational hazardous exposure to a hand eczema with a multifactorial
background may vary from 1 to 99% (Figure 1). However, what proportion shall be required to
be considered a significant contribution? Or, in other words, when is the hand eczema an OHE?
There is no obvious answer to this question and, furthermore, there is no simple way to estimate
the contribution of a single factor. This assessment is also influenced by the definition of OHE.
As mentioned before, the medical and medico-legal definitions may differ. For example, in Sweden
the legislation recognizes hand eczema as occupational if the arguments against such an interpretation
are not significantly stronger than the arguments in favor (25% in favor of an occupational origin
is sufficient). The reason for this benevolence is a wish to exclude the possibility that OHE is
incorrectly assessed as a nonoccupational hand eczema due to the imperfectness of the dermatological discipline. However, this liberal legislation has meant that most hand eczemas (including
many endogenous ones) have been approved as OHE. The official statistics on OHE is Sweden,
therefore, is not directly comparable to statistics on OHE based on a more strictly medical definition
of the diagnosis.

In patients with chronic hand eczema with a multifactorial background the significance of an
occupational factor and other contributing factors can be estimated and presented as in the left bar
in Figure 2. However, the relative significance of these factors may vary from time to time (Figure

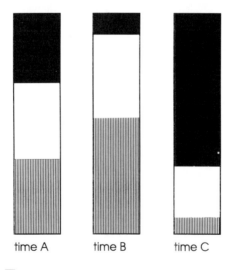

time A   time B   time C

■ occupational hazardous exposure
   non-occupational hazardous exposure
▥ endogenous factor (dermatitis)

FIGURE 2.   Hand eczema with a multifactorial background. The relative significance of contributing factors and the variation of relative significance from time to time.

2). What shall then be required to be considered an OHE? Is the contribution of the occupational hazardous exposure occurring just once above a certain level sufficient to justify a diagnosis of OHE? Is it the average contribution of the occupational hazardous exposure over a certain period that shall be above a certain level to enable a diagnosis of OHE? In the latter case, how is the average contribution assessed?

There are no simple and obvious answers to all the questions asked in this section. The assessment of the relative significance of the various factors contributing to a hand eczema with a multifactorial background, and their variation from time to time, is one of the most demanding tasks for a dermatologist and requires experience, skill, and a broad knowledge of potentially hazardous exposures, both occupational and environmental. To ensure a reasonable accuracy in the assessments, the contributing factors have to be identified and the course of the hand eczema has to be followed with regard to the variation in activity of the endogenous factor and the variation of the exogenous hazardous exposures, preferably during periods when it is possible to eliminate exposures, one at a time. Obviously, this is a time-consuming and laborious task which is more or less insurmountable. Thus, usually preventive and, when necessary, rehabilitative measures have to be initiated based on cruder estimates of the relative significance of the contributing factors than those which might have been possible to achieve after a more extended and extensive investigation.

5. Endogenous Dermatitis

A person with endogenous dermatitis can get hand eczema as a manifestation of this dermatitis (Table 1). Of course, a person with endogenous dermatitis can also get an exogenous hand eczema indistinguishable from an exogenous hand eczema in a person without endogenous dermatitis.

It is conceivable to consider a person with an endogenous dermatitis, for example atopic dermatitis, to have two major skin types: (1) normal skin, and (2) diseased skin. The diseased skin can be subdivided into: (2a) clinically manifested eczematous skin, and (2b) macroscopically normal but microscopically diseased skin ("preeczematous"). If a worker with an endogenous dermatitis is occupationally exposed to an irritant or sensitizer, the exposure may be insufficient to cause dermatitis on completely normal skin but sufficient to produce dermatitis on already diseased skin (Figure 3). Already existing eczema (2a), will be aggravated, and in preeczematous skin (2b), the emerging eczema will most likely have the features of endogenous dermatitis so the possibility of a significant contribution of an occupational hazardous exposure will easily be overlooked. However, if such a patient is followed, with regard to the course of the eczema and its relationship to

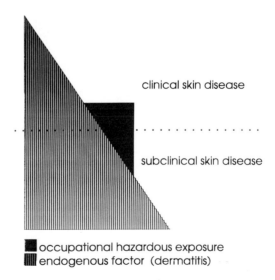

clinical skin disease

subclinical skin disease

■ occupational hazardous exposure
|||| endogenous factor (dermatitis)

FIGURE 3.   Figurative presentation of the skin in a person with endogenous dermatitis and the significance of an occupational hazardous exposure.

his work, the significance of the occupational hazardous exposure will be obvious. The incidence of this combination (2b) is not known. The author has had some patients with endogenous dermatitis clinically, including lesions on the hands and face which initially looked like and were considered as manifestations of endogenous dermatitis, but where exposure to a sensitizer (for example, epoxy resin, Kathon CG, resin based on phenol and formaldehyde, and colophony) has been shown to be responsible for the macroscopic eczematous lesions on the hands and face, but not for the other eczematous lesions on the body.

Anyway, these cases emphasize the need and necessity of considering and assessing the possible contribution of exogenous hazardous exposures for any hand eczema. For a patient with chronic hand dermatitis with a multifactorial background, it is important to know the approximate relative significance of the contributing factors. Although sometimes of minor significance for hand eczema, the exogenous hazardous exposure may be the only factor that can be altered and thus permanently change the severity of the eczema, and is therefore of utmost importance for the patient. Before rehabilitating a person with hand eczema, it is also important to know the relative significance of the various contributing factors in order to give proper vocational guidance and to have realistic expectations on the outcome of the rehabilitation.

6. Nonoccupational Hazardous Exposure

Another situation in which it is hard to determine whether (or what proportion) a hand eczema is occupationally originated concerns those patients who have the same type of hazardous exposure both occupationally and nonoccupationally. This issue will be discussed under two subtitles, sensitizers and irritants.

a. *Sensitizers*
When a patient is sensitized to a compound present only at work, it is usually no problem to determine whether this hypersensitivity and exposure to the sensitizer is responsible for the hand eczema under investigation. However, some sensitizers such as nickel, chromate, rubber allergens, and formaldehyde, as well as some other preservatives, are ubiquitous. If there is a significant occupational exposure to such a sensitizer in a person developing hand eczema and the investigation shows sensitization to this occupational sensitizer, an OHE is likely. However, generally there is also a nonoccupational exposure to a ubiquitous sensitizer. Sensitization is the initial and crucial step in the development of allergic contact dermatitis, and if it was occupationally induced all subsequent and unavoidable exposure to the sensitizer causing hand eczema should be considered a consequence and complication of the OHE and thus compensated for as such, although the occupational exposure may have ceased. After sensitization, nonoccupational exposure may be sufficient to maintain or elicit a dermatitis, since fewer molecules are required for this than for the induction of sensitization. Decisive in the assessment of any clinical relevance for this nonoccupational exposure is (1) the strength of hypersensitivity in the sensitized individual, and (2) the type of nonoccupational exposure to the sensitizer; i.e., will this nonoccupational exposure provide the necessary number of molecules of the sensitizer within the skin to maintain or elicit an allergic contact dermatitis.[49] This sounds obvious and simple, but for the individual patient it can be hard and sometimes impossible to rule out significant exposure to a ubiquitous sensitizer — partly because of imperfect knowledge of the presence of the sensitizer in the environment, but also because of the insufficient possibilities for chemical analysis of the environment.

A different situation arises when a subject, already nonoccupationally sensitized, enters a job where there is exposure to the sensitizer. Once again, decisive in the assessment of clinical relevance for the occupational hazardous exposure is the type of dermatitis, its localization, and course with regard to the occupational exposure. An eczema which heals when the person is off work and then reappears when back at work should be considered to be an OHE, independent of predisposing factors. This corresponds to the situation where a subject without hand eczema but with an atopic constitution gets a job with exposure to irritant factors and a subsequent development of hand eczema.

In Sweden, about 10% of the females are nickel hypersensitive mainly due to ear piercing with nickel-containing objects.[54] Of course, many of these females will enter jobs where they have exposure to nickel in coins, cutting fluids, etc. When these women get hand eczema it is a risk to overdiagnose an occupational allergic contact dermatitis from nickel. Again, the diagnosis can not solely rely on the knowledge of a potential hazardous exposure, but it has to be known or shown that the exposure provides the necessary number of molecules within the skin to elicit a dermatitis, and that the type of eczema, its anatomical distribution, and course are consistent with what is expected from the hazardous exposure.

b. Irritants

Generally, many women work part time since they also have the main responsibility for the family. Their housewife job includes exposure mainly to irritants, but usually the legislation does not recognize this exposure as occupational. Thus, when a woman with small children and a part-time job as a cleaner gets a suspected exogenous hand eczema, it can be very hard to determine the significance of the occupational exposure to the irritants. Also, during sick leave the woman often has to take care of the children and the family, so exposure to irritants will thus continue at home. Therefore, the eczema will not heal but can improve. If such an improvement is followed by a deterioration when back at work, and this sequence of events is repeated more than once, it can be concluded that occupational exposure to the irritants is significant and partly responsible for the eczema and therefore a diagnosis of OHE is justified.

A similar situation with both occupational and nonoccupational exposure to irritants sometimes occurs in men. For a machinist exposed to cutting fluids, the major hobby and leisure-time activity can be the repairing of cars and motorcycles. When a hand eczema develops and the investigation, including patch testing, makes a diagnosis of irritant hand eczema likely, it is again hard to determine the significance of the occupational exposure. However, in this case it is easier to let the person temporarily abandon the leisure-time exposure. Thereafter, assessment of the significance of the occupational exposure can be made when working as well as when off work, if necessary.

7. Postoccupational Eczema

When a person gets OHE it does not necessarily mean that the person has to change jobs. Knowledge of the incriminating factor can imply a change in the work procedure in such a way that the exposure is eliminated or diminished. For other persons with an obvious OHE, it might be impossible to eliminate or diminish the occupational hazardous exposure. However, sometimes workers can not change jobs due to sociomedical reasons or factors related to the labor market, or if the present profession is their dream job, and they may decide to continue despite having weak symptoms. For years, hand eczema can behave as expected; i.e., disappear when the hazardous exposure ceases and reappear when the exposure is resumed. However, suddenly or slowly, the hand eczema can change character and become an eczema which with regard to type, localization, and course is indistinguishable from an endogenous dermatitis.[2,55] This persistent hand eczema has been called postoccupational eczema[2] (maybe postexogenous is more appropriate) and it will continue although the hazardous exposure has terminated. Obviously, from a theoretical point of view it can always be argued that the patient with OHE coincidentally happened to also get another type of hand eczema or that a dormant endogenous dermatitis was awakened by the OHE. However, after having followed such patients in which the dermatitis has developed like this, it is easily conceived that the previous and obvious OHE has influenced the transition into an ''endogenous'' type of eczema in a decisive manner.

Anyway, this area needs more exploration with scientific investigations to determine the significance of OHE or any other exogenous, long-lasting hand eczema in the development of chronic hand eczema of the ''endogenous'' type. Furthermore, if there is a causal connection between the primary OHE and the later hand eczema of the ''endogenous'' type, the likelihood for this transition should be established. When taking care of patients with OHE the outcome of various situations should be known in order to give the patient as much reliable information as possible about the future development of the eczema.

IV. SUMMARY

OHE is common enough to expect a wide knowledge of this condition from dermatologists. To arrive at a diagnosis of OHE, two major prerequisites have to be fulfilled: (1) identification of hazardous exposure, and (2) establishment of a relationship between the hazardous exposure and the eczema. Many hand eczemas have a multifactorial background, which means that occupational hazardous exposure can both cause and provoke an eczema as well as aggravate a preexisting eczema. The relative significance of the occupational hazardous exposure for the hand eczema can be hard to determine and the relative significance may also vary from time to time. It is possible that OHE in some persons can develop into a persistent hand eczema, although exposure to the original hazardous factor has ceased and has not been replaced by another hazardous factor. This is an area requiring further exploration with a scientific approach.

REFERENCES

1. Meding, B., Epidemiology of hand eczema in an industrial city, *Acta Derm. Venereol.*, Suppl. 153, 1, 1990.
2. Wall, L. M. and Gebauer, K. A., A follow-up of occupational skin disease in Western Australia, *Contact Dermatitis*, 24, 241, 1991.
3. Peltonen, L., Nickel sensitivity in the general population, *Contact Dermatitis*, 5, 27, 1979.
4. Menné, T., Borgan, Ö., and Green, A., Nickel allergy and hand dermatitis in a stratified sample of the Danish female population: an epidemiological study including a statistic appendix, *Acta Derm. Venereol.*, 62, 35, 1982.
5. Coenraads, P., Nater, J. P., and van der Lende, R., Prevalence of eczema and other dermatoses of the hands and arms in the Netherlands. Association with age and occupation, *Clin. Exp. Dermatol.*, 8, 495, 1983.
6. Malten, K. E., Fregert, S., Bandmann, H.-J., et al., Occupational dermatitis in five European dermatology departments, *Berufsdermatosen*, 11, 181, 1963.
7. Rycroft, R. J. G., Occupational dermatoses, in *Textbook of Dermatology*, 5th ed., Champion, R. H., Burton, J. L., and Ebling, F. J. G., Eds., Blackwell Scientific, Oxford, 1992, 755.
8. Fisher, A. A. and Adams, R. M., Occupational dermatitis, in *Contact Dermatitis*, 3rd ed., Fisher, A. A., Ed., Lea & Febiger, Philadelphia, 1986, 486.
9. Mathias, C. G. T. and Morrison, J. H., Occupational skin diseases, U.S. Results from the Bureau of Labor Statistics annual survey of occupational injuries and illnesses 1973 through 1984, *Arch. Dermatol.*, 124, 1519, 1988.
10. Mathias, C. G. T., Prevention of occupational contact dermatitis, *J. Am. Acad. Dermatol.*, 23, 742, 1990.
11. National Institute for Occupational Safety and Health, Prevention of occupational skin disorders: a proposed national strategy for the prevention of dermatological conditions. 1, *Am. J. Contact Dermatitis*, 1, 56, 1990.
12. Wall, L. M. and Gebauer, K. A., Occupational skin disease in Western Australia, *Contact Dermatitis*, 24, 101, 1991.
13. Hogan, D. J., Dannaker, C. J., and Maibach, H. I., The prognosis of contact dermatitis, *J. Am. Acad. Dermatol.*, 23, 300, 1990.
14. Fregert, S., Occupational dermatitis in a 10-year material, *Contact Dermatitis*, 1, 96, 1975.
15. Church, R., Hand eczema in industry and the home, in *Essentials of Industrial Dermatology*, Griffiths, W. A. D. and Wilkinson, D. S., Eds., Blackwell Scientific, Oxford, 1985, 85.
16. National Institute for Occupational Safety and Health, Prevention of occupational skin disorders: a proposed national strategy for the prevention of dermatological conditions. Part 2, *Am. J. Contact Dermatitis*, 1, 116, 1990.
17. Burrows, D., Industrial dermatitis today and its prevention, in *Essentials of Industrial Dermatology*, Griffiths, W. A. D. and Wilkinson, D. S., Eds., Blackwell Scientific, Oxford, 1985, 12.
18. Mathias, C. G. T., The cost of occupational skin disease, *Arch. Dermatol.*, 121, 332, 1985.
19. Braun-Falco, O., Plewig, G., Wolff, H. H., and Winkelmann, R. K., Dermatitis and eczema, in *Dermatology*, Springer-Verlag, Berlin, 1991, 316.
20. Burton, J. L., Eczema, lichenification, prurigo and erythroderma, in *Textbook of Dermatology*, 5th ed., Champion, R. H., Burton, J. L., and Ebling, F. J. G., Eds., Blackwell Scientific, Oxford, 1992, 537.

21. Mathias, C. G. T., Contact dermatitis and worker's compensation: criteria for establishing occupational causation and aggravation, *J. Am. Acad. Dermatol.*, 20, 842, 1989.
22. Emmett, E. A., Phototoxicity and photosensitivity reactions, in *Occupational Skin Disease*, 2nd ed., Adams, R. M., Ed., W. B. Saunders, Philadelphia, 1990, 184.
23. Lane, G., Dennie, C. G., Downing, J. G., Foerster, H., Oliver, E. H., and Sulzberger, M., Industrial dermatoses, *J. Am. Med. Assoc.*, 118, 613, 1942.
24. Emmett, E. A., General aspects of occupational dermatoses, in *Dermatology in General Medicine*, 3rd ed., Fitzpatrick, T. B., Eisen, A. Z., Wolf, K., et al., Eds., McGraw-Hill, New York, 1987, 1567.
25. Calnan, C. D. and Rycroft, R. J. G., Rehabilitation in occupational skin disease, *Trans. Coll. Med. S. Afr.*, Suppl. 25, 136, 1981.
26. Fregert, S., Occupational contact dermatitis, in *Manual of Contact Dermatitis*, 2nd ed., Munksgaard, Copenhagen, 1981, 86.
27. Freeman, S., Diagnosis and differential diagnosis, in *Occupational Skin Disease*, 2nd ed., Adams, R. M., Ed., W. B. Saunders, Philadelphia, 1990, 194.
28. Rietschel, R. L., Patch testing in occupational hand dermatitis, *Dermatol. Clin.*, 6, 43, 1988.
29. Wilkinson, D. S., Some causes of error in the diagnosis of occupational dermatoses, in *Essentials of Industrial Dermatology*, Griffiths, W. A. D. and Wilkinson, D. S., Blackwell Scientific, Oxford, 1985, 47.
30. Foussereau, J., Benezra, C., and Maibach, H. I., Allergic history and indications of occupational allergic dermatitis, in *Occupational Contact Dermatitis, Clinical and Chemical Aspects*, Munksgaard, Copenhagen, 1982, 15.
31. Bruze, M. and Emmett, E. A., Occupational exposures to irritants, in *Irritant Contact Dermatitis*, Jackson, E. M. and Goldner, R., Eds., Marcel Dekker, New York, 1990, 81.
32. Gellin, G. A., Physical and mechanical causes of occupational dermatoses, in *Occupational and Industrial Dermatology*, 2nd ed., Maibach, H. I., Ed., Year Book Medical Publishers, Chicago, 1987, 88.
33. Malten, K. E., Thoughts on irritant contact dermatitis, *Contact Dermatitis*, 7, 238, 1981.
34. de Groot, A. C., *Patch Testing. Test Concentrations and Vehicles for 2800 Allergens*, Elsevier, Amsterdam, 1986.
35. Kaaman, T. and Torssander, J., Dermatophytide — a misdiagnosed entity, *Acta Derm. Venereol.*, 63, 404, 1983.
36. Mathias, C. G. T., Post-traumatic eczema, *Dermatol. Clin.*, 6, 35, 1988.
37. Wilkinson, D. S., Discoid eczema as a consequence of contact with irritants, *Contact Dermatitis*, 5, 118, 1979.
38. Veien, N. K., Menné, T., and Maibach, H. I., Systemically induced allergic contact dermatitis, in *Exogenous Dermatoses*, Menné, T. and Maibach, H. I., Eds., CRC Press, Boca Raton, FL, 1991, 267.
39. Mali, J. W. H., Uber einen Fall von dyshidrotischem Ekzem durch Chromat, *Hautarzt*, 11, 27, 1960.
40. Storck, H., Ekzem durch Inhalation, *Schweiz. Med. Wochenschr.*, 608, 1955.
41. Nakayama, H., Niki, F., Shono, M., and Hada, S., Mercury exanthem, *Contact Dermatitis*, 9, 411, 1983.
42. Wuthrich, B., Berufsdermatosen per inhalationem oder ingestionem, *Berufsdermatosen*, 25, 141, 1977.
43. Dooms-Goossens, A. and Deleu, H., Airborne contact dermatitis: an update, *Contact Dermatitis*, 25, 211, 1991.
44. Maurer, T., *Contact and Photocontact Allergens*, Marcel Dekker, New York, 1983.
45. *Animal Models in Dermatology. Relevance to Human Dermatopharmacology and Dermatotoxicology*, Maibach, H. I., Ed., Churchill Livingstone, Edinburgh, 1975.
46. Fregert, S., Publications of allergens, *Contact Dermatitis*, 12, 123, 1985.
47. Bruze, M., Sensitizers in resins based on phenol and formaldehyde, *Acta Derm. Venereol.*, Suppl. 119, 1, 1985.
48. Cronin, E., Clinical patterns of hand eczema in women, *Contact Dermatitis*, 13, 153, 1985.
49. Bruze, M., What is a relevant contact allergy?, *Contact Dermatitis*, 23, 224, 1990.

50. Guidotti, T. L., Cortez, J. H., Abraham, H. L., et al., Occupational and Environmental Health Committee of the American Lung Association of San Diego and Imperial Counties. Taking the occupational history, *Ann. Intern. Med.,* 99, 641, 1983.
51. Adams, R. M., Job descriptions with their irritants and allergens, in *Occupational Skin Disease,* 2nd ed., Adams, R. M., Ed., W. B. Saunders, Philadelphia, 1990, 578.
52. Bruze, M., Trulsson, L., and Bendsöe, N., Patch testing with ultrasonic bath extracts, *Am. J. Contact Dermatitis,* 3, 133, 1992.
53. Rycroft, R. J. G., Looking at work dermatologically, *Dermatol. Clin.,* 6, 1, 1988.
54. Larsson-Stymne, B. and Widström, L., Ear piercing — a cause of nickel allergy in schoolgirls?, *Contact Dermatitis,* 13, 289, 1985.
55. Burrows, D., Prognosis and factors influencing prognosis in industrial dermatitis, *Br. J. Dermatol.,* 105 (Suppl. 21), 65, 1981.

19

Hairdressers' Eczema

Beate Pilz and Peter J. Frosch

CONTENTS

0-8493-7355-7/94/$0.00 + $.50

I. INTRODUCTION

Hairdressers undoubtedly have an increased risk of developing an occupational dermatitis. Continual exposure to numerous irritants and allergens as well as to frictional forces and microclimatic changes are some of the factors causing hand dermatitis. In many patients the condition worsens progressively, in spite of correct diagnosis and various measures of treatment, leading to repeated sick leaves and, finally, surrender of the profession. The costs for medical care, and particularly for the retraining of the (usually) young patient, are substantial. The socioeconomic aspect, together with the personal suffering from the disease, and certain clinical features, justify a special chapter in a book on hand eczema.

II. PREVALENCE

Despite the fact that this is one of the most common occupational skin diseases, there are only a few reports providing detailed data. In most studies, a population of hairdressers seeking medical help is described in regard to clinical features and the results of patch testing. In a few studies, the number of hairdressers is related to the total population of patients with hand eczema or, even less precise, to patients with contact dermatitis. In Bäurle's[1] group of 683 patients with hand eczema, studied in Germany during the years 1981 through 1984, hairdressers represented only 4% of the group. In a questionnaire study, Stovall and associates[41] found that 50% of 405 responding hairdressers reported some type of cutaneous problem. In this group of patients, 10% were stated to have continued skin problems.

Rivett and Merrick[35] mailed 230 questionnaires to stylists, with only 66 (29%) responders. Among those, 30% reported a skin condition of the hands, and in 8 patients the skin condition had interfered significantly with their work. In a group of trainees — 94 completed questionnaires of 128 mailed — 70 (74%) had a skin condition of the hands, 49 had sought medical advice, and 10 had been referred to a dermatologist. Of all stylists who completed the questionnaire, 42% had left hairdressing, but only 14% of these named the skin condition as the reason — 50% of the leavers had simply left for better paying work. The authors point out that the prevalence rate of 30% could be an overestimate because of the poor return from the trainee group and the fact that those with a skin condition would probably be more likely to respond than those without. The results are also based on the subjective opinions of the hairdressers. However, the data indicate that occupational dermatitis is even more common among trainee hairdressers than some studies have suggested.[27]

In an epidemiologic study (questionnaire) of hand eczema, 13.5% of 74 hairdressers had a 1-year period prevalence of hand eczema in their occupation.[30] In this study, hairdressers had the highest frequency of occupational changes due to their skin disease (18% of hairdressers; 8% of all patients with hand eczema).

Cronin and Kullavanijaya[6] reported that of 33 apprentices examined in a hairdressing salon in London, 30 had "some cutaneous problem"; 39% of the cases were mild, 39% moderate, and 12% severe.

In Finland, Hannuksela and Hassi[25] examined 32 hairdressers working in small salons. As many as 22 of the 32 subjects were found to have hand dermatitis, nail disorders, or callosities on the fingers, while the remaining 10 had no signs of occupational disorders. The disorders caused some discomfort, but required no absence from work.

Although these prevalence rates are useful and show the eminent role of hairdressers in the field of occupational dermatitis, more exact figures for incidence rates are needed. The number of patients must be related to the total number of employees in the area studied. For metal workers, such figures have been provided recently by Diepgen et al.[10] In cooperation with state medical authorities (Staatlicher Gewerbearzt) and insurance institutions the number of occupational dermatitis cases in this trade was calculated to be 11.9/10,000 metal workers in North Bavaria. For hairdressers in the same region the incidence was calculated to be 242/10,000. In comparison to metal workers, this is an alarming factor of 20. It is extremely difficult to obtain accurate figures of this type, however, only accurate figures can provide meaningful information on the occurrence of a disease in a population at risk. This is a prerequisite for adequate preventive measures.

III. CLINICAL FEATURES

The clinical findings show large individual variations and depend on the type and duration of the dermatitis.

A.   Irritant Contact Dermatitis

This is most frequently seen in apprentices during the first weeks after entering the profession. An acute irritant contact dermatitis develops, with redness on the dorsum of the hand and the back of the proximal fingers. The finger webs are often affected, too. Another favored site of irritation is the finger skin under rings — it is now the fashion to wear several rings on one or more fingers and hairdressers in particular seem to be fond of this trend. Many of them do not take off the rings during work. After an exposure-free weekend, scaling is noted. Inflammatory papules may coalesce to infiltrated plaques on the back of the hands, spreading to the lateral aspect of the fingers and palms. At this stage some patients develop so-called hardening, and the dermatitis does not progress despite continued exposure to the irritants. In others, the dermatitis worsens and causes considerable discomfort with severe scaling, fissures, and vesicles. This chronic irritant contact dermatitis must always raise the suspicion of a contact allergy. For further information on the clinical aspects and pathogenesis of irritant contact dermatitis the reader is referred to a recent review by Frosch.[16]

B.   Allergic Contact Dermatitis

The hallmark of this type of contact dermatitis is the presence of numerous vesicles associated with papules and intensive itching. Recurrence of objective and subjective symptoms develops rapidly within hours of exposure after a longer rest period. The weekend is usually not sufficient to clear all lesions.

If a contact allergy to one or more occupational allergens has developed, the skin of the whole hand is usually abnormal and in a chronic eczematous stage. The lesions may spread to the proximal ventral forearms, and in cases with a high degree of sensitization, even further to the face and other parts.

On rare occasions, a finger tip dermatitis (pulpitis) may be noticed due to contact with glyceryl monothioglycolate when the strength of the permanent wave is checked with the unprotected hand before applying the fixative.

In former times, when scissors were mainly made from nickel alloys, the eczema was localized to the areas with intimate contact (palm, thumb, and ring finger). However, nowadays scissors are primarily made from stainless steel and the grips are covered with plastic.

C.   Atopic Hand Dermatitis

This type of dermatitis is described in detail elsewhere in this book. Briefly, the eczematous lesions follow a bizarre pattern in the palms and on the lateral aspects of the fingers. Bouts of vesiculation with intensive itching also occur in exposure-free intervals and may be precipitated by mental or physical stress.

D.   Hybrids

As has been pointed out by some Scandinavian authors,[32,36] a combination of the main types of contact dermatitis — allergic and irritant — as well as associations with atopy must be kept in mind. At a single time point of examination — even with a careful workup, including patch testing and screening for atopy — it may be impossible to make the correct diagnosis in a difficult case. After observing the course and reexamining the clinical pattern, however, an experienced dermatologist will be able to mark the case as atopic (endogenous), irritant (without atopy), contact allergy, or a combination of the three types.

E.   Cheiropompholyx

The eruption of little vesicles along the lateral and palmar aspect of the fingers (in severe cases, also in the palms) and associated usually with itching but not with visible inflammatory changes, is called cheiropompholyx or (genuine) dyshidrosis. This condition may be a sign of atopy but also definitely occurs in nonatopic subjects. The vesicles dry within few days under the formation of fine areolar scaling.

This condition is frequent among young people and, although not related to the sweat glands, often occurs in hot humid climates. Of the 74 hairdressers studied by Czarnecki,[7] 42 had already experienced this disease before entering the profession and 26 afterwards. These figures seem rather high and await further confirmation by other investigators.

F. Hyperhidrosis

It has been frequently stated that hairdressers suffer from hyperhidrosis, and this may result from the various chemicals they are in contact with. To date, there is no scientific proof that any of the substances typical to this trade increases the production of sweat. Czarnecki[7] reported a figure of 70% in regard to hyperhidrosis of the hands and feet, but pointed out that this condition had already existed before entering the profession in the majority of the cases.

G. Nail Changes

In chronic hand eczema various nail changes are observed: transverse ridges (most common), distal onycholysis, and loss of cuticle with thickened, infiltrated nail folds. Hannuksela and Hassi[25] described softening of the nails, subungual pseudomembrane, maceration, and an upward curving of the distal nail plates of the left hand. These changes were mainly seen in hairdressers doing permanent wave without gloves 1 to 20 times per week. In hairdressers, dark brown pigmentation may be seen if gloves are not regularly worn when dyeing the hair.

H. Pilonidal Sinus

This is a typical feature of hairdressers primarily engaged with cutting the hair of customers. The freshly cut hairs penetrate the skin like thorns, leading to foreign body granulomas and even deep sinuses. In female hairdressers, these lesions can develop in the periareolar region of the breast.[2,22,23]

I. Callosities

Scissors and combs may induce hyperkeratotic plaques in the palm, thumb, and on the dorsal aspect of the ring finger, usually more pronounced on the right side due to dexterity.

IV. CAUSATIVE FACTORS

A. Wet Work

Continuous exposure to water damages the skin considerably. This factor has been neglected in explaining the pathogenesis of irritant contact dermatitis and has become fully appreciated only recently. The stratum corneum's barrier function is impaired and inflammatory mediators are released from keratinocytes and possibly also from keratinous material itself. Patients with an atopic hand eczema frequently experience an exacerbation with a new burst of vesicles shortly after exposure to a wet environment.

B. Irritants

In hairdressing the skin is not only exposed to water but also to a number of irritants which intensify cutaneous damage.

Shampoos must be considered to be major irritants, particularly in apprentices, because shampooing is their major task in the first period of employment. Manufacturers of shampoos have definitely improved on mildness[28] and an irritant dermatitis in a customer after regular use is extremely rare. However, even mild surfactants might irritate the skin of the hands of a young hairdresser after shampooing 10 to 30 times a day.[6] Daily short-term exposure (30 min) to the model surfactant, sodium lauryl sulfate, damages the stratum corneum, even at low concentrations (1% aqueous), and leads to a drastic increase in transepidermal water loss.[18]

Permanent waving and bleaching solutions are further irritants to be considered because most hairdressers handle these agents without gloves. The old, cold permanent wave solution, containing ammonium thioglycolate as the major active ingredient, used to have a rather high pH of 10 to 11. Nowadays, they are calibrated to pH 8 to 9. Although pH is not the only factor determining the irritancy of a material, a high or extremely low pH will certainly have a deleterious effect on the skin, particularly if there is repeated or prolonged exposure. The new acid permanent wave solution with glyceryl monothioglycolate (GMTG) as the active ingredient has a pH of 5 to 6, which is that of normal skin.

C. Friction and Pressure

Frictional forces have been underestimated in the pathogenesis of irritant contact dermatitis.[31] This is also true for hairdressers' eczema. The fingers are constantly rubbed against the customer's hair and various instruments (comb, clips, hairnet, etc.). To normal skin these shearing forces may be minimal, but to diseased skin this will undoubtedly contribute to further damage, resulting in erosions and fissures.

Pressure due to holding and moving various instruments, particularly scissors, will lead to callosities in disposed individuals as described above.

D. Thermal Changes

The skin of a hairdresser is exposed to drastic changes in temperature due to hot and cold water when shampooing the hair. A hot air flow reaches the skin for several minutes when the hair is styled. The stratum corneum's capacity for retaining water depends not only on the content of epidermal lipids but is also a function of the ambient temperature and humidity. Dryness, scaling, and fissuring of the skin and nails is therefore also related to the microclimatic changes, and is not only a consequence of chemical irritants.

E. Allergens

1. Hairdressing Chemicals

Data on the frequencies of sensitization to allergens in hairdressers vary considerably from country to country, and even from center to center in the same country. The rank order of sensitizers depends very much on the chemicals used and on the various techniques applied in the salons when hair is dyed and waved. Most hairdresser salons are small businesses with few employees and the owner determines the style of work. It depends on him whether his employees wear gloves when dyeing or applying permanent wave liquids. If he is convinced of the value of preventive measures, this will carry on down to the junior hairdressers. If he is not, and even prevents employees from using gloves for high-risk procedures, then it is very likely that a high sensitization rate in this salon will ensue.

Until recently, the only studies reported were from single centers with low numbers of hairdressers derived from a relatively small geographic area.[6,26,40] In 1992, the combined experience in Italy of a large panel of 302 hairdressers from 9 centers was reported. Occupationally relevant sensitizations were found in 61% of the studied patients. Among hair dyes, *p*-phenylenediamine (PPD) showed the highest proportion of allergic reactions, followed by the acid permanent wave ingredient glyceryl monothioglycolate (GMTG), and the hair bleach ammonium persulfate (APS). A relatively low frequency of sensitization was found for ammonium thioglycolate, resorcinol, and pyrogallol (Table 1).

Concerned about the rising figures of sensitization to GMTG, particularly on the basis of the results of the German Contact Dermatitis Research Group — 38% positive in hairdressers[14] — the European Environmental and Contact Dermatitis Research Group (EECDRG) decided to collect their data to obtain an ad hoc survey of the present situation in Europe. The retrospective study involved 9 centers and 809 hairdressers.[17] Results obtained with the hairdressers' series of Trolab/

**TABLE 1   Positive Patch Test in Hairdressers Tested With the Hairdressers' Series
(Trolab/Hermal) and PPD as Reported on the Basis of Two Large Multicenter
Studies Conducted By the Italian Contact Dermatitis Research Group[24] and the
European Environmental and Contact Dermatitis Research Group[17]**

	Italian CDRG[a] pos/tested		European ECDRG[b] pos/tested	
Material (pet)				
ONPPD 1%	24/302	7.9%	33/798	4.2%
(*o*-Nitro-*p*-Phenylenediamine)				
Resorcinol 2%	4/302	1.3%	2/354	0.6%
PTD 1%	40/302	13.2%	59/781	7.6%
(*p*-Toluenediamine sulfate)				
GMTG 1%	34/302	11.3%	151/809	18.7%
(Glyceryl monothioglycolate)				
AMT 2.5%	15/302	5.0%	31/809	3.8%
(Ammonium thioglycolate)				
APS 0.25%	34/302	11.3%	66/809	8.2%
(Ammonium persulfate)				
PADH 0.25%	32/302	10.6%	13/365	3.6%
(*p*-Aminodiphenylamine hydrochloride)				
Pyrogallol 1%	4/302	1.3%	6/781	0.8%
PPD (base) 1%	50/302	16.7%	120/809	14.8%
(*p*-Phenylenediamine)				

[a]   Series comprised of 302 patients from 9 centers.
[b]   Series comprised of 809 patients from 9 centers.

Hermal (Reinbek, Germany) are shown in Table 1. The data also include those for PPD (base) of
the standard series.

In the EECDRG study, the rank order of the leading allergens was as follows: GMTG (19%),
PPD (15%), APS (8%), PTD (8%), ONPPD (4%), AMT (4%), and PADH (4%) (Table 1). The
frequency of sensitization showed marked regional variations, particularly to GMTG, which was
highest in Germany (51%), followed by Spain (22%), and U.K. (19%). The figures were much
lower in Denmark (8.5%), Finland (2.4%), and France (0%, only 11 patients).

The conclusion from these two large multicenter trials is that the present major sensitizers are
the hair dyes of the PPD type and its derivatives. According to Cronin,[4] cross-reactions occur with
other related hair dyes, such as *p*-toluenediamine, *p*-aminodiphenylamine, 2,4-diaminoanisole, and
o-aminophenol. Other authors[29,39] found cross-reactions in PPD-sensitized patients to benzocaine,
procaine, sulfonamides, and PABA sunscreens.

The active ingredient in the acid permanent wave solution, GMTG, is a problem sensitizer in
some locations in Europe. This may be related to high frequencies of usage in the salons and/or
variations in the usage of protective garments. In Finland, acid permanent wave solutions are rarely
used, whereas in Germany they are by far more frequently applied than the old alkaline permanent
wave solutions with AMT. In Denmark most hairdressers wear gloves when dyeing or permanent
waving, in Germany they are usually used only for dark hair dyes. In Italy only 12.5% of 240
hairdressers wore gloves for permanent waving, and 51% wore them for dyeing.[24] Nevertheless,
it is important to realize that the alkaline permanent wave products which have been in use since
the 1940s are definitely lower in sensitization frequency in comparison to the recently introduced
acid permanent wave products. Although accurate figures in regard to the number of exposed
hairdressers and number of sensitized hairdressers are missing for all these hairdressing chemicals,
it is obvious that the sensitization risk for GMTG must be higher than that for AMT.

2.   Other Sensitizers

a.   Nickel

Many hairdressers are allergic to nickel. This is now the leading allergen in females worldwide
and is attributed mainly to ear piercing and the wearing of costume jewelry with a high nickel

content. Although not firmly established by investigation, it is the common experience of dermatologists today that nickel is not a primary occupational allergen in hairdressers. Most female hairdressers report a history of intolerance to costume jewelry before entering the trade. The objects handled by a hairdresser in a modern salon are mainly of plastic or stainless steel. In former times, scissors, hairclips, and combs were nickel-plated. There is scientific evidence that nickel ions are more readily released from metallic objects when immersed in permanent wave solutions or bleaches.[8] However, it has not been shown that there is actually an increased nickel exposure to hairdressers, nor that this would lead to an exacerbation of hand eczema in nickel-sensitized individuals.

In the older literature, it has been stated that hairdressers and housewives are exposed to nickel and cobalt from detergents.[3,32] Since then, the content of these metals has been reduced to a range of a few ppm and it is now even less likely that they may play a role in the development of hand eczema, neither in hairdressers nor in housewives. However, a study under modern scientific standards is needed to prove this assumption.

If a hairdresser is sensitized to nickel, however, the dermatologist should carefully investigate the possibility of occupational nickel exposure. Using the DMGO test, one may find in the salon one or more objects with a high nickel content. This may be an old scissors or even another object that is not a typical hairdresser's utensil but handled while at work (e.g., a cashier's machine).

b. Formaldehyde

As for nickel, there is now considerable uncertainty whether this is a relevant allergen for hairdressers. In most countries, shampoos and other hair preparations no longer contain formaldehyde due to intensive public campaigns against this preservative. In the U.K., and in individual salons in other countries, however, this allergen may still be relevant. For every formaldehyde-sensitized patient, additional information about the handled products should be obtained from the manufacturer. According to Cronin,[5] there are still many hidden sources of formaldehyde exposure and — at least in the London area — many hand eczema cases benefit from totally avoiding formaldehyde-containing products.

c. Cocamidopropylbetaine

This surfactant is widely used in shampoos and also in other cosmetic products. In a German multicenter study of 178 hairdressers, this compound was found to be positive in 5% of all cases. Some of the positive reactions may be irritative ones. The allergen might be either cocamidopropylbetaine itself, or the impurity, amidoamine.[34]

d. (Chloro)methylisothiazolinone

This chemical is present in Kathon CG and Euxyl K 100 and has been widely used in shampoos and in various leave-on cosmetics. Due to the high sensitizing frequencies reported from various countries, most manufacturers are now using other preservatives. In a hairdresser highly sensitive to CMI/MI who has frequent contact with shampoos this might still be a relevant allergen. Therefore, as with formaldehyde, such a patient should be advised to use only CMI/MI-free shampoos, both at work and for personal use.

e. Fragrances

Fragrances are ubiquitous, and in a highly sensitized subject an effort must be made to avoid them completely. In the hairdressing trade most articles are perfumed. So far, there is insufficient evidence for the assumption that hairdressers are sensitized primarily to fragrances by the products used at work. In an individual case it may be relevant, even if the source of sensitization is nonoccupational.

F. Immediate Type Reactions

If hairdressers complain of shortness of breath, swelling of the eyelids, or even generalized urticaria during or after work, the possibility of immediate type reactions to various materials must be ruled out. A major cause is ammonium persulfate found in hair bleaches.[13] This material caused occupational asthma in bakers when it was added to flour as a bleaching agent. Banned from the food industry, surprisingly, it is still used in the hairdressing trade.

Further sources of immediate type allergic reactions may be latex gloves and the hair dye, henna. Henna is used frequently in India and other Asian countries. On rare occasions it can cause a contact allergy.[33] Frosch and Hausen[15] described a 19-year-old hairdresser with a high degree of sensitization to various types of henna. She developed anaphylactic symptoms even when being in the room where other colleagues worked with the material. When extracts from lawson, the main ingredient of henna, were studied by thin-layer chromatography and skin tested, 2-hydroxy-1,4-naphthochinone and the red dye remained negative, whereas an extract from black and brown henna produced strong reactions.

Hair sprays frequently cause nonspecific irritative reactions of the bronchial system, particularly in atopics.[38]

V. DIAGNOSIS

The diagnosis must be based on history, clinical findings, and the results of patch testing. When patch testing, the standard series and the supplementary series for hairdressers (Hermal/Trolab, Reinbek; Chemotechnique, Malmo) should be used. The authors do not recommend routine testing with shampoos and other materials hairdressers use because false positive irritant reactions may occur. This may be done only if the suspicion of a missed allergen is raised after negative tests with both the standard and hairdressers' series. Adequate controls are mandatory.

In Germany, most dermatologists perform careful screening for atopy (prick tests with common inhalant allergens, total IgE level, and Phadiatop/SX-1 screening for specific IgE). This is helpful in supporting an endogenous character of the hand dermatitis, particularly in preparing expert opinions for legal compensation claims.

In patients with asthma, prick tests with various materials are indicated after a careful history (APS, henna, etc.).

VI. TREATMENT

This is covered in other chapters. There are no specific aspects in hairdressers' eczema in this regard.

VII. PROGNOSIS

In irritant contact dermatitis the prognosis, in general, is good. This is particularly true for the acute type, frequently seen in young apprentices during the first weeks of work. The skin may accommodate to the various irritative factors and show the signs of hardened skin: slight erythema, thickening, and scaling. At this stage, regular use of skin emollients is very helpful. The usage of so-called barrier creams (skin protective creams) is controversial. If a patient has not used anything before, some benefit will result from nearly any type of barrier cream. There is a lack of well-controlled clinical studies supporting the claims of various manufacturers. Only recently, a guinea-pig model and a human bioassay for quantifying the efficacy of this product line were published.[18,20,21] In these studies the following products have been found effective against the standard anionic detergent, sodium lauryl sulfate: Taktosan Salbe (Stockhausen, Krefeld), Reamin (Wella, Darmstadt), and Atrix (Beiersdorf, Hamburg).

Most shampoos nowadays contain the less-irritating laurylether sulfates, sulfosuccinates, and nonionic detergents.

The prognosis decreases in cases of atopic hand eczema and, particularly, if a contact allergy to one or more hairdressing chemicals is present. Even with good dermatological care and compliance of the patient, the irritants and allergens cannot be completely avoided. The long-term usage of gloves frequently increases skin damage due to maceration of the skin. Patients with a dyshidrotic type of eczema experience intense itching and a new bout of vesiculation.

These patients must leave their occupation and should be retrained for a new, clean, dry job. It is extremely important to make a carefully diagnostic workup and inform the patient about all details of the disease. As a recent study has shown, the prognosis of patients with hand eczema is strongly dependent on the degree of knowledge of their diseases.[11,12] The legal aspects for the handling of occupational dermatitis cases show a great variation among various European countries. This subject has been reviewed recently.[19]

VIII. PREVENTION

The main goal must be a safer working place; the number of irritants and allergens in the hairdressing salon must be reduced to the minimum. Hairdressing preparations must be scrutinized by predictive assays and usage tests in regard to their skin compatibility. Even preparations with a low irritating potential may build up to a clinical disease under repetitive long-term conditions. Therefore the mildest shampoos of modern technology should be used by hairdressers. Allergens such as GMTG pose a special hazard for hairdressers and less-sensitizing alternatives should be sought immediately. The same holds true for the hair dyes.

Young hairdressers frequently are not well informed about the hazards in their profession. They need detailed instructions regarding the potential irritants and sensitizers and how to reduce direct contact time with the skin. Gloves are still underused in hairdressing salons. Metallic objects should not contain nickel because many hairdressers are entering the trade already sensitized by costume jewelry.

Special attention should be given to regular skin care with bland emollients and barrier creams. This must be undertaken from the first day on, and not after a dermatitis has already developed.

On the basis of several studies on hand eczema we know that atopics are at special risk. However, at this moment it is still unclear how atopy should be defined, because the criteria varied in these studies. The authors recommend the use of the score for atopy developed by Diepgen et al.[9] Furthermore, it has not been clearly shown that exclusion of atopics will lead to a marked decrease in the occurrence of hand eczema in hairdressers. Ethical considerations speak against such a preselection of trainees.

REFERENCES

1. Bäurle, G., *Handekzeme*, Schattauer, Stuttgart, 1986.
2. Bowers, P. W., Roustabouts' and barbers' breasts, *Clin. Exp. Dermatol.*, 7, 445, 1982.
3. Clemmensen, O. J., Menné, T., Kaaber, K., and Solgaars, P., Exposure of nickel and the relevance of nickel sensitivity among hospital cleaners, *Contact Dermatitis*, 7, 14, 1981.
4. Cronin, E., *Contact Dermatitis*, Churchill Livingstone, Edinburgh, 1980, 137.
5. Cronin, E., Formaldehyde is a significant allergen in women with hand eczema, *Contact Dermatitis*, 25, 276, 1991.
6. Cronin, E. and Kullavanijaya, P., Hand dermatitis in hairdressers, *Acta Derm. Venereol.*, 59 (Suppl. 85), 47, 1979.
7. Czarnecki, N., Zur Klinik und Pathogenese des Friseurekzems, *Z. Hautkr.*, 52(1), 1, 1977.
8. Dahlquist, D., Fregert, S., and Gruvenberger, B., Release of nickel from plated utensils in permanent liquids, *Contact Dermatitis*, 5, 52, 1979.
9. Diepgen, T. L., Fartasch, M., and Hornstein, O. P., Kriterien zur Beurteilung der atopischen Hautdiathese, *Dermatosen*, 39(3), 79, 1991.
10. Diepgen, T. L., Fartasch, M., and Schmidt, A., Epidemiology of occupational dermatoses in North Babaria, *Contact Dermatitis*, in press.
11. Edman, B., The usefulness of detailed information to patients with contact allergy, *Contact Dermatitis*, 19, 43, 1988.
12. Hogan, D. J., Dannaker, C. J., and Maibach, H. I., The prognosis of contact dermatitis, *J. Am. Acad. Derm.*, 23(2), 300, 1990.
13. Fisher, A. A. and Dooms-Goossens, A., Persulfate hair bleach reaction, *Arch. Dermatol.*, 112, 1407, 1976.
14. Frosch, P. J., Aktuelle Kontaktallergene, *Hautarzt*, 41 (Suppl. 10), 129, 1989.
15. Frosch, P. J. and Hausen, B. M., Allergische Reaktionen vom Soforttyp auf das Haarfärbemittel Henna, *Allergologie*, 9(8), 351, 1986.
16. Frosch, P. J., Cutaneous irritation, in *Textbook of Contact Dermatitis*, Rycroft, R. J. G., Menné, T., Frosch, P. J., and Benezrea, C., Eds., Springer-Verlag, Berlin, 1992, 28.
17. Frosch, P. J., Burrows, D., Camarasa, J. G., et al., Allergic reactions to a hairdressers' series: results from nine European centres, *Contact Dermatitis*, 28, 180, 1993.
18. Frosch, P. J., Kurte, A., and Pilz, B., Evaluation of skin barrier creams. III. The repetitive irritation test (RIT) in humans, *Contact Dermatitis*, in press.

19. Frosch, P. J. and Rycroft, R. J. G., International legal aspects of contact dermatitis, in *Textbook of Contact Dermatitis,* Rycroft, R. J. G., Menné, T., Frosch, P. J., and Benezra, C., Eds., Springer-Verlag, Berlin, 1992, 751.

20. Frosch, P. J., Schulze-Dirks, A., Hoffmann, M., and Axthelm, I., Evaluation of skin barrier creams. II. Ineffectiveness of a popular "skin protector" against various irritants in the repetitive irritation test of the guinea pig, *Contact Dermatitis,* in press.

21. Frosch, P. J., Schulze-Dirks, A., Hoffmann, M., Axthelm, I., and Kurte, A., Efficacy of skin barrier creams. I. The repetitive irritation test (RIT) in the guinea pig, *Contact Dermatitis,* in press.

22. Gannon, M. X., Crowson, M. C., and Fielding, J. W. L., Periareolar pilonidal abscesses in a hairdresser, *Br. Med. J.,* 297, 1641, 1988.

23. Grobe, J. W., Pilonidal-sinus bei einem Friseur, *Dermatosen,* 26, 190, 1978.

24. Guerra, L., Tosti, A., Bardazzi, F., et al., Contact dermatitis in hairdressers: the Italian experience, *Contact Dermatitis,* 26, 101, 1992.

25. Hannuksela, M. and Hassi, J., Hairdresser's hand, *Dermatosen,* 28(5), 149, 1980.

26. Holness, D. L. and Nethercott, J. R., Dermatitis in hairdressers, *Dermatol. Clin.,* 8(1), 119, 1990.

27. James, J. and Calnan, C. D., Dermatitis in ladies hairdressers, *Trans. St. John's Hosp. Dermatol. Soc.,* 42, 19, 1959.

28. Kästner, W. and Frosch, P. J., Hautirritation verschiedener anionischer Tenside im Duhrig-Kammer-Test am Menschen im Vergleich zu in vitro- und tierexperimentellen Methoden, *Fette, Seifen, Anstrichm.,* 83, 33, 1981.

29. MacKie, B. S. and MacKie, L. E., Cross sensitization in dermatitis due to hair dyes, *Aust. J. Dermatol.,* 7, 189, 1964.

30. Meding, B., Epidemiology of hand eczema in an industrial city, *Acta Derm. Venereol.,* Suppl. 153, 1990.

31. Menné, T., Frictional dermatitis in post-office workers, *Contact Dermatitis,* 9, 172, 1983.

32. Nilsson, E., Mikaelsson, B., and Andersson, S., Atopy, occupational and domestic work as risk factors for hand eczema in hospital workers, *Contact Dermatitis,* 13, 216, 1985.

33. Pasricka, J. S., Gupta, R., and Panjawani, S., Contact dermatitis to henna (Lawsonia), *Contact Dermatitis,* 6, 288, 1980.

34. Peter, C. and Hoting, E., Contact allergy to cocamidopropyl betaine, *Contact Dermatitis,* 26, 282, 1992.

35. Rivett, J. and Merrick, C., Prevalence of occupational contact dermatitis in hairdressers, *Contact Dermatitis,* 22, 304, 1990.

36. Rystedt, I., Atopic background in patients with occupational hand eczema, *Contact Dermatitis,* 12, 247, 1985.

37. Savaides, A., Schultz, T., and Salce, L., The evaluation of gloves for protection against cosmetic ingredients, *J. Soc. Cosmet. Chem.,* 41, 267, 1990.

38. Schlueter, D. P. et al., Airway response to hair spray in normal subjects and subjects with hyperreactive airways, *Chest,* 75, 544, 1979.

39. Schonning, L. and Hjorth, N., Cross sensitization between hair dyes and rubber chemicals, *Dermatosen,* 17, 100, 1969.

40. Storrs, F. J., Permanent wave contact dermatitis: contact allergy to glyceryl monothioglycolate, *J. Am. Acad. Dermatol.,* 11, 74, 1984.

41. Stovall, G. K., Levine, L., and Oler, J., Occupational dermatitis among hairdressers: a multifactor analysis, *J. Occup. Med.,* 25, 871, 1983.

20

Skin Symptoms among Workers in the Fish Processing Industry

Lars Halkier-Sørensen and Kristian Thestrup-Pedersen

CONTENTS

I. INTRODUCTION

In Denmark, skin diseases rank as the third most common reported occupational disease, and 94%
of the cases are contact dermatitis.[1] However, among young people (≤25 years), occupational skin
diseases rank first. The single most commonly recognized occupational disorder is contact dermatitis.[1] Therefore, occupational contact dermatitis causes many socioeconomic problems.

The most important group of exposure sources are detergents, water, metals, food products,
and rubber. The food industry ranks third overall, and the second most important single occupation
within the food industry is the fish processing industry (FPI).[1] When one evaluates all single
occupations in Denmark, the FPI ranks twelfth among industries reporting occupational skin disorders. Furthermore, fish products are among the 5% most frequently mentioned causes for occupational dermatitis among several hundred listed exposure sources.[1]

In the winters of 1985/86 and 1986/87 an increasing number of workers in the Danish FPI
complained of skin problems, which led to an investigation of three large factories. The investigation
consisted of

1. An interview and a clinical examination
2. Studies with various fish products in volunteers to imitate the situation in the FPI
3. Comparison of clinical symptoms and experimental results
4. Skin tests with the protein/lipid fractions and the various degradation products in fish, and
   examination of bacteria and algae
5. Studies on the effect of cold exposure on itch and erythema
6. Skin physiological measurements among workers in the FPI during and after work
7. Studies on the effect of cold on barrier recovery

II. SUBJECTIVE COMPLAINTS AND CLINICAL FINDINGS

The investigation took place in factories that mainly processed round fish (codfish [72%], haddock
[23%], and coalfish and whiting [≤5%]). The fish were caught in the Baltic Sea, the North Sea,
the Arctic Ocean, the North and South Atlantic, and in Danish open seas (i.e., the Skagerak).
After being caught, the entrails were removed and the fish were stored on ice in the fishing boats
for a maximum of 14 days before landing. The fish were processed in the factories the same day
or after 1 or 2 days of storage on ice or in cold storage rooms; 86% of the supply was iced fish,
while 14% was delivered frozen by refrigerated vans. During processing in the factories the fish
products have a temperature of 2 to 6°C. A total of 196 workers — 172 women and 24 men —
participated in the study. Their mean age was 31 years, and their average length of employment
in the factories was 5 years. The workers were exposed to juice from fish boxes, remaining entrails,
slime/skin, fish juice from fillets, fish meat, cold, and water. They washed their hands, on average,
20 to 25 times a day.

A total of 80% (156) of the workers had on some occasion experienced skin problems during
contact with fish. The predominant symptoms were itching, redness, and stinging (Table 1), thus
belonging to contact urticarial symptoms. The symptoms were located on the forearms, the back
of the hands, and on the face and neck, but only seldom on the palms and fingers although these
areas were in direct contact with the fish products[2] (Table 2). Some of the workers complained of
itching or worsening of an itch after a hot shower following work. The skin symptoms, in general,
were mild to moderate and of short duration, and seldom interfered with the working capacity of
the employees. A total of 89% of the fillet workers, controllers, weighers, and wrappers (''clean''
production) stated that fish juice was responsible for the skin symptoms, and only 7% mentioned
the meat.[3] The employees working at the machines suspected contaminated juice from the fish
boxes, remaining entrails, and slime/skin (''dirty'' production). There were 12% who complained
of symptoms from the eyes (itching and redness), and 17% had symptoms from the upper respiratory
tract, mainly sneezing in the morning.

During the investigational period skin changes were observed in 11%, mostly an urticarial or
reddish rash on the volar aspect of the forearms. Only 2% had eczema.[2] However, some of the

TABLE 1　The Frequency of Skin Symptoms Among 156 Workers Employed in the Fish Processing Industry

Skin symptoms	n	%
Itch	136	87
Redness	100	64
Sting	61	39
Papules	24	15
Burning	16	10
"Acne"	13	8
Others	—	<8

Modified from Halkier-Sørensen, L. and Thestrup-Pedersen, K., *Contact Dermatitis,* 19, 206, 1988. With permission.

workers stated that they developed dry skin (chapping) on the fingers and palms shortly (30 to 60 min) after work that lasted for hours.

It was not possible to relate the symptoms to fish caught in specific areas, but the frequency of skin symptoms increased during the winter, when the workload is higher and the fish are richer in proteins.

During a 10-year period less than 1% of the 4000 employees had left their job because of skin problems. Most of the workers who stopped working on the FPI did so because they found another job, moved to another area, or found the work too hard. Others were laid off because of scarcity of the raw materials.

III. EXPERIMENTAL STUDIES WITH VARIOUS FISH PRODUCTS

As mentioned, itching, erythema, and stinging were anamnestically the predominant symptoms[2] (Table 1). In order to investigate whether the fish products possess the capacity to induce these symptoms, and to imitate the situation in the FPI regarding storage time, etc., skin reactivity to various fish products was studied under different conditions. Scratch tests were performed in 145 volunteers (101 women and 44 men, mean age 34 years) on the volar aspect of the forearms, where skin symptoms most often occurred. Saline 0.9% and histamine 3 mg/ml (0.3%) were used as

TABLE 2　The Location of Skin Symptoms (n = 156)

Location	%
Forearm	70
Volar	67
Dorsal	3
Face/neck[a]	60
Hands (dorsal)	26
Finger webs	5
Fingers	4
Hands (palmar)	3

[a]　10% had symptoms on the face only.

From Halkier-Sørensen, L. and Thestrup-Pedersen, K., *Contact Dermatitis,* 19, 206, 1988. With permission.

No. reactions

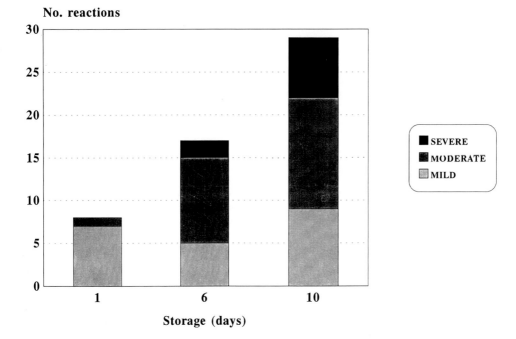

Storage (days)

FIGURE 1. Artificial storage of fillets in a refrigerator (2°C) for 10 days. Scratch tests were performed on 11 volunteers after 1, 6, and 10 days of storage. Notice that the number and severity of reactions are related to time of storage.

negative and positive controls. Reading was performed after 20 min. Most tests were performed with codfish, because it formed the majority (72%) of the production.

Fillets were collected in a randomized way from the conveyer belt, and 82 volunteers were tested with fish juice and meat; 45% reacted with itching, erythema, and/or stinging. Fish juice caused 87% of the reactions. Most reactions were mild or moderate (88%), and erythema and itching were the predominant symptoms (85%).[3]

An increasing post-mortem age of fish was obtained by storing the fillets in a refrigerator (2°C) for 10 days. Tests were performed with juice and meat after 1, 6, and 10 days on 11 volunteers. The results clearly demonstrate that the number and severity of the reactions are related to the time of storage (Figure 1). Erythema and itching were again the predominant symptoms (87%). Whealing was observed only after storage for 10 days.[3]

To imitate the actual situation in the FPI, iced fish with a post-mortem age of 1 to 2, 5 to 7, and 10 to 12 days (organoleptic quality assessment) were collected in the factories, and volunteers were tested with the various fish products the same day, or on day 3 (stored in a cold storage room at 2°C) to imitate the weekend situation. Tables 3 and 4 show how itching and erythema are related to the post-mortem age of the various fish products and storage through the weekend. Notice that totally fresh fish (1 to 2 days old) hardly cause any skin reaction in spite of a damaged skin barrier (scratch). The total number of stinging reactions caused by the same fish, as mentioned in Tables 3 and 4, were 11 (7 mild, 3 moderate, 1 severe) on day 1 and 20 (15 mild, 1 moderate, 4 severe) after "the weekend"; 88% of the reactions were itching and erythema, and severe itch reactions were seen more often than severe erythema.[3] The results demonstrate that the post-mortem age of the fish is of great importance for the frequency and severity of skin reactions, and that fish stored through the weekend make reactions worse. Objective measurements for erythema (laser Doppler and "paper"-size) confirmed the subjective readings (mild, moderate, severe), and showed that the reactions to fish products were mild to moderate compared to histamine 0.3% (Tables 3 and 4).[3]

Testing with entrails clearly demonstrated that contamination with juice from the stomach and gall bladder was of importance: 85% of the reactions were itching and erythema, and severe itch reactions occurred often.[3]

TABLE 3 Itch in Response to Different Fish Products in 39 Volunteers

Material	Post-mortem age (days)	Day 1 test			Day 3 test		
		No. tested	No. of reactions	(%)	No. tested	No. of reactions	(%)
Fish juice	1–2	23	1 (1, 0, 0)	4	24	4 (4, 0, 0)	16
Fish meat		23	1 (1, 0, 0)	4	24	6 (3, 3, 0)	25
Fish juice	5–7	23	11 (2, 5, 4)	48	24	18 (3, 7, 8)	75
Fish meat		23	2 (1, 1, 0)	9	24	6 (2, 3, 1)	25
Fish juice	10–12	12	5 (3, 1, 1)	42	12	9 (0, 2, 7)	75
Fish meat		12	1 (0, 1, 0)	8	12	2 (0, 0, 2)	17
Skin	1–2	8	0 (0, 0, 0)	0	10	0 (0, 0, 0)	0
Skin	10–12	8	5 (1, 2, 2)	63	10	7 (3, 3, 1)	70
Slime	4–5	7	1 (1, 0, 0)	14	7	1 (0, 1, 0)	14
Slime	10–12	7	4 (3, 1, 0)	57	10	7 (2, 3, 2)	70
Contaminated juice from fish boxes	10–12	7	6 (0, 2, 4)	86	10	10 (2, 0, 8)	100
Total no. of reactions			37 (13, 13, 11)	24		70 (19, 22, 29)	42
Control (NaCl 0.9%)					39	0 (0, 0, 0)	0
Control (histamine 0.3%)					24	24 (0, 3, 21)	100

Note: Scratch tests were performed on days 1 and 3 in order to imitate a weekend situation. The test products were refrigerated at 2°C in between. The results are given as the number of participants who reacted, followed by parentheses indicating the number who had mild, moderate, or severe reactions. The results show the relation between the post-mortem age of the fish and the number and severity of reactions, and the change caused by storage.

From Halkier-Sørensen, L. and Thestrup-Pedersen, K., *Contact Dermatitis*, 21, 172, 1989. With permission.

TABLE 4   Erythema in Response to Different Fish Products in 39 Volunteers

Material	Post-mortem age (days)	Day 1 test			Day 3 test		
		No. tested	No. of reactions	(%)	No. tested	No. of reactions	(%)
Fish juice	1–2	23	0 (0, 0, 0)	0	24	1 (1, 0, 0)	4
Fish meat		23	0 (0, 0, 0)	0	24	2 (2, 0, 0)	8
Fish juice	5–7	23	15 (6, 9, 0)	65	24	20 (7, 8, 5)	83
Fish meat		23	2 (1, 0, 1)	9	24	11 (5, 5, 1)	50
Fish juice	10–12	12	7 (1, 6, 0)	58	12	9 (1, 5, 3)	75
Fish meat		12	0 (0, 0, 0)	0	12	4 (4, 0, 0)	33
Skin	1–2	8	0 (0, 0, 0)	0	10	0 (0, 0, 0)	0
Skin	10–12	8	6 (4, 2, 0)	75	10	9 (3, 6, 0)	90
Slime	4–5	7	0 (0, 0, 0)	0	7	2 (2, 0, 0)	29
Slime	10–12	7	6 (3, 3, 0)	86	10	6 (3, 1, 2)	60
Contaminated juice from fish boxes	10–12	7	6 (0, 2, 4)	86	10	10 (2, 2, 6)	100
Total no. of reactions			42 (15, 22, 5)	27		74 (30, 27, 17)	44
Control (NaCl 0.9%)					39	0 (0, 0, 0)	0
Control (histamine 0.3%)					24	24 (0, 2, 22)	100

Note: Scratch tests were performed on days 1 and 3. The products were refrigerated at 2°C to imitate a weekend situation. The results are given as the number of participants who reacted followed by parentheses indicating the number who had mild, moderate, or severe reactions. The results show the relation between the post-mortem age of the fish and the number and severity of reactions, and the change caused by storage.

From Halkier-Sørensen, L. and Thestrup-Pedersen, K., *Contact Dermatitis*, 21, 172, 1989. With permission.

TABLE 5   The Relative Frequency of Itching, Redness, and Stinging Obtained Anamnestically Among Workers in the Fish Processing Industry and By Scratch Test With Various Fish Products in Volunteers

Complaints	Anamnestically (workers)		Scratch tests (volunteers)	
	n	(%)	n	(%)
Itching	136	46	163	40
Redness	100	34	182	44
Stinging	61	20	64	16
Combined itching and redness		80		84

Modified from Halkier-Sørensen, L. and Thestrup-Pedersen, K., *Contact Dermatitis*, 19, 206, 1988 and 21, 172, 1989. With permission.

Also, the reactivity to juice from the fish boxes was significantly related to the post-mortem age of the fish. Reaction to old, contaminated juice from the fish boxes was very pronounced (see also Section V.A).[3]

Nearly all reactions disappeared within 1 h. The cumulative number of reactions to all the various fish products was 163 for itching, 182 for erythema, and 64 for stinging (see also Section IV and Table 5). Itching and erythema were the predominant symptoms (84%), and 75% of all reactions were mild to moderate. Severe itch reactions (40%) occurred more often than severe erythema (17%). Itching and erythema caused by histamine 0.3% were much more pronounced: all responses being moderate or severe (0, 10, and 90%). Closed patch tests with fish products (1 to 6 h), and application of fish juice to undamaged skin for hours on the volar aspect of the forearm, did not result in any reaction. However, in a patient with atopic dermatitis, application of fish juice on the forearm resulted in itching and erythema. Furthermore, when scratches were performed during work on the volar aspect of the forearm in asymptomatic fillet workers, 50% complained of itching and erythema after 20 min. The above-mentioned observations indicate that a defective skin barrier seems to be necessary for the symptoms to occur.

IV.   COMPARISON OF SUBJECTIVE AND EXPERIMENTAL RESULTS

The relative frequency of itching, redness, and stinging registered by workers in the FPI,[2] and results obtained by scratch tests with various fish products in volunteers,[3] are shown in Table 5. As can be seen, there is a reasonable correlation between the anamnestic and experimental results. Itching and redness were the predominant symptoms (approximately 80%). In both cases, fish juice caused reactions much more often than fish meat. The skin symptoms were mild to moderate, and disappeared within a short time.

V.   CAUSE OF THE SKIN SYMPTOMS

Tests with various fish products (Section III) revealed that skin irritancy was related to the post-mortem age of the fish. In order to further describe which compounds in fish impart skin irritancy, scratch tests were performed with the lipid and protein fraction of fish juice, high and low molecular weight compounds, and with degradation compounds known to accumulate in fish during storage on ice. Bacteriological studies and studies for algae were also included. The tests were performed among 75 volunteers — the same participants who also took part in the study of skin reactivity to various fish products (Section III).

A. Lipid and Protein Fraction

Only the protein fraction of fish juice led to skin reactions. The skin reactivity to the protein fraction was positive-correlated to the post-mortem age of the fish (Table 6). The severe erythematous reactions caused by the protein fraction of old, contaminated juice from fish boxes were larger than usual, having an effect close to that of histamine.[4]

B. High and Low Molecular Weight Compounds

Raw fish juice was filtered through an Amicon ultrafiltration cell. Scratch tests were performed with the filtered compounds of <1500 Da, 1500 to 10,000 Da, and >10,000 Da. Mainly, fractions with molecules >10,000 Da resulted in positive reactions (Table 7). The relative number of severe reactions was also greater in this fraction.[4]

C. Protein Concentration and Peptide Pattern

The average concentration of protein in raw fish juice was 8.5 g/l, while the fraction <2000 Da only contained 0.4 g/l. There were no differences in the peptide pattern in fish juice known to have caused skin symptoms and in nonirritant control samples. The average pH of the fish products was 6.5.[4]

D. Degradation Products

Different low molecular weight degradation products, known to accumulate in fish stored on ice for a maximum of 2 weeks, were dissolved in concentrations equal to or ten times the maximum concentration given in textbooks (Table 8); 45 volunteers were tested with these compounds. The concentrations of the different degradation products in fish samples collected in the factories were measured and compared to the maximum allowed concentrations (Table 8).

All tests with degradation compounds within the relevant concentration range were negative. When using concentrations that were ten times higher, it appeared that NH_3, trimethylamine (TMA), dimethylamine (DMA), lactate, formaldehyde, and some of the amino acids possessed skin irritancy properties. The measured concentrations of degradation products in fish products (juice and meat) were all within limits of acceptability (Table 8). Only traces of the biogenic amines, histamine and cadaverine (Table 8), were found in fish juice known to have caused skin symptoms.[4]

E. Bacteria and Algae

A total of 200 samples for bacteriological examination were collected from various fish products (Table 9). The investigations were carried out in 1987–88, and therefore attempts to isolate *Listeria* were not performed. Samples known to have caused itching or irritation of the skin did not differ from nonirritant samples, and furthermore, fewer bacterial species were isolated from fillets and fish juice ("clean" production line — Table 9), although skin symptoms often occurred among workers in the "clean" production line. Toxic algae were not isolated from the slime.[4]

VI. THE EFFECTS OF COLD EXPOSURE ON ITCH AND ERYTHEMA

As mentioned in Section II, symptoms were not found on skin areas directly in contact with fish, but were mostly localized to the volar aspect of the forearms and the backs of the hands. The skin surface temperature on the fingers and palms of the employees was less than 20°C, whereas the temperature on the back of the hands and on the forearms was between 25 and 30°C (Table 10). In an attempt to imitate the situation in the FPI, the influence of cold exposure on itch, erythema, and wheal in response to histamine scratch tests was studied in 14 volunteers.[5] Cooling of the skin to less than 20°C was induced by application of an ice cube for 30 min on the inside of the forearm. This abolished itch and reduced the intensity of erythema by approximately 50% and the size of the erythema by approximately 20% (Figures 2 to 4). The wheal reaction was unaffected by cooling.[5] Furthermore, cooling abolished itch and reduced erythema in response to other inflammatory

TABLE 6 Reactivity to the Lipid and Protein Fractions of Fish Juice From Fillets and Juice From the Boxes

Material	Post-mortem age (days)	Fraction	No. Tested	Stinging	Itching	Erythema	Total no. of reactions	No. reacted	(%)
Fish juice	1–2	Lipid	14	0 (0, 0, 0)	0 (0, 0, 0)	1 (1, 0, 0)	1	1	36
		Protein	14	2 (1, 1, 0)	2 (2, 0, 0)	1 (1, 0, 0)	5	5	
Fish juice	5–7	Lipid	14	1 (1, 0, 0)	0 (0, 0, 0)	0 (0, 0, 0)	1	1	85
		Protein	14	4 (3, 4, 0)	7 (3, 3, 1)	12 (8, 3, 1)	23	12	
Fish juice	10–12	Lipid	14	1 (1, 0, 0)	0 (0, 0, 0)	0 (0, 0, 0)	1	1	93
		Protein	14	5 (4, 1, 0)	8 (1, 5, 2)	12 (6, 4, 2)	25	13	
Contaminated juice from fish boxes	10–12	Lipid	8	0 (0, 0, 0)	0 (0, 0, 0)	0 (0, 0, 0)	0	0	100
		Protein	8	2 (0, 2, 0)	5 (0, 1, 4)	8 (2, 3, 3)	15	8	
Total no. of reactions				15 (10, 5, 0)	22 (6, 9, 7)	34 (18, 10, 6)			
Control (NaCl 0.9%)			14	0 (0, 0, 0)	0 (0, 0, 0)	0 (0, 0, 0)			

Note: As can be seen, only the protein fraction is of importance. The numbers in parentheses indicate mild, moderate, or severe reactions, respectively.

From Halkier-Sørensen, L. and Thestrup-Pedersen, K., *Contact Dermatitis*, 21, 172, 1989. With permission.

TABLE 7 Scratch Tests Performed on 50 Volunteers With Fish Juice After Ultrafiltration

Mol wt	No. of tests	Positive tests n	Positive tests %	Stinging	Itching	Redness	Total no. of reactions
>10,000	120	81	68	18 (11, 4, 3)	53 (10, 21, 22)	71 (26, 26, 19)	142 (47, 51, 44)
10,000–1,500	120	42	35	5 (5, 0, 0)	29 (17, 8, 4)	23 (16, 7, 0)	57 (38, 15, 4)
<1,500	120	36	30	8 (7, 1, 0)	23 (11, 6, 6)	21 (14, 4, 3)	52 (32, 11, 9)
Control (NaCl 0.9%)	50			0 (0, 0, 0)	0 (0, 0, 0)	0 (0, 0, 0)	0 (0, 0, 0)

Note: Parentheses indicate mild, moderate, and severe reactions, respectively.

From Halkier-Sørensen, L. et al., *Contact Dermatitis*, 24, 94, 1991. With permission.

TABLE 8   The Maximum Concentration of Different Degradation Products in Cod Stored on Ice for ≤2 Weeks and the Measured Values

Products	No. of samples	Max. concentration	Units	Measured values
Trimethylamine oxide (TMAO)	28	120	mg N/100 g	40 (0.1–90)
Trimethylamine (TMA)	6	15	mg N/100 g	4 (3–7)
Dimethylamine (DMA)	6	10	mg N/100 g	12 (9–16)
Ammonia		30	mg N/100 g	—
Formaldehyde	16	4	mg/100 g	1.8 (0.1–5.3)
Inosine monophosphate (IMP)	15	5	μmol/g	0.8 (0–2.9)
Inosine	15	4.5	μmol/g	2.6 (0.2–4.4)
Hypoxanthine	15	5.5	μmol/g	2.8 (0.7–5.1)
Histidine	6	10	mg/100 g	6 (3–8)
Anserine		150	mg/100 g	—
Taurine	6	375	mg/100 g	150 (125–169)
Glycine	6	175	mg/100 g	46 (33–70)
Arginine	6	10	mg/100 g	6 (5–8)
Alanine	6	125	mg/100 g	52 (37–71)
Lysine	6	40	mg/100 g	22 (9–33)
Histamine	6	—	μmol/ml	<0.01
Cadaverine	6	—	μmol/ml	<0.05
Creatine		400	mg/100 g	—
Lactate		500	mg/100 g	—
Dimethylsulfide		5	μg volatile sulfide/100 g	
TVN[a]	28	35	mg N/100 g	26 (0–172)
K-value[b]	15	70–100	%	83 (57–100)

[a]   TVN = total volatile nitrogen (NH_3, TMA, DMA).

[b]   K-value: expression of freshness (see Reference 12).

From Halkier-Sørensen, L. et al., *Contact Dermatitis*, 24, 94, 1991. With permission.

TABLE 9 Distribution of Bacterial Strains Isolated from Cod (86.4%) and Haddock (13.6%)

Culture medium	Incubation temperature/time	Genera	"Dirty" production[a]	"Clean" production[b]
Blood agar base (Gibco) + 5% calf blood	20°/48 h	Streptococcus[c]	+	+
	37°/24 h	Lactobacillus[c]	+	−
		Corynebacterium[c]	+	+
		Aeromonas	+	+
		Vibrio	+	+
		Enterobacteria	+	−
		Flavobacterium	+	−
Marine agar (Difco) + 5% calf blood	20°/48 h	Streptococcus	+	−
		Lactobacillus	+	−
		Corynebacterium	+	−
		Moraxella	+	−
		Aeromonas	+	+
		Vibrio	+	+
		Enterobacteria	+	−
		Pseudomonas	+	+
Thiosulfate, citrate, bile salt, sucrose agar (TCBS, Difco)	20°/48 h	Plesiomonas	+	−
	37°/24 h	Vibrio	+	+
MacConkey agar (Gibco)	20°/48 h	Enterobacteria	+	−
		Aeromonas	+	+
No. of samples (total 200)			**169**	**31**

[a] Samples taken from the bottom of the hold in the fishing boats, juice from fish boxes, slime/skin, and belly.

[b] Samples taken from the fillets and fish juice after filleting.

[c] Gram-positive, all others are Gram-negative.

From Halkier-Sørensen, L. et al., *Contact Dermatitis*, 24, 94, 1991. With permission.

TABLE 10   Finger, Hand, and Forearm Skin Temperatures (°C) Among 143 Workers Employed in the Fish Processing Industry

Location	n_1	With protection*	n_2	Without protection
Volar				
3rd Finger	190	23.9 (4.4)	94	22.8 (3.9)
Hand	190	29.2 (2.3)	94	27.0 (2.8)
Forearm	121	31.2 (1.4)	163	30.0 (2.0)
Dorsal				
3rd Finger	190	25.4 (4.3)	94	24.0 (3.7)
Hand	190	29.6 (1.8)	94	27.9 (2.2)
Forearm	121	31.0 (1.6)	163	29.9 (1.9)

Skin Temperature (°C) Measured Directly at the Working Table

Location	n_3	Without protection	n_4	Controls
Volar				
3rd Finger	43	17.3 (2.4)	58	29.5 (3.2)
Hand	30	19.9 (3.8)	58	32.1 (1.4)
Forearm	10	28.0 (1.8)	58	32.8 (0.9)
Dorsal				
3rd Finger	18	16.7 (2.1)	58	30.6 (2.7)
Hand	37	24.1 (2.6)	58	32.1 (1.2)
Forearm	10	28.6 (2.2)	58	32.4 (1.0)

Note: n = number of measurements, figures in parentheses = standard deviation.

From Halkier-Sørensen, L. and Thestrup-Pedersen, K., *Contact Dermatitis*, 24, 345, 1991. With permission.

*   Protection: gloves and/or plastic sleeves.

substances such as LTC4 and C5$_a$, and also in response to fish juice. These findings seem important in order to explain why contact urticarial symptoms in the FPI seldom occur on the fingers and palms (temperature <20°C), although these areas are in direct contact with the fish products.

VII.   SKIN PHYSIOLOGICAL MEASUREMENTS

Although dry skin (chapping) or eczema seldom occur among workers in the FPI during work periods, some of the workers complained of temporarily dry skin on the fingers and hands 30 min to 1 h after a working day.

The skin surface temperature (digital thermometer, Ellap type TRD, probe diameter 12 mm); transepidermal water loss (TEWL) (Evaporimeter EP1, Servomed, Stockholm); and electrical capacitance (Corneometer CM420, Schwartzhaupt, Germany) were measured on the left and right side and on the volar and dorsal aspect of the tip of the third finger, the middle of the hand, and the forearm among workers in the FPI. The results on the fingers were compared with workers in other occupations. Because it took 5 to 7 min to perform all measurements, and because skin temperature increased very rapidly among workers in the FPI when exposure to the cold fish products was stopped, measurements also were performed directly at the working table. Furthermore, the skin blood flow (laser Doppler flowmeter, Periflux, Perimed, Sweden), skin temperature, TEWL, and electrical capacitance were followed at various intervals for 1 h after the working day in 10 employees.[7]

The workers in the FPI have very low skin surface temperature and TEWL, and high electrical capacitance on the fingers and palms at their working position, compared to control persons (Tables 10 to 12). A significant positive correlation was found between the skin temperature and TEWL in all measured areas (p <0.001–0.01), a significant negative correlation between the temperature

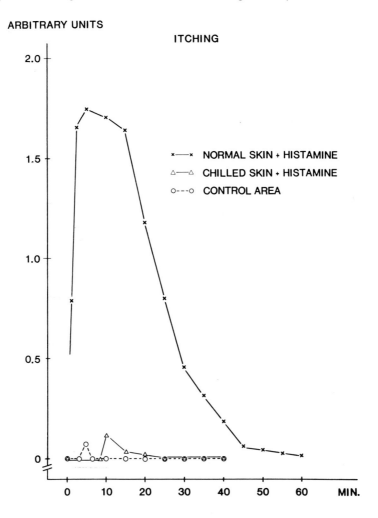

FIGURE 2.   Itch in response to histamine (3 mg/ml) on chilled and normal skin, using an arbitrary scale from 0 to 3, reflecting none, mild, moderate, and pronounced responses. The intensity of itch on chilled and normal skin differed significantly (sign test, 10 min, $p < 0.001$). The intensity of itch on chilled skin compared to the control (saline) did not differ. The values indicate mean values. (From Halkier-Sørensen, L. and Thestrup-Pedersen, K., *Contact Dermatitis*, 21, 179, 1989. With permission.)

and the electrical capacitance on the fingers and palms ($p < 0.001$–0.01), and a significant negative correlation between the capacitance and TEWL on the fingers ($p < 0.01$ — regression analysis) (Figures 5 to 7). The relationship between temperature and TEWL and between the temperature and capacitance was similar (parallel regression lines) on the right and left side and on the volar and dorsal aspect, and independent of whether the employees used protection (gloves, plastic sleeves) or not (parallel regression lines).[6] The relationships between the skin temperature-TEWL values and between the skin temperature-capacitance values on the fingers among workers in the respective occupations are shown in Figures 8 and 9. It can be seen that the various occupational groups are linear positive (TEWL-temperature values) or linear negative (capacitance-temperature values) correlated. The temperature-TEWL relationships in the respective groups were identical on the volar and dorsal aspect ($p = 0.83$) and the slope was identical in all groups ($p = 0.18$) (slope = 1.87, SE = 0.14, natural logarithms) (Figure 10) indicating a similar temperature-TEWL

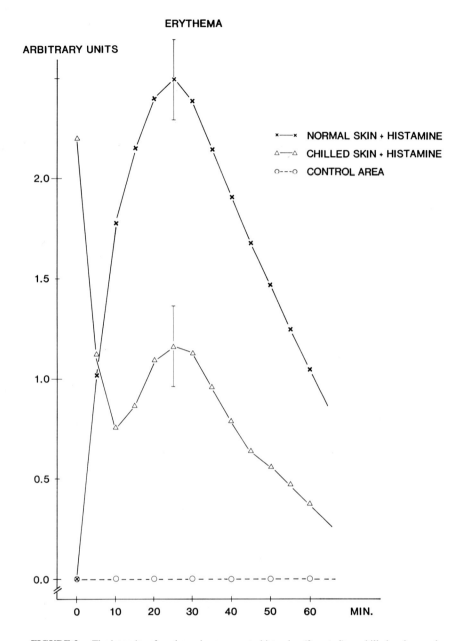

FIGURE 3.   The intensity of erythema in response to histamine (3 mg/ml) on chilled and normal
skin, using an arbitrary scale from 0 to 3, reflecting none, mild, moderate and
pronounced responses. Saline was used as control. The intensity of erythema on
chilled skin was significantly lowered (paired *t*-test, 25 min, *p* <0.001). The values
indicate mean values and standard errors of mean (SE). (From Halkier-Sørensen,
L. and Thestrup-Pedersen, K., *Contact Dermatitis,* 21, 179, 1989. With permission.)

dependence in all groups (regression analysis).[6] Therefore, differences in the levels (or interception
on the TEWL axis) between the respective occupations and controls and between the various groups
might indicate damage to the skin. The relationship between temperature and capacitance in the
respective groups was also identical on the volar and dorsal aspect (*p* = 0.92), but the slope was
not identical in all groups (*p* <0.0004) (regression analysis).[6]

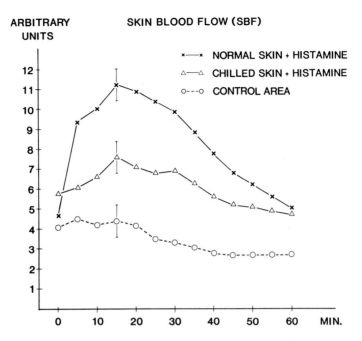

FIGURE 4. Measurements of the skin blood flow (SBF), performed by means of a laser Doppler flow meter, showing that the SBF in response to histamine (3 mg/ml) was significantly lowered in chilled skin (paired *t* test, 15 min, *p* <0.001). The difference between chilled skin and the control (saline) was also significant (*p* <0.001). The values indicate mean values and standard errors of mean (SE). (From Halkier-Sørensen, L. and Thestrup-Pedersen, K., *Contact Dermatitis*, 21, 179, 1989. With permission.)

To collect information on seasonal variations, the skin temperature, TEWL, and capacitance were followed at intervals of 6 to 7 weeks from March to January. The skin temperature was constant (*p* = 0.15) through the period, while TEWL was significantly lower (*p* <0.001) and the capacitance significantly higher (*p* <0.01) during the summer season (analysis of varians). The workload is higher in the FPI during the winter season. A more defective barrier during winter, making penetration by polypeptides easier, could explain why skin symptoms (contact urticaria) occur more often during the 6 months of winter in the FPI. Furthermore, the fish are richer in proteins during winter.[6]

Measurements performed during the hour after work showed that the skin blood flow, skin surface temperature, and TEWL increased markedly to values above normal within 10 to 15 min, while the electrical capacitance decreased to subnormal values (Figure 11a to 11d).[7] The skin blood flow and TEWL normalized within 1 h, while the capacitance showed only a slight tendency toward normalization during the observation period. The high TEWL and the low capacitance after work can explain why some of the workers experienced dry skin after work.[7]

A significantly linear positive relationship was found between the respective temperature-TEWL values in the various groups. More important is the observation that the slope of the temperature-TEWL relationships based on natural logarithms on both axes was identical (*p* = 0.18) in all groups.[6] One of the essential factors dictating the rate of TEWL is the skin surface temperature. Therefore, to facilitate inter- and intrasubject comparisons, a formula has been proposed to convert TEWL at any given skin surface temperature to a standard reference temperature of 30°C: log $TEWL_{30}$ = log $TEWL_T$ + a(30 − T), where a is the slope.

However, the previously calculated slopes differ significantly, being 0.084 and 0.035, respectively.[8,9] The skin temperatures among workers in the various groups ranged from 15 to 35°C.

TABLE 11   Finger, Hand, and Forearm TEWL (g/m²h) among 143 Workers Employed in the Fish Processing Industry

Location	n_1	With protection*	n_2	Without protection
Volar				
3rd Finger	190	40.0 (23.3)	94	40.7 (19.3)
Hand	190	35.1 (15.0)	94	38.5 (14.2)
Forearm	121	10.8 (9.0)	163	9.6 (6.6)
Dorsal				
3rd Finger	190	23.1 (15.9)	94	25.9 (15.2)
Hand	190	12.5 (9.3)	94	11.0 (7.6)
Forearm	121	7.5 (5.8)	163	7.0 (4.6)

TEWL (g/m²h) Measured Directly at the Working Table

Location	n_3	Without protection	n_4	Controls
Volar				
3rd Finger	20	13.6 (8.8)	58	62.6 (21.1)
Hand	11	22.6 (5.1)	58	45.3 (17.4)
Forearm	10	7.7 (2.2)	58	8.0 (4.3)
Dorsal				
3rd Finger	11	9.1 (6.5)	58	28.4 (14.3)
Hand	11	19.6 (6.2)	58	13.3 (9.4)
Forearm	10	6.7 (2.2)	58	5.6 (3.3)

Note: n = number of measurements, figures in parentheses = standard deviation.

From Halkier-Sørensen, L. and Thestrup-Pedersen, K., *Contact Dermatitis,* 24, 345, 1991. With permission.

*   Protection: gloves and/or plastic sleeves.

Using common logarithms and with the data plotted semilogarithmically (TEWL) the slope of the resulting line was 0.030 (SE = 0.023),[10] and approximates the lowest of the previously reported slope values (0.035).[9] Using the above-mentioned equation (slope = 0.030), for conversion of TEWL among workers in the FPI to a common reference temperature of 30°C, it appeared that the TEWL on the dorsal aspect of the fingers was significantly higher than normal controls.[10] These results suggest that workers in the FPI actually may have a barrier defect masked by the low skin temperature during work.

VIII.   THE EFFECT OF COLD EXPOSURE ON SKIN BARRIER RECOVERY

Some of the employees in the FPI complained of dry skin or chapping on the fingers and palms after work. This suggested that the workers in the FPI may have a defect in barrier function (perhaps caused by prolonged hydration, excessive handwashing — 20 to 25 times a day — and/or by inhibition of the metabolic processes necessary for barrier homostasis/recovery during long-term exposure to cold), which, however, is masked by the low skin temperature, resulting in low TEWL rates and high capacitance during work. To imitate the situation in the FPI, hairless mice were exposed to ice (water) for hours (skin temperature 10 to 15°C) after breaking the barrier with acetone.[11] Immediately after cold exposure, the low skin temperature misleadingly suggested barrier recovery (low TEWL). However, 15 min after rewarming, TEWL increased dramatically, followed by a gradual decrease to pre-cold exposure values over 1 to 2 h. Thereafter, the barrier recovered normally. Electron microscopic examination immediately after cold exposure revealed abnormal morphology of almost all nascent lamellar bodies (LBs) and paucity of the secreted LB material

TABLE 12   Finger, Hand, and Forearm Capacitance (a.u.) among 143 Workers Employed in the Fish Processing Industry

Location	n_1	With protection*	n_2	Without protection
Volar				
3rd Finger	190	71.1 (16.1)	94	73.8 (18.8)
Hand	190	82.4 (19.9)	94	85.0 (19.3)
Forearm	121	100.6 (11.9)	163	91.7 (13.9)
Dorsal				
3rd Finger	190	54.9 (14.4)	94	60.9 (19.8)
Hand	190	92.8 (15.0)	94	91.3 (18.0)
Forearm	121	89.6 (12.8)	163	81.2 (18.7)

TEWL (g/m²h) Measured Directly at the Working Table

Location	n_3	Without protection	n_4	Controls
Volar				
3rd Finger	12	95.8 (15.5)	58	78.2 (14.3)
Hand	12	116.1 (13.2)	58	88.2 (18.6)
Forearm	10	91.7 (5.8)	58	91.6 (9.9)
Dorsal				
3rd Finger	12	70.4 (13.7)	58	45.5 (11.1)
Hand	12	107.3 (13.5)	58	81.4 (12.1)
Forearm	10	81.5 (8.4)	58	75.7 (14.9)

Note: n = number of measurements, figures in parentheses = standard deviation, a.u. = arbitrary units.

From Halkier-Sørensen, L. and Thestrup-Pedersen, K., *Contact Dermatitis,* 24, 345, 1991. With permission.

*   Protection: gloves and/or plastic sleeves.

at the SG-SC interface. After 1 h of cold exposure, the majority of nascent LBs displayed normal morphology.[11]

Exposure to warm water (33°C) after barrier abrogation only slightly affected barrier recovery (TEWL) compared to air (normal recovery) and the LBs had normal morphology. When normal skin was exposed to ice (water) the LBs were not affected, but hydration led to structural changes in the stratum corneum (hydration damage), resulting in slightly elevated TEWL.

The results show that cold exposure after barrier disruption totally blocks the normal formation of LBs and barrier recovery, and provides an explanation for the clinical syndrome in the FPI.[11]

IX. COMMENTS AND CONCLUSIONS

In Denmark, the fish processing industry (FPI) ranks as twelfth among occupations with reported occupational contact dermatitis.[1] The workers are exposed to various fish products, water, and cold.

A. Skin Symptoms

This investigation confirms that itching and erythema (Table 1) often occur among workers in the FPI during contact with fish.[2] However, the observed skin symptoms, in general, were mild to moderate and of short duration, and seldom interfered with the working capacity of the employees.[2] The skin symptoms were mainly localized to the volar side of the forearms, face/neck, and back of the hands (Table 2).[2]

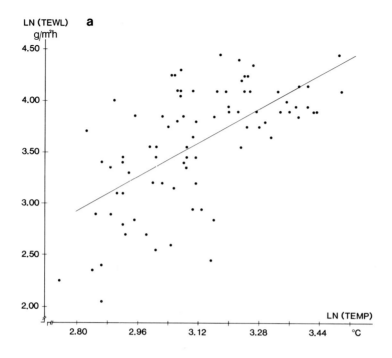

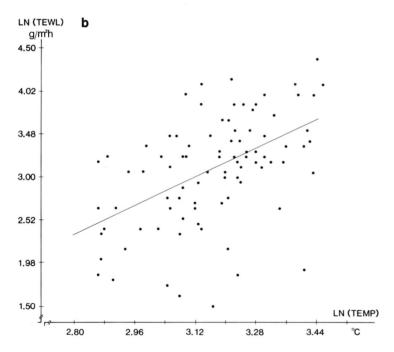

FIGURE 5. Relationship between skin surface temperature and transepidermal water loss (TEWL) expressed logarithmically (natural) among workers in the fish processing industry. Measurements performed on the volar (slope = 2.09, SE = 0.27, $p <0.001$) (a) and dorsal (slope = 2.10, SE = 0.36, $p <0.001$) (b) aspect of the tip of the 3rd finger (no protection) (regression analysis). (From Halkier-Sørensen, L. and Thestrup-Pedersen, K., *Contact Dermatitis*, 24, 345, 1991. With permission.)

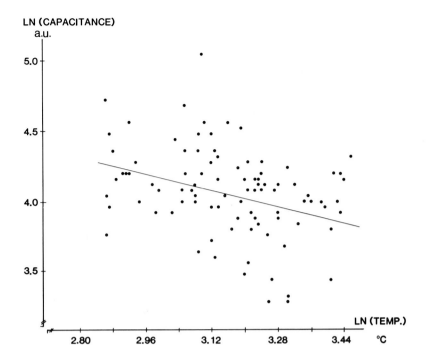

FIGURE 6. Relationship between skin surface temperature and capacitance, expressed logarithmically (natural), among workers in the fish processing industry. Measurements performed on the dorsal aspect of the tip of the 3rd finger (no protection); slope = −0.69 (SE = 0.20, p <0.001). The slope on the volar aspect (not shown) was −0.48 (SE = 0.15, p <0.01) (regression analysis). (From Halkier-Sørensen, L. and Thestrup-Pedersen, K., *Contact Dermatitis*, 24, 345, 1991. With permission.)

Experimental studies[3] with the various fish products showed that all fish products were capable of causing irritant skin reactions (Tables 3 and 4). The predominant symptoms were itching and erythema.[3] The frequency and severity of the reactions caused by the fish products were significantly related to the post-mortem age of the fish, and the storage time in the factories (Figure 1, Tables 3 and 4). However, in general, the reactions were mild to moderate compared to histamine 0.3%.[3] The experimental results were in accordance with the subjective complaints among workers in the FPI (Table 5).

Only the protein fraction, and mainly the high molecular weight compounds (>10,000 Da), of fish juice caused symptoms (Table 6 and 7).[3,4]

The major post-mortem changes are due to autolysis and activity of Gram-negative bacteria.[12] Bacterial activity may therefore accelerate the degradation of some compounds.[12] Fish muscle proteinases (mainly neutral proteinases) lead to hydrolysis of large muscle proteins[13,14] and the various fragments accumulate in the fish juice (the fillets lose 5 to 10% of their weight when kept in plastic pails for 2 to 4 days). Also, contamination with digestive enzymes may contribute to hydrolysis of fish muscle proteins.[15] Trypsin and pepsin themselves can cause keratinolysis in human skin,[16,17] thereby reducing the barrier function.

Tests with low molecular weight degradation compounds (Table 8) were all negative,[12] and the concentrations of the compounds were within limits of acceptability.[4] Only traces of the biogenic amines, histamine and cadaverine,[18] were found.[4]

The microflora from fish known to have caused skin symptoms and from controls did not differ. Furthermore, fewer bacterial species were isolated from fillets and fish juice ("clean" production line) (Table 9) although skin symptoms often occur among fillet workers.[4] The genera found on the skin of the examined species were similar to the flora of the Atlantic salmon.[19]

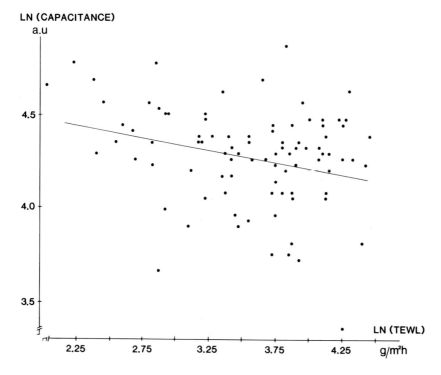

FIGURE 7. Relationship between electrical capacitance and transepidermal water loss (TEWL), expressed logarithmically (natural), among workers in the fish processing industry. Measurements performed on the volar aspect of the tip of the 3rd finger (no protection); slope = −0.13 (SE = 0.05, p <0.01) (regression analysis). (From Halkier-Sørensen, L. and Thestrup-Pedersen, K., *Contact Dermatitis*, 24, 345, 1991. With permission.)

The reactivity to totally fresh fish products was very low (Tables 3 and 4) and, even for old fish products, a defective skin barrier was necessary for a reaction to occur.[3] However, small wounds, scratches, and slight excoriations are not uncommon among workers in the FPI, and as mentioned, juice from the stomach contains trypsin and pepsin, which cause keratinolysis.[16,17]

If denatured protein fragments (polypeptides) are the main cause of the skin symptoms, it explains why only totally fresh fish possess extremely low irritant properties, even on damaged skin (scratch test).[3] This is well known among the workers in the FPI; who say "the old fish bite". The first symptoms is often an itch and very slight erythema. If left untouched, the itch may disappear within minutes, but if the skin is scratched, severe erythema occurs. This phenomenon is called "burning eczema".

The post-mortem age of the fish, and a defect barrier, are essential factors for the skin symptoms to occur. However, individual susceptibility may also influence the results; i.e., it has been shown that raw fish products induce an urticarial reaction in 55% of nonatopic and 71% of atopic persons.[20,21]

Skin symptoms from contact with fish have been described before,[20-23] and protein contact dermatitis from food items is often caused by fish products in kitchen personnel.[22] Though immunologic contact urticaria to fish has been described,[24] most reactions are nonallergic, probably caused by penetration of protein fragments and liberation of histamine and/or other inflammatory mediators.[4]

B. Cold and Location of the Symptoms

One observation from the study was that the skin symptoms were not found on skin areas (fingers and palms) that were directly in contact with the fish products.[2] The temperature of the fingers

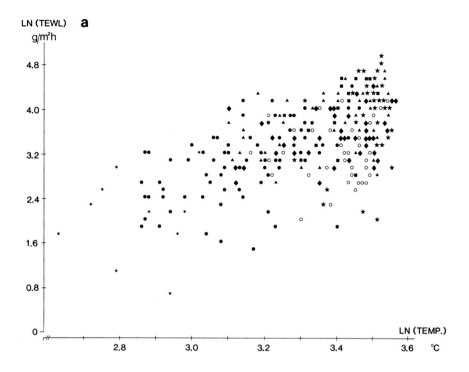

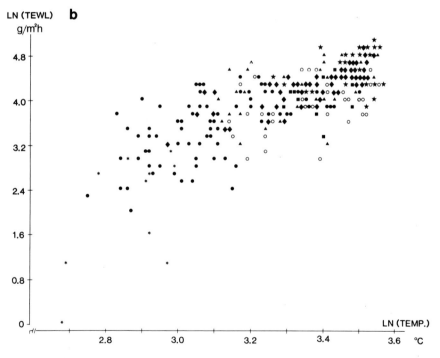

FIGURE 8. Relationship between the respective skin temperature-TEWL values of the various occupations, expressed logarithmically (natural). Measurements performed on the dorsal (a) and volar (b) aspect of the tip of the 3rd finger. *, fish processing industry at the working position; ●, fish processing industry; ▲, cleaners; ○, normal controls; ■, gut cleaners; ★, metal workers; and ◆, coincidence points. (From Halkier-Sørensen, L. and Thestrup-Pedersen, K., *Contact Dermatitis,* 24, 345, 1991. With permission.)

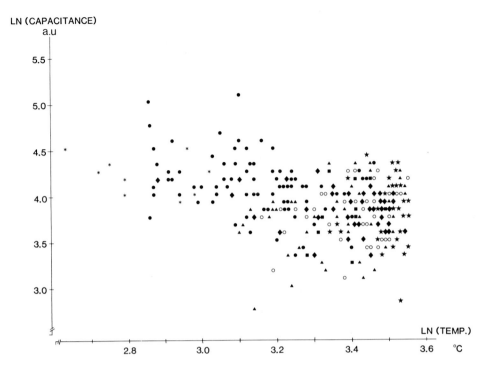

FIGURE 9. Relationship between the respective skin temperature-capacitance values of the various occupations, expressed logarithmically (natural). Measurements performed on the volar aspect of the tip of the 3rd finger. *, fish processing industry at the working position; ●, fish processing industry; ▲, cleaners; ○, normal controls; ■, gut cleaners; ★, metal workers; and ◆, coincidence points. (From Halkier-Sørensen, L. and Thestrup-Pedersen, K., *Contact Dermatitis, 24*, 345, 1991. With permission.)

and palms was less than 20°C during work, and cooling of the skin to less than 20°C completely abolished itch and reduced erythema by approximately 50%.[5] This suggests that the peripheral nerve fibers, and/or mediators involved in the transmission of itch,[25] and the axon reflex mediating the flare reaction,[26] are blocked or inhibited by low skin temperatures. Others have shown that the mean temperature at which itch disappears is about 19°C, and that changes in skin temperature have a marked influence on itch intensity.[27] Itching, therefore, cannot arise on the fingers and palms (<20°C) during work, but only on the warmer skin on the back of the hands and forearms (25 to 30°C). The effects of thermal stimulation on itch explain why some of the workers observed itching or worsening of the itch after a hot shower following work.[27]

The average histamine levels in the various skin areas (palm, back of the hand, and forearm) are comparable,[28] and this supports the observation that the skin temperature, and not differences in the level of skin histamine, is an important factor for the location of the symptoms among workers in the FPI.[5]

C. Skin Physiological Measurements and Barrier Function

The skin physiological measurements (Figures 5 to 7) confirmed, from a practical point of view, the observations from earlier experimental studies of a linear relationship between temperature and TEWL[8,9,29] and the observation of an inverse relationship between TEWL and skin hydration in scaly dermatoses.[30-35] As a new finding, the measurements showed that the capacitance (Figure 6) is sensitive to changes in skin temperature.[6] Furthermore, a linear positive relationship was found between the respective temperature-TEWL values and a linear negative relationship between the respective temperature-capacitance values (Figures 7 to 9) in the various groups.[6] The calculated

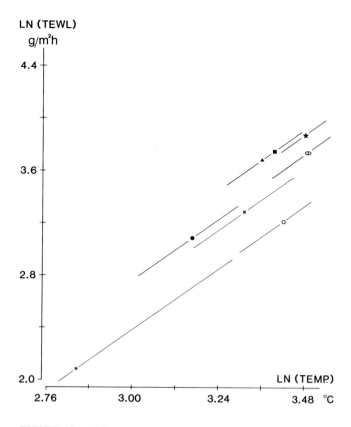

FIGURE 10. Differences in levels (or interception on the TEWL axis and comparison at the same temperature) between the respective groups and controls and between the various occupations, expressed logarithmically (natural). The observed differences in levels may indicate damage to the skin barrier, but environmentally related variables may also affect the level. Measurements performed on the dorsal aspect of the tip of the 3rd finger. The slope = 1.87 (SE = 0.14) was identical in all 8 groups (p = 0.18) (regression analysis). *, fish processing industry at the working position; ●, fish processing industry; ▲, cleaners; ○, normal controls; x, nurses; ■, gut cleaners; ø, office workers with indoor climate syndrome; and ★, metal workers. (From Halkier-Sørensen, L. and Thestrup-Pedersen, K., *Contact Dermatitis*, 24, 345, 1991. With permission.)

slope based on 887 paired measurements of the temperature and TEWL, for conversion of TEWL to a common reference temperature of 30°C, was 0.030,[10] and approximates the lowest of the previously calculated slopes for conversion of TEWL to a common reference temperature.[8,9]

Dry skin or chapping seldom occurred during work. However, 30 to 60 min after work some of the employees complained of dry skin on the hands. Skin physiological measurements showed that the skin temperature was very low during work, resulting in a low TEWL and a high capacitance (Tables 10 to 12, Figure 11), thereby protecting the skin against drying.[6,7] Furthermore, wet work hydrates the skin. After work, the TEWL increased to values above normal, while the capacitance decreased to values below normal (Figure 11).[7] The skin physiological measurements, therefore, are in accordance with the clinical findings among workers in the FPI.

These observations suggested a defect barrier function, which, however, is masked by the low skin temperature during work. During the last decade, the essential role of lipids in the regulation

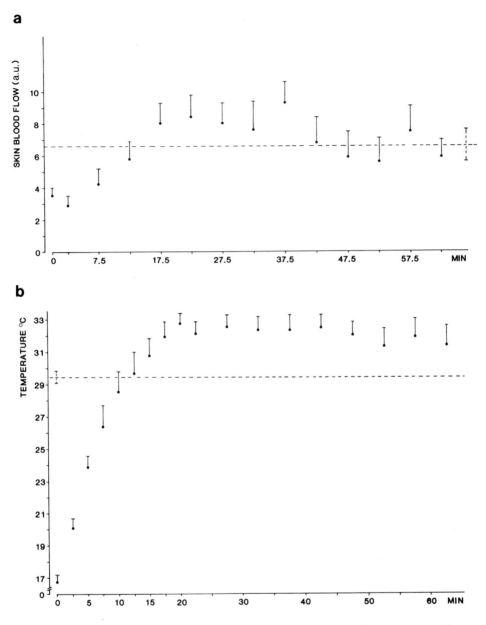

FIGURE 11. Volar 3rd finger measurements of (a) skin blood flow, (b) skin surface temperature, (c) transepidermal water loss (TEWL), and (d) electrical capacitance in 10 fillet workers at their working position (0 min) and the changes during the first h (2.5 to 62.5 min) after a working day. Broken lines represent normal controls. Mean and SEM. (From Halkier-Sørensen, L. and Thestrup-Pedersen, K., *Contact Dermatitis*, 25, 19, 1991. With permission.)

of stratum corneum barrier function,[34-38] and the role of lipids in the water-holding properties of the stratum corneum[39] have been described. Experimental studies in hairless mice showed that cold exposure, after barrier abrogation, totally blocked the normal formation of lamellar bodies (LBs) and barrier recovery.[11] These results provide an explanation for the clinical findings of dry skin on the hands among workers in the FPI after work. Hydration of normal skin led to structural changes in the stratum corneum resulting in slightly elevated TEWL, and hydration damage may contribute to changes in barrier function.

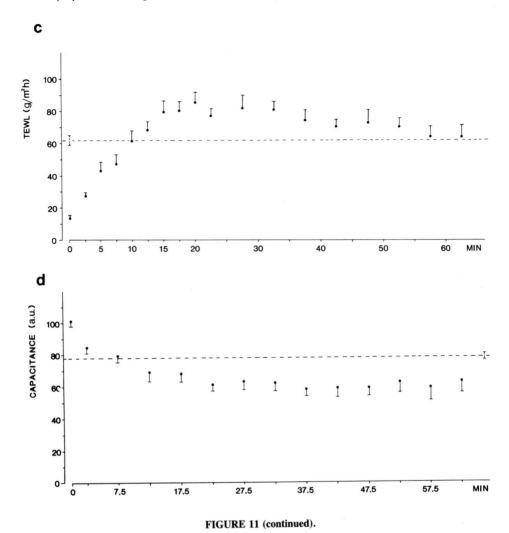

FIGURE 11 (continued).

In order to reduce the frequency of skin symptoms in the FPI (1) the fish should be processed in the factories as fast as possible after the catch, (2) juice in the fish boxes should be removed before processing, and (3) emollients and protective clothing should be used. Pollutants, bacteria, algae, or volatile amines do not seem to play an important role in the occurrence of contact urticarial symptoms from fish.

REFERENCES

1. Halkier-Sørensen, L., Haugaard-Petersen, B., and Thestrup-Pedersen, K., Occupational dermatitis in Denmark 1984–91. Book of Abstracts, 1st Congr. Eur. Soc. Contact Dermatitis, 37, October, 1992.
2. Halkier-Sørensen, L. and Thestrup-Pedersen, K., Skin temperature and skin symptoms among workers in the fish processing industry, *Contact Dermatitis*, 19, 206, 1988.
3. Halkier-Sørensen, L. and Thestrup-Pedersen, K., Skin irritancy from fish is related to its postmortem age, *Contact Dermatitis*, 21, 172, 1989.
4. Halkier-Sørensen, L., Heickendorff, L., Dalsgaard, I., and Thestrup-Pedersen, K., Skin symptoms among workers in the fish processing industry are caused by high molecular weight compounds, *Contact Dermatitis*, 24, 94, 1991.

5. Halkier-Sørensen, L. and Thestrup-Pedersen, K., The relevance of low skin temperature inhibiting histamine-induced itch to the location of contact urticarial symptoms in the fish processing industry, *Contact Dermatitis,* 21, 179, 1989.

6. Halkier-Sørensen, L. and Thestrup-Pedersen, K., The relationship between skin surface temperature, transepidermal water loss and electrical capacitance among workers in the fish processing industry: comparison with other occupations. A field study, *Contact Dermatitis,* 24, 345, 1991.

7. Halkier-Sørensen, L. and Thestrup-Pedersen, K., Skin physiological changes in employees in the fish processing industry immediately following work. A field study, *Contact Dermatitis,* 25, 19, 1991.

8. Grice, K., Sattar, H., Sharratt, M., and Baker, H., Skin temperature and transepidermal water loss, *J. Invest. Dermatol.,* 57, 108, 1971.

9. Mathias, C. G. T., Wilson, D. M., and Maibach, H. I., Transepidermal water loss as a function of skin surface temperature, *J. Invest. Dermatol.,* 77, 219, 1981.

10. Halkier-Sørensen, L., Thestrup-Pedersen, K., and Maibach, H. I., Equation for conversion of transepidermal water loss (TEWL) to a common reference temperature: what is the slope?, *Contact Dermatitis,* in press.

11. Halkier-Sørensen, L., Elias, P. M., Menon, G., Thestrup-Pedersen, K., and Feingold, K. R., Skin function changes among workers in the fish processing industry: comparison with barrier function and recovery in hairless mice after long-term cold exposure, *J. Invest. Dermatol.,* 96, 621, 1991.

12. Huss, H. H., Fresh fish — quality and quality changes (FAO Fisheries Ser. No. 29). Food and Agriculture Organization. Danish International Development Agency, Rome, 1988.

13. Makinodan, Y., Yokoyama Y., Kinoshita, M., and Tokyohara, H., Characterization of an alkaline proteinase of fish muscle, *Comp. Biochem. Physiol.,* 87B, 1041, 1987.

14. Makinodan, Y., Hirotsuka, M., and Ikeda, S., Neutral proteinase of carp muscle, *J. Food Sci.,* 44, 1110, 1979.

15. Hjelmeland, K. and Res, J., Fish tissue degradation by trypsin type enzymes, in *Advances in Fish Science and Technology,* Fishing Books, London, 1979, 456.

16. Bjelland, S., Gildberg, A., and Volden, G., Degradation of human epidermal keratin by fish pepsin, *Arch. Dermatol. Res.,* 280, 119, 1988.

17. Bjelland, S., Hjelmeland, K., and Volden, G., Degradation of human epidermal keratin by cod trypsin and extracts of fish intestines, *Arch. Dermatol. Res.,* 280, 469, 1989.

18. Kalusen, N. K. and Lund, E., Formation of biogenic amines in herring and mackerel, *Z. Lebensm. Unters. Forsch.,* 82, 4569, 1986.

19. Horsley, R. W., The bacterial flora of the Atlantic Salmon (*Salmon salar,* L.) in relation to its environment, *J. Appl. Bacteriol.,* 36, 377, 1973.

20. Beck, H.-I. and Nissen, B. K., Type-I reactions to commercial fish in non-exposed individuals, *Contact Dermatitis,* 9, 219, 1983.

21. Beck, H.-I. and Nissen, B. K., Contact urticaria to commercial fish in atopic persons, *Acta Derm. Venereol.,* 63, 257, 1983.

22. Hjorth, N. and Roed-Petersen, J., Occupational protein contact dermatitis in food handlers, *Contact Dermatitis,* 2, 28, 1976.

23. Kavli, G. and Moseng, D., Contact urticaria from mustard in fish-stick production, *Contact Dermatitis,* 17, 153, 1987.

24. Melino, M., Toni, F., and Riguzzi, G., Immunologic contact urticaria to fish, *Contact Dermatitis,* 17, 182, 1987.

25. Fjellner, B., Experimental studies and clinical pruritus. Studies on some putative peripheral mediators. The influence of ultraviolet light and transcutaneous nerve stimulation, *Acta Derm. Venereol.,* Suppl. 97, 5, 1981.

26. Czarnetzki, B. M., *Urticaria,* Springer-Verlag, Berlin, 1986, 5.

27. Fruhsdorfer, H., Hermanns, M., and Latzke, L., The effects of thermal stimulation on clinical and experimental itch, *Pain,* 24, 259, 1986.

28. Zacahariae, H., Skin histamine, in *Spectrofluorometric Studies on Normal and Diseased Skin,* Munksgaard, Copenhagen, 1965.

29. Thiele, F. A. and Van Senden, K. G., Relationship between skin temperature and the insensible perspiration of the human skin, *J. Invest. Dermatol.,* 47, 307, 1966.

30. Tagami, H. and Yoshikuni, K., Interrelationship between the water barrier and reservoir function of pathologic stratum corneum, *Arch. Dermatol.,* 121, 624, 1986.

31. Thune, O., Nilsen, T., Hanstad, K., Gustavsen, T., and Dahl, H. L., The water barrier function of the skin in relation to the water content of stratum corneum, pH and skin lipids, *Acta Derm. Venereol.,* 68, 277, 1988.

32. Werner, Y. and Lindberg, M., Transepidermal water loss in dry and clinically normal skin in patients with atopic dermatitis, *Acta Derm. Venereol.,* 65, 102, 1986.

33. Blichmann, C. and Serup, J., Hydration studies on scaly hand eczema, *Contact Dermatitis,* 16, 155, 1987.

34. Elias, P. M., Epidermal lipids, barrier function, and desquamation, *J. Invest. Dermatol.,* 80 (Suppl. 6), 44, 1983.

35. Grubauer, G., Feingold, K. R., Harris, R. M., and Elias, P. M., Lipid content and lipid type as determinants of the epidermal permeability barrier, *J. Lipid Res.,* 30, 89, 1986.

36. Grubauer, G., Elias, P. M., and Feingold, K. R., Transepidermal water loss: the signal for recovery of barrier structure and function, *J. Lipid Res.,* 30, 323, 1989.

37. Elias, P. M. and Menon, G. K., Structural and lipid biochemical correlates of the epidermal permeability barrier, in *Advances in Lipids Research,* Vol. 24, Elias, P. M., Ed., Academic Press, San Diego, 1991.

38. Feingold, K. R., The regulation and role of epidermal lipid synthesis, in *Advances in Lipids Research,* Vol. 24, Elias, P. M., Ed., Academic Press, San Diego, 1991.

39. Imikawa, G. and Hattori, M., A possible function of structural lipids in the water-holding properties of the stratum corneum, *J. Invest. Dermatol.,* 84, 282, 1985.

21

Occupational Dermatitis by Metalworking Fluids

Edith M. De Boer and Derk P. Bruynzeel

CONTENTS

0-8493-7355-7/94/$0.00 + $.50

I. METALWORKING

During industrial fabrication of hard materials, usually metals, metalworking fluids (MWF) are widely used as coolants and lubricants. In metalworking procedures frictional heat is generated due to the pressure between the chip and the tool of the machine, and the deformation of metal. This heat can be reduced, on the one hand, by cooling the workpiece and the tool with a liquid and, on the other hand, by reducing the friction with a lubricant. The temperature at the tip of the tool can become very high. Therefore the tool wears quickly, causing a diminishing of the accuracy of the cut and of the finish of the workpiece. Particles of swarf may even become welded to the tool, thus increasing the friction.[1] Figure 1 shows schematically the cutting of metal.

The main function of MWF is to reduce the frictional heat between the tool and from the workpiece. Furthermore, MWF improves the surface finish of the workpiece and removes the swarf, thus prolonging the life of tools and reducing the consumption of power.[1] As long as metalworking has been done by mankind, MWF have been used. The earliest coolants and lubricants were plain water and animal fat. A disadvantage of water is its corrosiveness to iron and steel and its lack of lubricating properties. In the 18th century, soap-water was used in metalworking, which had some lubricant and anticorrosive effect.

The application of animal fat as a lubricant also has its disadvantages: lard becomes rancid very quickly. With the discovery of mineral oil, used alone or in combination with animal fat, the stability of the product and its lubricating properties improved. By coincidence, it was found that the addition of sulfur improved the cutting properties still further. A historical review of the use of MWF is given by Crow.[1]

A problem occurs when, due to high pressure between the tool and the workpiece, the cutting oil is squeezed out. For this purpose, extreme-pressure additives are used. They are activated by great heat and then combine with the metal surface. In this way a solid lubricant is formed by these salts of sulfur and/or chlorine. They may be used in very high concentrations and are then very effective in heavy-duty cutting procedures. A disadvantage is their high cost.

II. METALWORKING FLUIDS (MWF)

A. Types of MWF

Nowadays, MWF can be divided into two groups: neat oils and soluble oils (Table 1). Neat oils, or insoluble oils, are undiluted oils, mostly mineral, and usually contain extreme-pressure additives and sometimes other additives. Soluble oils, or water-based metalworking fluids, always contain water. Three subgroups of soluble oils can be distinguished: the first group are the classic soluble oils that contain 50 to 80% mineral oils and may contain a high concentration of extreme-pressure additives; the second group, which are the most commonly used soluble oils and are "semisynthetic", oil-in-water emulsions that contain mineral oils in a concentration of 5 to 10% and therefore

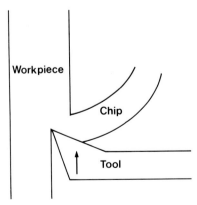

FIGURE 1.   The heat production is highest
at the tip of the tool.

TABLE 1 Types and General Composition of MWF: Substances that Might be Present in Neat Oils and Water-Based Fluids

MWF	Type	Possible Components
Neat oil	Insoluble oils	Mineral oil, extreme-pressure additive, corrosion inhibitors, antifoams, dyes, fragrances
Water-based fluids	Soluble oils Semisynthetic solutions Synthetic solutions	Mineral oil, emulsifiers, stabilizers, extreme-pressure additives, corrosion inhibitors, antifoams, preservatives, dyes, fragrances

From De Boer, E. M., Ph.D. thesis, Free University Amsterdam, 1989. With permission.

need a considerable amount of emulsifiers; and the third group which are not really soluble oils as they contain no oils — they are called aqueous solutions or ''synthetic'' solutions. They always contain large amounts of emulsifiers and anticorrosives. They lack lubricating properties and are used for grinding only.

Neat oils are used undiluted, as they are delivered by the producer. Water-based MWF are delivered as a concentrate, and are diluted with water to 1 to 10% before use.

B. Composition of MWF

A list of possible ingredients of MWF is given in Table 2. The composition of MWF is not constant in time as a result of adaptation to specific purposes, and as there are numerous producers of MWF using their own formulas for the production of MWF this list does not pretend to be complete. All

TABLE 2 Additives of Dermatological Significance in MWF

Additive	Possible chemicals	Remarks
Emulsifiers	Abietic acid	In colophony
	Coconut diethanolamide	
	Oleic acid	
	Tall oil	In colophony
	Petroleum sulfonate	
	Soap	
	Ethoxylates	
Hard-water stabilizers	Copolymers of olefinic oxides	
Extreme-pressure additives	Sulfur, chlorine, and phosphorus compounds	
	Dipentene	
Corrosion inhibitor	Mercaptobenzotriazole	
	Hydrazine sulfate	Also emulsifier
	Sodium sulfonate	Also emulsifier
	Sodium nitrite	
	Di/Triethanolamine	
	p-tert-Butylbenzoic acid	
Antifoams	Silicones	
	Waxes	
Preservatives	See Table 3	
Coupling agents	Propylene glycol	Also lubricant/preservative
	Triethylene glycol	
	Xylenol	
	Cresylic acid	
Miscellaneous	Tricresylphosphate	Antiwear agent
	Dimethyldithiocarbamate	Antioxidant
	Dyes	
	Fragrances	

water-based MWF are prone to bacterial colonization. The presence of bacteria, also nonpathogens, cause splitting of the emulsion due to a diminishing of the pH and destruction of the surfactants. In contrast to neat oils, water-based MWF generally circulate in a reservoir and are thus used for a long period of time, making them even more vulnerable to bacterial growth. Therefore, all water-based MWF contain preservatives or biocides.

A peculiar problem in the estimation of the use of biocides is the nomenclature used. Some producers do not apply the name biocide but refer to their products as "biostabilizers" or "conditioners". The use of biocides is not constant; often, newer types of biocides replace the conventionally used substances. A change of components is often not a reason to change the name of an MWF, which might be confusing to the user.

Almost all biocides have an irritant effect on the skin when used in a high concentration.[4-6] The influence of biocides on the skin is always related to the other irritant components of the fluids, e.g., the emulsifiers or the soap-like components. The use of biocides adds to the adverse effect on the skin of the fluid as a whole, especially when the concentration is high. This may happen when dilution has not been performed properly or when extra biocides are added to a fluid already containing a biocide. The induction of contact allergic dermatitis has been described as due to many kinds of biocides. Some biocides have a higher sensitizing potential than others. A problem is that many reports on contact allergy are case reports, thus a conclusion on epidemiology is difficult.

In Table 3, a list of the main biocides used in MWF is given with both the generic and some of the trade names. Publications on the occurrence of contact sensitization in metalworkers are indicated as far as possible.

C. Maintenance of MWF

Neat oils do not require much care. Usually, they are used only once. When they circulate from a reservoir, simple replacement is mostly sufficient.

In contrast, water-based fluids usually circulate in a system, and require care, not only during the preparation of a fluid, but also during the whole period they are in use. The concentrate that is purchased from the manufacturer has to be diluted with water to the user's concentration (1 to 10%). During the cutting procedure the concentration is likely to change as water evaporates owing to the heat generated by the cutting. As a result of pollution, bacteria may grow freely in the fluid and cause the emulsion to "break". The growth of bacteria in cutting fluids causes a decrease in pH by the production of acids. The fluids become rancid. After addition of a biocide the pH will again rise to a normal value for cutting fluids (about pH 8 to 10). When the concentration of biocides is unintentionally increased excessively, the pH may rise somewhat more.

Extra exposure to biocides occurs when system cleaners are added to the fluids and circulate while the work continues. System cleaners contain a high concentration of biocides and are used to clean the machine once in a while. In some plants this is done once every 3 months and in others not more than once in 2 years. The system cleaners are added to the reservoir of the machine and circulate for about 1 to 3 days. Working during this period means exposure to a high concentration of biocides. Pollution with particles of metal may also occur, as they may stay in the fluid, even after filtration. In open systems pollution with all kinds of things may occur, such as cigarettes, coffee, and fruit peelings.

D. Exposure to MWF

Exposure of the skin may occur when preparing the dilution, during filling of the machine, the placing of the workpiece and the tools, the procedure itself, and the removal, cleaning, and measuring of the workpiece and tools. The parts of the body that are exposed to fluids, of course, are predominantly the hands and forearms. However, considerable exposure may occur in the face and neck as the fluids spatter and evaporate. The latter is especially so with cutting fluids, although not as often with neat oils. Contamination with MWF may also occur when a hand wet with MWF is used to wipe the face. In the same way, the anogenital region may be exposed to MWF. Furthermore, leaning against a wet machine may soak the clothes at waist or thigh height. Putting a wet rag, used for wiping MWF, into a pocket is another source of exposure.

TABLE 3 Biocides Occurring in MWF

Generic name	Trade name	Reference to contact sensitization in metalworkers
Group I		
Formaldehyde and/or Formaldehyde releasers		7–23
Triazines		
Hexahydro-1,3,5-tris(2-hydroxyethyl)-s-triazine	Grotan BK	
	Glokill 77	
	Triadine 10	
	Onyxide 200	
	Bacillat 35	
	Bakzid 80	
Hexahydro-1,3,5-triethyl-s-triazine	Bactocide THT	
	Di Baktolan 34	
	Vancide TH	
Hexamine derivatives		24
1-(3-Chloroallyl)-3,4,7-triaza-1-azonia-adamantane	Dowicil 75[a]	
1-(3-Chloroallyl)-3,5,7-triaza-1-azonia-adamantane	Dowicil 100, 200[a]	
	Quaternium 15	
	Preventol D1	
"Benzylhemiformal derivative"	Preventol D2	
1-Carboxymethyl-3,5,7 triaza-1-azoniatricyclodecane	Busan 1024	
Imidazoles		[b]
N,N-methylene bis-[5'-(1-hydroxymethyl)-2,5-dioxo-4-imidazolidinyl urea]	Germall 115	
	Biopure 100	
	Euxyl K200	
1-Monomethyloldimethylhydantoin	Dantoin 685	
Aliphatic derivatives[c]		25
2,2-Dibromo-3-nitrilopropionamide	Dow Antimicrobial 7287, 8536, XD 8254, XD 8254 DPNPA Biosperse 240, 244	
Tris(hydroxymethyl)nitromethane = 2-(hydroxymethyl)-2-nitro-1,3-propanediol[d]	Tris Nitro	
2-Bromo-2-nitropropanediol[d]	Onyxide 500	
	Bronopol	
	Myacide S1	
Acetamides		26–28
Chloromethyl acylaminomethanol = n-hydroxymethylchloroacetamide	Grotan HD2	
	Parmetol K50	
	Preventol D3	
"Cyclic aminoacetal"	Bakzid	
Others		13
Tetrahydro-3,5-dimethyl-2H-1,3,5-thiadiazine-2-thione	Chemviron D3T	
	Protectol TDE	
	Busan 1058	

TABLE 3   Biocides Occurring in MWF (continued)

Generic name	Trade name	Reference to contact sensitization in metalworkers
5-Ethyl-1-aza-3,7-dioxa-bicyclooctane	Bioban CS-1246	
4,4 Dimethyl-1-oxa-3-azacy-cyclopentane	Bioban CS-1135	

Group II

Benzisothiazolones		8,29–31
2-n-Octyl-4-isothiazolin-3-one	Grotan TK2	
	Skane M8	
	Kathon 893, 4200, LM	
1,2-benzisothiazolin-3-one = benzisothia-zolone = BIT	Proxel GXL (proxel CRL = BIT + ethylenediamine)	
5-Chloro-2-methyl-4-isothiazolin-3-one +	Kathon CG, 886 MW	
2-Methyl-4-isothiazolin-3-one		

Group III

Phenols		32–34
o-Phenylphenol	Dowicide A, 1	
	Preventol O extra	
2,4,5-Trichlorophenol	Dowicide B, 2	
4-Chloro-3-methylphenol = p-chloro-m-cre-sol	Preventol CMK	
2,3,4,6-Tetrachlorophenol + pentachloro-phenol	Dowicide 6	
2,2-Methylene-bis(4-chlorophenol) = dichlo-rophene	Preventol GD	
	Panacide C	
p-Chloro-m-xylenol = chloroxylenol	Dettol	
Anilides		
3,4',5-Tribromosalicylanilide + 3,5'-dibro-mosalicylanilide	Tuasal 85	

Group IV

Morpholines		8,13,35
4-(2-Nitrobutyl)morpholine + 4,4-(2-ethyl-2-nitrotrilene) dimorpholine[d]	Bioban-1487	

Group V

Ethylenediamine		7,8,9,34,36

Group VI

Others		22,37
Pyridine derivatives		
1-Hydroxy-2(1H)pyridinethione = (2-pyri-dinethiol-1-oxide):zinc or sodium com-plexes	Zinc Omadine Sodium Omadine	
Dithiocarbamates		[b]
Potassium dimethyl dithiocarbamate	Busan 85	
Sodium dimethyl dithiocarbamate + sodium dimercaptobenzothiazole	Vancide 51	
Potassium N-hydroxymethyl-N-methyldi-thiocarbamate + sodium dimercaptoben-zothiazole	Busan 52	

TABLE 3   Biocides Occurring in MWF (continued)

Generic name	Trade name	Reference to contact sensitization in metalworkers
Quaternary ammonium compounds		
Benzalkonium chloride	Querton KKBCL[b]	
	Docligen 226	
	Zephirol	
	Barquat MB50	
Cyanates		[b]
Methylene bisthiocyanate	Biosperse 284	
	Metasol T-10	
	Cytox 3522	
	Chemviron T-9	
	Slimicide A	
Dioxanes		[b]
6-acetoxy-2,4-dimethyl-*m*-dioxane	Giv-Gard DXN	
	Dioxin	
Ethylene(dimethylimino)ethylene	Busan 77	[b]
2-(Thiocyanomethylthio) benzothiazol	Busan 30	[b]
	Tolcide C30	
5-Bromo-5-nitro-1,3-dioxan	Bronidox L	[b]

[a]   Confusion in nomenclature of Dowicil 75 and 100.
[b]   No data found about sensitization to these biocides in MWF.
[c]   This group of biocides is sometimes classified as a separate group, as formaldehyde release may not be the most important working mechanism.
[d]   This substance also has the capacity of nitrite release.

From De Boer, E. M., Ph.D. thesis, Free University Amsterdam, 1989. With permission.

Exposure is not always dependent on the degree of automation, as one would expect. Fast-working, computerized machines often require replacements of workpieces at short intervals, increasing the risk of exposure. Only fully automatic machinery that delivers completely cleaned and dried end products guarantees a minimum exposure.

III.   DERMATITIS FROM METALWORKING FLUIDS

The presentation of skin changes due to contact with MWF is very variable. Contact with neat oils may lead to folliculitis and oil acne. Occasionally irritant reactions occur and contact sensitization is extremely rare.[2,38] The use of old-fashioned neat oils regularly induced hyperpigmentation, keratoses, and cancer of the skin. Nowadays this problems is solved, as polycyclic aromatic hydrocarbons are removed by improved refinery techniques.

Exposure to soluble oils may partly cause other health hazards. Due to the abundant evaporation that occurs when spraying the fluids, a mist of water-based MWF may reach the bronchial system and cause CARA-like complaints. Another problem may occur as nitrites and secondary or tertiary amines react in the fluids to form the carcinogenic nitrosamines. In the modern soluble oils, formation of nitrosamines is minimized or absent.

The use of soluble oils may cause a wide range of skin problems. In the early stages the skin may become dry and rough, with a slight erythema and a fine chapping. Van Neste and co-workers call this condition a rough dermatitic skin if it is caused by irritation of the skin.[39,40] A fine, sometimes follicular erythema may develop, progressing to papular eczema, often patchy or nummular. Frequently, the dermatitis starts at the dorsa of the hands above the metacarpo-phalangeal joints, in the fingers and the webs, but the palms are also often involved.

A diffuse dermatitis of the hands may occur. The dermatitis may also show the clinical pattern of a dyshidrotic eczema.[43] The periungual skin is often involved in the process, showing slight erythema and fine cracks in the cuticles up to a manifest chronic paronychia with disappearance of the cuticles.[44] Not uncommon is the presence of dermatitis on the wrists and forearms.[41]

A. Etiology of Dermatitis

MWF dermatitis often has a multifactorial origin. Trauma makes the skin more accessible to both allergens and irritants. In an epidemiological study in the Netherlands among 286 metalworkers, almost half of the workers had mechanical injuries on their hands.[44]

B. Allergic Contact Dermatitis

The percentage of contact sensitization found in patch testing ranges from 20 to 48%.[3,42,45] These varying percentages depend on the differences in the design of the study. Lowest percentages are found by investigators who examine a whole group of nonselected workers on only one occasion. The highest percentages are found in departments of occupational dermatology, who get these patients from other centers or factories.

Reports about sensitization in metalworkers often concern only small numbers of sensitized operators and are mostly an allergy to a component of soluble oils. Biocides are usually mentioned as allergens, and sensitization to stabilizers and corrosion inhibitors is less often reported.[46,47] In the biocides that cause sensitization, the group including formaldehyde and formaldehyde releasers is important. These biocides are commonly used in soluble oils. Sensitization has often been observed, especially to hexahydro-1,3,5-tris (2-hydroxyethyl)-triazine (Grotan BK) and to a far lesser extent to 2-bromo-2-nitropropane-1,3-diol (Bronopol), and 1-(3-chloroallyl) hexaminiumchloride (Dowicil 200 = Quaternium 15).[1,17,19,21]

Besides the formaldehyde group, the other most important biocides are isothiazolinones, phenols, morpholins, and "biostatic" agents such as complexes of alkanolamineborate (Table 3).

It is important to realize that the frequency in which these components are used in different countries can differ considerably. Furthermore, there are some trends in the use of several components. Another confusing factor is the widespread use of the same biocides for industrial and cosmetic products, making it unclear whether sensitization occurred at work or at home.

A special problem may occur in the case of an allergy to a soluble oil. In the case of a positive reaction to the suspected fluid, patch tests with the separate components sometimes appear negative. In such cases identification of the allergen is impossible as several unknown reaction products can form in the fluid itself. This makes reliable testing very difficult.[48-50]

C. Irritant Contact Dermatitis

Workers with extensive contact to MWF more often have irritant dermatitis than workers with limited exposure. Exposure to soluble oils, compared with neat oils, causes more irritant dermatitis, including paronychia.[44] MWF contains several potentially irritating components such as mineral oils, organic acids, amines, emulsifiers, preservatives, and others. Water-based MWF have an especially complicated composition and they are alkaline: pH 8 to 10. As a result of the heat produced during the cutting procedure the fluid may become more concentrated and some components may reach an irritant concentration. Also, the pH may rise, which leads to a further augmentation of the irritancy of the fluid. Adding extra biocides or other chemicals such as system cleaners and antifoams will also contribute to the ultimate irritant potential of the water-based fluids.

Metalworkers are exposed to other hazards at work besides MWF.[42] Aggressive degreasers are used for cleaning the workpieces.[24,44] Contact of the hands of the operators with these mostly organic solvents, although often avoidable, is not unusual. The use of hand cleaners also adds to the damage to the skin when aggressive detergents or granules for scrubbing are used, especially if such agents contain organic solvents. Additionally, considerable exposure to all kinds of irritants and allergens at home is common, as metalworkers are often enthusiastic handicraftsmen.

IV. EPIDEMIOLOGY OF DERMATITIS IN METALWORKERS

A. Prevalence

The prevalence of contact dermatitis due to MWF is not well known. Most literature focuses on causal and epidemic events. These patient histories and publications from specialized occupational centers are important for determining which components in MWF cause sensitization.

Epidemiological studies among large groups of metalworkers are more scarce. Rycroft[42] investigated the workers in one plant during the course of a year and found that 33% of the workers more or less had contact dermatitis. An epidemiological study in the Netherlands in 10 plants among 286 workers showed a prevalence of dermatitis of 14%. Only 42% of all workers had no skin abnormality at all; 31% showed minor changes, such as a dry, rough skin with erythema and some periungual erythema. Another 13% had more severe erythema, induration and scaling, and chronic paronychia, and the prevalence of frank eczema was 14%.[44] In a separate study, out of 49 metalworkers exposed to MWF, 32% had minor changes, 6% had definite skin changes (major), while 6% had frank eczema.[51] Out of 27 metalworkers not exposed to MWF, the figures, respectively, were 48%, 7%, and 0%. In a control group of 47 office workers, 94% had a normal skin, 4% had a dry rough skin, and 2% had eczema.

In Singapore in 21 small-scale metal factories, 6.6% of 751 workers had a skin disorder on the hands, being confirmed as dermatitis in 4.5%. Most workers were exposed to neat oils and less to soluble oils. Concomitant exposure to solvents was favorable for the development of dermatitis.[24]

Histories of epidemics clearly show the multifactorial origin of the dermatological problems.

B. Epidemic Outbreaks of Dermatitis

Some reports describe more-or-less sudden outbreaks of skin disorders in factory workers exposed to MWF. Epidemic outbreaks of dermatitis caused by adding excessive amounts of formaldehyde-releasing biocides are described. Contact allergy to these biocides was demonstrated in several patients.[14,15,17] Weidenbach and Rakoski described an outbreak of dyshidrotic eczema among a considerable proportion of workers in a plant due to contact with water-based MWF.[52] Contact sensitization was not demonstrated.

In our own epidemiological study we encountered the same phenomenon seen in other epidemics of dermatitis. We were told in several factories that sudden, small outbreaks of dermatitis had taken place, often resulting in experiments with new biocides and MWF.[4] Characteristic of these outbreaks is that a group of workers in a factory, seemingly without any special problem, suddenly develop more-or-less severe eczema. The cause remains unclear and it is usually the cutting fluid that is held responsible, which is then removed from the reservoirs of the machines. The machines are then cleaned, and work is continued with some other cutting fluid. This sometimes solves the problem as it attracts the attention of the workers to the maintenance of the machines and the MWF. In the beginning, the dilution of the cutting fluid will be done accurately, the machines will be kept clean, and everyone will take care to work without unnecessary exposure to MWF. Hence, this irrational act of changing of the cutting fluid may lead to a lessening of the irritant dermatitis. This procedure often fails when several cutting fluids are used at the same time in a factory. These fluids have to be diluted differently; some fluids might require additives and others not. This might lead to confusion. Moreover, when workers have developed a contact sensitization to some component of MWF, usually a biocide, changing fluids without paying attention to the exact composition of the new MWF may not be problem solving.

V. THERAPY AND PREVENTION

A. General Measures

The most important advice to metalworkers is to limit contact with MWF as much as possible. Usually, the use of protective gloves is too dangerous and also appears not to be very effective.

Contact with MWF due to leaning on the machine or from wet cloths in the pocket is easily avoidable. By using screens around the machines, wearing impermeable aprons, and using disposable rags, exposure may be limited to some extent. Crucial is the limitation of other irritant and damaging influences on the skin, as the etiology of soluble oil dermatitis is multifactorial.[52] Protective gloves can be used while cleaning the machine, to avoid scratching and cutting of the skin. Direct skin contact with degreasers used for the work piece is very common, but often unnecessary in metalworkers. When cleaning the hands after work the mildest soap appropriate for this special purpose should be advocated. The use of aggressive soaps, sometimes with granules which grind the skin, should be limited. After work, emollient creams may help to restore the fat lost during the day, provided that they contain no irritants and preferably no biocides, at least not those which are also used in MWF. Barrier creams, which are much more expensive to use, have not demonstrated a barrier effect against detergents in these circumstances.

The general advice to metalworking factories is to use only a limited number of MWF, and to choose MWF that need no further addition of biocides or other components. The dilution of the fluid should be done properly and checked adequately. In case of contact sensitization to one or more of the components of MWF, it is sometimes possible to use a metalworking fluid without these or related compounds. Sometimes it is difficult to change a MWF on an entire workfloor just because one individual is allergic to some components.

B. Handling an Individual Worker with Hand Dermatitis

A thorough history of the dermatitis and insight into the daily exposure to all kinds of stimuli is important. Additional information on the specific circumstances on the workfloor and exact data on the chemicals used can usually best be obtained from the plant manager.

Patch testing should be performed with the European standard series, a special MWF series, and the plant's MWF in proper dilutions. It is recommended to patch test neat oils as is and diluted 50% in olive oil, water-based fluids 50, 10, and 3% in water, and use MWF as obtained from the floor. In case of positive reactions, control tests should be performed.

C. Preemployment Examination

A preemployment estimation of the risk of the development of dermatitis of the hands is tricky. A history of atopy, especially of atopic skin disease in the past or at present, seems to make the skin more vulnerable to irritant influences. Some authors plead that individuals with atopic skin disease should be advised not to become metalworkers.[54-56]

Patch tests as a routine before employment are not advisable as they have no predictive value. The future possible allergy has not yet developed. Patch tests can be useful in cases of existing dermatitis before employment.

In persons with psoriasis, mechanical injuries may aggravate existing lesions and induce new lesions (Koebner phenomenon). A history of psoriasis of the hands is a contraindication for working with irritant substances and for exposure to considerable mechanical trauma.

VI. PROGNOSIS

The prognosis of chronic dermatitis of the hands is unfavorable. This also applies to dermatitis caused by MWF. In a recent study, a questionnaire was used to evaluate 100 machine operators tested for soluble oil dermatitis more than 2 years before.[57] A poor prognosis, both for those who had continued to work with soluble oils and those who stopped, was observed. No significant difference was seen between both groups. Of those who had continued, 78% still suffered from eczema, as did 70% of those who had stopped. Only 25% were healed. It appears that there is a group of workers who heal quickly if cessation of contact is made before the dermatitis exists longer than 3 months; others develop chronic eczema. No factor could be identified to distinguish those with the more favorable prognosis.

In another follow-up study among 40 patients with soluble oil dermatitis who were sent a questionnaire up to 2½ years later, 45% were healed.[58] Only one person had stopped work because of dermatitis, but two others had been made redundant and two took early retirement.

TABLE 4 The Relationship of Exposure to MWF at Work and the Presence of Dermatitis in 10 Metalworkers With Allergic Contact Dermatitis (5) or Irritant Contact Dermatitis (5) as Obtained From a Questionnaire

Exposure to MWF	Persistent dermatitis		Dermatitis healed	
	+	−	+	−
Allergic dermatitis	3	1[a]	1[b]	—
Irritant dermatitis	3		1	1
Total	6	1	2	1

[a] Unfit to work, but dermatitis spreads.
[b] Avoiding one soluble oil.

Our department used a questionnaire for 13 metalworkers tested 1 to 3 years before. Ten nonforeigners replied. The three nonresponders had irritant dermatitis. The course of the dermatitis in relation to fulltime exposure to MWF at work is shown in Table 4.

None of these figures gives an optimistic impression on the prognosis of hand dermatitis. In a study on the outcome of occupational dermatitis in 230 workers (all kinds of occupations) after a mean period of 5 years, it was shown that workers with a better understanding of their skin disease had a better prognosis.[59] A good education with respect to skin exposure and preventive measures is important in hazardous professions like metalworking.

VII. EXPERIMENTAL INVESTIGATIONS

A. Experiments with Animals

The effect of repeated application of a cutting oil on guinea pigs and the influence of barrier creams has been studied.[60] During a 6-week period, 4 days a week, cutting oils were applied under occlusion on test sites on the shaved flanks of guinea pigs. Before application of the MWF some test sites were treated with barrier creams. Skin irritation was assessed by a visual score and the measurement of skin water loss. Considerable irritation due to the cutting oil was observed. It was a striking finding that the skin sites pretreated with barrier cream showed significantly more irritation. In a similar experiment,[61] emollient creams applied after removal of a cutting oil also appeared to aggravate the irritant effect.

B. Experiments with Healthy Volunteers

The irritant effect of repeated application on the forearms, after stripping of the stratum corneum, of 2 neat oils and 3 water-based MWF in user's concentration was assessed in 13 healthy volunteers by a visual score and the measurement of skin blood flow by Laser Doppler Flowmetry for a period of 5 days.[62] The MWF caused, in general, marginal skin irritation — the water-based MWF being more irritant than the neat oils. A similar experiment with some components of the MWF indicated an emulsifier and a corrosion inhibitor as the most irritant of the components.[62]

C. Experiments with Healthy Metalworkers

In 54 newly recruited metalworkers, skin water loss was measured on several sites on the hands and forearms weekly for a period of 12 weeks.[63] Skin water loss increased considerably in workers exposed to neat oils and somewhat in those exposed to soluble oils, in comparison to nonexposed workers. One would expect to find the opposite. This investigation was done in a warm climate; this might have influenced the results.

Preemployment screening for contact sensitization to nickel, cobalt, and chromium among pupils of a metal industry school has been advocated.[64] A relation with dermatitis has not been studied. In our opinion, contact sensitization to metals is not a major problem in metalworkers; Coenraads found that metalworkers with metal allergy often perform their job without a problem of the skin.

However, sensitization may occur from metal leached out into cutting fluids.[65] Preemployment testing is only useful in persons suspected of having a contact sensitization or having dermatitis.

REFERENCES

1. Crow, K. D., The engineering and chemical aspects of soluble coolant oils, *Br. J. Dermatol.*, 105 (Suppl. 21), 11, 1981.
2. Foulds, I. S., Dermatitis from metalworking fluids, *Clin. Exp. Dermatol.*, 15, 157, 1990.
3. Grattan, C. E. H., English, J. S. C., Foulds, I. S., and Rycroft, R. J. G., Cutting fluid dermatitis, *Contact Dermatitis*, 20, 372, 1989.
4. De Boer, E. M., Occupational Dermatitis by Metalworking Fluids, Ph.D. thesis, Free University, Amsterdam, 1989.
5. Shennan, J. L., Selection and evaluation of biocides for aqueous metal-working fluids, *Tribol. Int.*, 16, 317, 1983.
6. De Groot, A. C. and Bos, J. D., Preservatives in the European standard series for epicutaneous testing, *Br. J. Dermatol.*, 116, 289, 1987.
7. Angelini, G. and Meneghini, C. L., Dermatitis in engineers due to synthetic coolants, *Contact Dermatitis*, 3, 219, 1977.
8. Alomar, A., Conde-Salazar, L., and Romaguera, C., Occupational dermatoses from cutting oils, *Contact Dermatitis*, 12, 129, 1985.
9. Fisher, A. A., Allergic contact dermatitis of the hands due to industrial oils and fluids, *Cutis*, 23, 131, 1979.
10. Schneider, W., Huber, M., Kwoczek, J. J., Popp, W., Schmitz, R., and Tronnier, H., Weitere Untersuchungen zur Frage der Hautverträglichkeit hoch verdünnter Kühlmittel, *Berufs-Dermatosen*, 13, 65, 1965.
11. Dahl, M. G. C., Patch test concentrations of Grotan BK, *Contact Dermatitis*, 7, 607, 1981.
12. Dahlquist, I. and Fregert, S., Formaldehyde releasers, *Contact Dermatitis*, 4, 173, 1978.
13. Dahlquist, I., Contact allergy to cutting oil preservatives Bioban CS-1246 and P-1487, *Contact Dermatitis*, 10, 46, 1984.
14. Rietschel, E., Erfahrungen aus der werksärztlichen Praxis über Hautschäden bei Nasschleifern, *Berufs-Dermatosen*, 12, 284, 1964.
15. Van Ketel, W. G., Grotans — een arbeidsdermatologisch onderzoek, *Nieuwsbrief Contactdermatol.*, 16, 232, 1983.
16. Keczkes, K. and Brown, P. M., Hexahydro,1,3,5,tris (2-hydroxyethyl) triazine, a new bactericidal agent as a cause of allergic contact dermatitis, *Contact Dermatitis*, 2, 92, 1976.
17. Van Ketel, W. G. and Kisch, L. S., The problem of the sensitizing capacity of some Grotans used as bactericides in cooling oils, *Dermatosen*, 31, 118, 1983.
18. Lange, H. and Prange, E., Erfahrungen mit einem neuartigen Konservierungsmittel für Bohrölemulsionen, *Berufs-Dermatosen*, 10, 269, 1962.
19. Fiedler, H. P., Formaldehyd. Formaldehyd-Abspalter, *Dermatosen*, 31, 187, 1983.
20. Harke, H. P., The sensitizing effect of preservatives for coolants, *Contact Dermatitis*, 3, 51, 1977.
21. Rycroft, R. J. G., Is Grotan BK a contact sensitizer?, *Br. J. Dermatol.*, 99, 346, 1978.
22. Van Hecke, E., Contact allergy in metal workers, *Contact Dermatitis*, 23, 241, 1990.
23. Grattan, C. E. H., English, J. S. C., Foulds, I. S., and Rycroft, R. J. G., Cutting oil dermatitis, *Br. J. Dermatol.*, 119 (Suppl. 33), 57, 1988.
24. Coenraads, P. J., Foo, S. C., Phoon, W. O., and Lun, K. C., Dermatitis in small-scale industries, *Contact Dermatitis*, 12, 155, 1985.
25. Robertson, M. H. and Stors, F. J., Allergic contact dermatitis in two machinists, *Arch. Dermatol.*, 188, 997, 1982.
26. Hjorth, N., N-methylol-chloracetamide, a sensitizer in coolant oils and cosmetics, *Contact Dermatitis*, 5, 330, 1979.
27. Hamann, K., Forcide 78 — another formaldehyde releaser in coolant oil, *Contact Dermatitis*, 6, 446, 1980.

28. Lama, L., Vanni, D., Barone, M., Patrone, P., and Antonelli, C., Occupational dermatitis to chloracetamide, *Contact Dermatitis*, 15, 243, 1986.
29. Alomar, A., Contact dermatitis from benzisothiazolone in cutting oils, *Contact Dermatitis*, 7, 155, 1981.
30. Brown, R., Concomitant sensitization to additives in a coolant fluid, *Contact Dermatitis*, 5, 340, 1979.
31. Pilger, C., Nethercott, J. R., and Weksberg, F., Allergic contact dermatitis due to a biocide containing 5-chloro-2-methyl-4-isothiazolin-3-one, *Contact Dermatitis*, 14, 201, 1986.
32. Adams, R. M., Allergic contact dermatitis due to *o*-penylphenol, *Contact Dermatitis*, 7, 332, 1981.
33. Adams, R. M., *p*-Chloro-*m*-xylenol in cutting fluids: two cases of contact dermatitis in machinists, *Contact Dermatitis*, 7, 341, 1982.
34. Crow, K. D., Peachy, R. D. G., and Adams, J. E., Coolant oil dermatitis due to ethylenediamine, *Contact Dermatitis*, 4, 359, 1978.
35. Wrangsjö, K., Martensson, A., Widström, L., and Sundberg, K., Contact dermatitis from Bioban P 1487, *Contact Dermatitis*, 14, 182, 1986.
36. Camarasa, J. M. G. and Alomar, A., Ethylenediamine sensitivity in metallurgic industries, *Contact Dermatitis*, 4, 178, 1978.
37. Tosti, A., Piraccini, B., and Brasile, G. P., Occupational contact dermatitis due to sodium pyrithione, *Contact Dermatitis*, 22, 241, 1990.
38. Rycroft, J. R. G., Cutting fluids, oil, and lubricants, in *Occupational and Industrial Dermatology*, Maibach, H. I. and Gellin, G. A., Eds., Year Book Medical Publishers, Chicago, 1982, chap. 26.
39. Van Neste, D., Masmoudi, M., Leroy, B., Mahmoud, G., and Lachapelle, J. M., Regression patterns of transepidermal water loss and of cutaneous blood flow values in sodium laurylsulfate induced irritation: a human model of rough dermatitic skin, *Bioeng. Skin*, 2, 103, 1986.
40. Van Neste, D., Mahmoud, G., and Masmoudi, M., Experimental induction of rough dermatitic skin in humans, *Contact Dermatitis*, 16, 27, 1987.
41. Rycroft, R. J. G., Soluble oil dermatitis, *Clin. Exp. Dermatol.*, 6, 229, 1981.
42. Rycroft, R., Soluble oil dermatitis, in *Essentials of Industrial Dermatology*, Griffiths, W. A. D. and Wilkinson, D. S., Eds., Blackwell Scientific, Oxford, 1985, chap. 7.
43. De Boer, E. M., Bruynzeel, D. P., and Van Ketel, W. G., Dyshidrotic eczema as an occupational dermatitis in metalworkers, *Contact Dermatitis*, 19, 184, 1988.
44. De Boer, E. M., Van Ketel, W. G., and Bruynzeel, D. P., Dermatoses in metalworkers. I. Irritant contact dermatitis, *Contact Dermatitis*, 20, 212, 1989.
45. Alomar, A., Conde-Salazar, L., and Romaguera, C., Occupational dermatoses from cutting oils, *Contact Dermatitis*, 20, 372, 1989.
46. Cronin, E., *Contact Dermatitis*, Churchill Livingstone, London, 1980, 840.
47. Kalimo, K., Jolanki, R., Estlander, T., and Kanerva, L., Contact allergy to antioxidants in industrial greases, *Contact Dermatitis*, 20, 151, 1989.
48. Shrank, A. B., Allergy to cutting oil, *Contact Dermatitis*, 12, 229, 1985.
49. Rycroft, R. J. G., Personal communication.
50. De Boer, E. M., Van Ketel, W. G., and Bruynzeel, D. P., Dermatoses in metalworkers. II. Allergic contact dermatitis, *Contact Dermatitis*, 20, 280, 1989.
51. Krijnen, R., Bruynzeel, D. P., and De Boer, E. M., Unpublished data.
52. Weidenbach, Th. and Rakoski, J., Gehäuftes Auftreten von dyshidrosiformen Handekzemen durch eine Öl-in-Wasser- Emulsion bei Metallarbeitern, *Dermatosen*, 33, 121, 1985.
53. Rycroft, R. J. G., Hand Hygiene, Occupational Safety and Health, 1987, 24.
54. Rystedt, I., Work-related hand eczema in atopics, *Contact Dermatitis*, 12, 164, 1985.
55. Rystedt, I., Atopic background in patients with occupational eczema, *Contact Dermatitis*, 12, 247, 1985.
56. Shmunes, E. and Keil, J., The role of atopy in occupational dermatoses, *Contact Dermatitis*, 11, 174, 1984.
57. Pryce, D. W., Irvine, D., English, J. S. C., and Rycroft, R. J. G., Soluble oil dermatitis: a follow-up study, *Contact Dermatitis*, 21, 28, 1989.

58. Grattan, C. E. H. and Foulds, I. S., Outcome of investigation of cutting fluid dermatitis, *Contact Dermatitis,* 20, 377, 1989.

59. Holness, D. L. and Nethercott, J. R., Is workers' understanding of their diagnosis an important determinant of outcome in occupational contact dermatitis?, *Contact Dermatitis,* 25, 296, 1991.

60. Goh, C. L., Cutting oil dermatitis on guinea pig skin. I. Cutting oil dermatitis and barrier cream, *Contact Dermatitis,* 24, 16, 1991.

61. Goh, C. L., Cutting oil dermatitis on guinea pig skin. II. Emollient creams and cutting oil dermatitis, *Contact Dermatitis,* 24, 81, 1991.

62. De Boer, E. M., Scholten, R. J. P. M., Van Ketel, W. G., and Bruynzeel, D. P., The irritancy of metalworking fluids: a Laser Doppler Flowmetry study, *Contact Dermatitis,* 22, 86, 1990.

63. Coenraads, P. J., Lee, M. P. H., and Pinnagoda, J., Changes in water vapor loss from the skin of metal industry workers monitored during exposure to oils, *Scand. J. Work Environ. Health,* 12, 494, 1986.

64. Kraus, S. M. and Muselinovic, N. Z., Pre-employment screening for contact dermatitis among the pupils of a metal industry school, *Contact Dermatitis,* 24, 342, 1991.

65. Einarsson, Ö., Kylin, B., Linstedt, G., and Wahlberg, J. E., Dissolution of cobalt from hard metal alloys by cutting fluids, *Contact Dermatitis,* 5, 129, 1979.

22

Dermatitis from Acrylates in Dental Personnel

Lasse Kanerva, Tuula Estlander, Riitta Jolanki, and Kyllikki Tarvainen

CONTENTS

I. INTRODUCTION

As early as 1948 Bradford[1] reported on a patient with stomatitis from a dental methacrylate prosthesis. The patient showed an allergic patch test reaction with the prosthesis. In 1954 Fisher[2] described two dentists with dermatitis on the right hand, mainly on the first fingers, and two dental technicians with dermatitis on both hands. The patients had occupationally been sensitized to methacrylates, and had positive patch test reactions to 100% methyl methacrylate (MMA). Three dentists and three dental technicians with allergic contact dermatitis from MMA were reported by Calnan and Stevenson.[3] The number of cases of occupational allergic contact dermatitis (ACD) caused by acrylates, however, was relatively low in the 1970s,[4] partly because of the awareness of the sensitizing capacity of acrylates,[4] but also because MMA was possibly not very sensitizing.[5]

The newer acrylates are much stronger sensitizers than MMA[5,6] and dental personnel seem to be at special risk to develop occupational allergy to acrylics. In the present report, we review our findings on occupational skin diseases caused by acrylics in dental personnel during 1974–1992.

II. MATERIAL AND METHODS

All the cases of occupational ACD detected in our Institute between January 1, 1974 and May 15, 1992 are reported here. The material is based on previous publications[7-10] complemented with more recent data. The skin and allergy tests used have been described in the appropriate publications and summarized in, e.g., Estlander[11] and Jolanki.[12] (Meth)acrylates have been tested as follows:

1. Before 1982 only methyl methacrylate (MMA) 10% w/w pet and substances brought in by the patients were tested when allergy to an acrylate was suspected.
2. In 1982–1985, seven acrylic compounds including MMA were used[15] (see Table 2).
3. Since September, 1985 we have used the (meth)acrylate series of Chemotechnique Diagnostics AB (Malmö, Sweden) containing 28 to 30 substances, including four epoxy acrylates (Tables 5 and 9).

The abbreviations of the acrylics in Tables 5 and 9 are used in the text. Because four patients were actively sensitized,[13] the test concentrations of EA, 2-HEA, and 2-HPA were lowered from 0.5 to 0.167% w/w pet since the beginning of 1987, and later to 0.1%. Because one further patient was sensitized, three acrylics (EA, 2-HEA, and 2-HPA) were deleted from the (meth)acrylate series starting in January, 1991.[14] Cyanoacrylate (2% pet, Epikon, Helsinki, Finland) was added to the (meth)acrylate series September 1, 1991 (previously in the plastics and glue series, see Reference 15). N,N-dimethylaminoethyl methacrylate (2%, pet) was added to the dental series starting in January, 1991.[16] The acrylic resins brought in by the patients were mostly tested at 1% w/w pet. Information on the contents of DCRs according to safety data sheets is shown in Table 7.

All the patients reported here have been compensated as having occupational diseases by insurance companies according to Finnish legislation.[11]

III. OCCUPATIONAL IRRITANT CONTACT DERMATITIS CAUSED BY ACRYLICS

Acrylics irritate, and occupational contact dermatitis may develop without allergy. The first case of occupational ICD was diagnosed in 1982, and since then six patients have been compensated as occupational ICD caused by acrylics (Table 1). A more detailed analysis of cases[1-4] (cases 1, 4, 5, and 7 in Estlander et al.[7]) was reported earlier.[7] All the patients were dental technicians and the causative acrylate was MMA.

COMMENT: a contributing factor in the development of ICD was the abundant hand washing (20 to 100 times a day).[7] Patch testing with acrylics was negative in all cases. Only one of the patients was atopic.

TABLE 1 Data of Six Dental Technicians (Patient 6 Was a Dental Technician Apprentice) with Occupational Irritant Contact Dermatitis Caused by Acrylics

Patient	1	2	3	4	5	6
Age (years)	41	43	41	42	37	20
Gender (m = male, f = female)	m	m	f	m	f	f
Exposure before onset of symptoms (years)	24	17	1	1	6	1 month
Duration of symptoms before examination (years)	1	6	23	9	1.5 months	1
Use of protective gloves with acrylic monomers	Never	Yes	Yes	Never	Occasionally	Occasionally
Atopy						
Patient	No	No	No	Yes	No	Yes
Family	No	Yes	Yes	No	No	Yes
Positive patch-test reactions	None	None	Nickel	None	Balsam of Peru	Chromate, *p-tert-*butylphenol-formaldehyde resin

Adapted from Estlander et al.[7]

IV. OCCUPATIONAL ALLERGIC CONTACT DERMATITIS CAUSED BY WORK WITH PROSTHESES

Four patients have developed ACD from work with prostheses (Table 2). Patients 1 to 3 (Table 2) were tested with an acrylic series of seven acrylics that we used from 1982 to 1985[7,13] and Patient 4 with the large methacrylate series that we have used since 1985.[9,13] All of the patients were women, and they had not used protective gloves. None of the patients were atopic, nor was there atopy in their family.

Patient 1 had worked as a dentist for 5 years, of which the last 2 years was as an orthodontist, before she started to develop pulpitis of finger 2 of the right hand. She was exposed to MMA liquid when she remodeled children's dental devices to achieve better fit. For this remodeling she used the normal two-component MMA system consisting of poly-MMA powder and MMA liquid (Table 3). After having developed fingertip symptoms she started to use her other, healthy fingers, on which dermatitis also developed (Figure 1). Gradually, she also developed fingernail changes before she was referred to us, suspected of having occupational mycosis of the nails. A dermatophyte culture of the fingernails was negative but MMA, BA, EA, and 2-HPMA gave allergic patch test reactions (Table 2). The reactions to BA, EA, and 2-HPMA probably represented cross-allergy with MMA, the only acrylate she had been exposed to. She has been able to work as an orthodontist by avoiding exposure to MMA liquid.

Patient 2 had worked as a dental technician apprentice for 1.5 years before she developed a vesicular hand dermatitis. The dermatitis was worse on the left hand. Her left hand was more exposed to MMA because she frequently had to fill small bottles from a larger bottle containing MMA liquid, and the liquid often spilled onto her left hand. She has worked part-time as a dental technician and been in our follow-up because of repeated episodes of hand dermatitis. In 1989 she was retested, and her green latex gloves gave an allergic patch test reaction. Our rubber chemical series, containing 30 rubber chemicals, was negative, as were the latex prick tests. The agent causing the allergic reaction thus remained unclear, possibly being the dyes.[17] In the dental series in 1989 she had an allergic patch test reaction with EGDMA, possibly because dimethacrylates may be used as cross-linking agents in the manufacture of prostheses, or because of a cross-reaction between MMA and EGDMA. Epoxy acrylates were negative on patch testing.

Patient 3 had had an irritant contact dermatitis of short duration during the beginning of her dental technician apprenticeship. Three years later the hand dermatitis worsened and patch testing showed her MMA allergy. She reacted both with liquid MMA and polymerized powder MMA

TABLE 2 Data of Four Patients Who Developed Allergic Contact Dermatitis from Working with Prostheses

Patient no.		1	2	3	4
Age		32	23	24	25
Occupation		Dentist	Dental technician apprentice	Dental technician	Dental worker
Exposure before sensitization (years)		2	1.5	3	2
Year of diagnosis		1982	1982	1983	1990
Localization of dermatitis		Fingertips	Fingertips, hands, face	Fingertips	
Patch test sessions		1	2	3	1
Patch tests					
Acrylics					
Butyl acrylate (BA)	1% pet	2+	2+	3+	Several (see text)
tert-Butyl acrylate (t-BA)	1% pet	–	–	1+	
Ethyl acrylate (EA)	1% pet	3+	2+	3+	
2-Ethylhexyl methacrylate (2-EHMA)	1% pet	–	–	–	
2-Hydroxypropyl methacrylate (2-HPMA)	1% pet	2+	2+	3+	
N-tert-butylacryl amide (N-t-BAA)	1% pet	–	–	–	
Methyl methacrylate (MMA)	1–10% pet	2+	2+	3+	
Own methacrylates					
Polymethacrylate powder	100%	ND[a]	ND	2+	–
Liquid acrylate monomer	1% pet	3+	2+	2+ Palavit G® 1%, 3+ Opaquer® 1%, 3+	2+ (2% pet)
Other positive acrylates		–	EGDMA 2+	EGDMA 2+ TREGDMA 2+	Several (see text)
Other positive patch tests		–	Rubber glove 2+	Formaldehyde 2+ Glutaraldehyde 2+ p-tert-Butylphenol-formaldehyde resin 3+ Dequalon 3+ Neomycin 3+ Bacitracin 3+	Own rubber glove Hexamethylenetetramine 2+ 1-3-Diphenylguanidine 1+

[a] ND = not done.

Adapted from Kanerva et al.[56]

TABLE 3 Components of the Powder and Liquid of an Acrylic Denture Base Material

Powder	Liquid
Poly(methyl methacrylate) or polymer	Methyl methacrylate or monomer
Organic peroxide initiator	Hydroquinone inhibitor
Titanium dioxide to control translucency	Dimethacrylate or cross-linking agent[a]
Inorganic pigments for color	Organic amine accelerator[b]
Dyed synthetic fibers for esthetics	

[a] A cross-linking agent is present if the manufacturer indicates that the material is a cross-linked acrylic.

[b] The amine is present only if the material is labeled as a product to be processed at room temperature. Some manufacturers list them as cold-curing or self-curing materials.

(Figure 2). Gradually, she developed recalcitrant hand dermatitis. She also had several other allergic patch test reactions (Table 2), of which sensitization to formaldehyde and glutaraldehyde was considered occupational. Six years later, she started secretarial studies.

Patient 4 was working in a dental technician's laboratory, first as an errand girl, but since 1991 she worked full time in the manufacture and repair of dental prostheses. Initially she did not use protective gloves, but since here hand dermatitis, which started from the fingertip of the right hand, she used latex gloves with textile under the gloves.

Her hand dermatitis started from the tip of the right forefinger, which later excoriated. Later the dermatitis spread to fingertips 1 to 3 on both hands. After a sick leave of 2.5 months, her fingertip dermatitis recovered. On patch testing, the Standard European series was negative but she had several positive patch test reactions with the (meth)acrylates as follows: BA 2 + ; EMA 2 + ; BMA 2 + ; 2-HEMA 3 + ; 2-HPMA 3 + ; EGDMA 3 + ; and MMA 2 + . Her own liquid

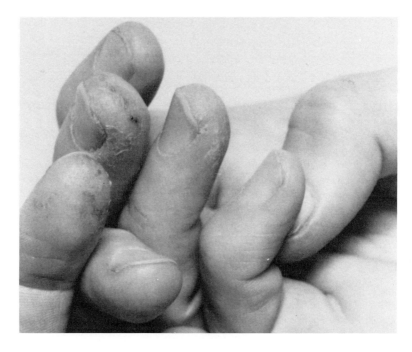

FIGURE 1. Fingertip dermatitis of orthodontist allergic to methyl methacrylate. The allergy and dermatitis developed in work where the orthodontist was remodeling children's dental devices for better anatomical fit, with two-component methyl methacrylate liquid and powder. Data on the orthodontist is given in Table 2 (Patient 1).

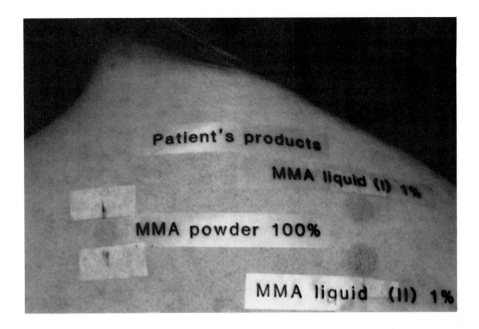

FIGURE 2. Both liquid and powder methyl methacrylate gave an allergic patch-test reaction in this dental technician (Table 2, Patient 3).

methacrylate preparations, tested at 2% pet gave 2+ reactions (De Tray Dentsply RR liquid; Special Tray liquid) while the corresponding powders were negative when tested as is (100%). Her own disposable glove gave a 2+ reaction when tested with a drop of water, but in acetone the piece of glove gave a negative reaction.

She was later retested with the plastics and glue series[15] containing 50 substances, as well as with the rubber series (30 substances); in these series hexamethylenetetramine gave a 2+ allergic patch test reaction, while 1,3-diphenylguanidine gave a 1+ allergic reaction, possibly explaining the rubber glove reaction.

COMMENT: Patient 3 reacted to both liquid MMA and polymerized MMA powder. The latter reaction is unusual, e.g., the patients of Fisher[2] did not react with the powder. It is evident that even the powder contained small amounts of uncured, i.e., nonpolymerized, MMA monomer and this caused the allergic reaction.

Patient 4, who was diagnosed to have an ACD by acrylics, recently showed allergic patch test reactions with several acrylics. Dental technicians also are currently using more modern light-cured acrylics, and it is evident that dental technicians are going to have the same type of acrylic reactions that have been demonstrated from DCR and dentin primers (see below).

V. OCCUPATIONAL ALLERGIC CONTACT DERMATITIS CAUSED BY DENTAL COMPOSITE RESINS

Data on the eight patients sensitized from dental composite resins are given in Tables 4 through 7. Patients 1 to 7 have been presented earlier.[9] Patient 8 was a dental nurse who had atopy in her family, and she herself had a possibly mild atopic dermatitis in childhood. She had been working for 16 years without skin symptoms, before finger and hand dermatitis started. Two patch test sessions revealed allergic patch test reactions to several acrylics (Table 5) and her own DCR (Delton, Table 6). She had earlier also used Silar, Silux, and Concise products. The last three products gave a doubtful patch test reaction (?+, 1% pet) which probably indicated allergy. The reactions were probably weak because the test concentration was low. She had also used the dentin primer, Scotchbond (see below), but this gave a negative patch test reaction.

TABLE 4 Characteristics of Eight Patients Sensitized to Dental Composite Resins (DCR)

Patient no.	1	2	3	4	5	6	7	8
Occupation	Dental nurse	Dental nurse	Dental nurse	Dental nurse	Dental nurse	Dental nurse	Dentist	Dental nurse
Sex	Female	Female	Female	Female	Female	Female	Female	Female
Year of diagnosis	1979	1982	1985	1986	1986	1987	1986	1990
Hand eczema since	1970	1982	1984	1984	1979	1974	1985	1989
Age (when diagnosis made)	60	22	20	34	28	41	41	50
Probable exposure time to DCR, before sensitization	1 yr	1 yr	3 mo	9 yr	1 yr	5 yr	14 yr	16 yr
Own/family atopy	−/−	+/−	−/−	+/+	−/+	+/+	−/+	+/+
Atopic dermatitis	No	No	No	Yes	No	Yes	No	Yes
Number of patch test sessions	3	1	5	3	4	3	2	2
Use and type of protective gloves	Yes, rubber	No	No	Yes, rubber	Yes, PVC	Yes, rubber	Yes, rubber	No
Localization of eczema	Fingers, both hands	Fingers, right hand	Fingers, both hands	Fingers, right hand, face	Fingers, both hands, face	Fingers, both hands, face	Fingers, both hands	Fingers, both hands

Adapted from Kanerva et al.[9]

TABLE 5   Patch Test Results of (Meth)acrylate Series and Epoxy Resin of Patients Sensitized to Dental Composite Resins

Compound		Conc. % (w/w)	Patient							
			1	2	3	4	5	6	7	8
Ethyl acrylate	(EA)	0.5–0.1	ND[a]	ND	–	1+	–	–	3+	–
Butyl acrylate	(BA)	0.5–0.1	ND	ND	–	2+	–	–	3+	?+
2-Ethylhexyl acrylate	(2-EHA)	0.5–0.1	ND	ND	–	–	–	–	–	–
2-Hydroxyethyl acrylate	(2-HEA)	0.5–0.1	ND	ND	–	2+	–	–	3+	?+
2-Hydroxypropyl acrylate	(2-HPA)	0.5–0.1	ND	ND	–	2+	–	–	3+	–
Methyl methacrylate	(MMA)	2–10	–	–	3+	–	–	–	2+	–
Ethyl methacrylate	(EMA)	2	ND	ND	3+	–	–	–	3+	–
n-Butyl methacrylate	(BMA)	2	ND	ND	–	–	–	–	2+	–
2-Hydroxyethyl methacrylate	(2-HEMA)	2	ND	ND	–	1+	–	2+	3+	–
2-Hydroxypropyl methacrylate	(2-HPMA)	2	ND	ND	–	2+	–	2+	3+	–
Ethylene glycol dimethacrylate	(EGDMA)	2	ND	ND	–	–	–	3+	2+	–
Triethylene glycol dimethacrylate	(TREGDMA)	2	ND	ND	–	3+	–	4+	2+	3+
1,4-Butanediol dimethacrylate	(BUDMA)	2	ND	ND	–	–	–	–	1+	–
Urethane dimethacrylate	(UEDMA)	2	ND	ND	–	–	–	–	–	–
2,2-Bis[4-(2-methacryloxyethoxy)phenyl]propane	(BIS-EMA)	1	ND	ND	–	3+	–	–	–	–
2,2-Bis[4-(methacryloxy)phenyl]propane	(BIS-MA)	2	ND	ND	–	–	–	–	–	–
2,2-Bis[4-(2-hydroxy-3-methacryloxypropoxy)phenyl]propane	(BIS-GMA)	2	ND	ND	4+	3+	2+	2+	–	–
1,4-Butanediol diacrylate	(BUDA)	0.1	ND	ND	–	2+	–	–	2+	2+
1,6-Hexanediol diacrylate	(HDDA)	0.1	ND	ND	–	2+	–	–	–	–
Diethylene glycol diacrylate	(DEGDA)	0.1	ND	ND	–	3+	–	–	2+	2+
Tripropylene glycol diacrylate	(TPGDA)	0.1	ND	ND	–	–	–	–	–	–
Trimethylolpropane triacrylate	(TMPTA)	0.1	ND	ND	–	–	–	–	–	–
Pentaerythritol triacrylate	(PETA)	0.1	ND	ND	–	–	–	–	–	?+
Oligotriacrylate 480	(OTA 480)	0.1	ND	ND	–	–	–	–	–	–
Epoxy diacrylate	(BIS-GA)	0.5	ND	ND	4+	2+	2+	2+	–	–
Urethane diacrylate (aliphatic)		0.1	ND	ND	–	–	–	–	–	–
Urethane diacrylate (aromatic)		0.1	ND	ND	–	–	–	–	–	–
Triethylene glycol diacrylate	(TREGDA)	0.1	ND	ND	–	3+	–	2+	3+	3+
N,N-Methylenebisacrylamid		1	ND	ND	ND	ND	ND	ND	ND	–
Tetrahydrofurfuryl methacrylate		2	ND	ND	ND	ND	ND	ND	ND	–
Epoxy resin		1	–	–	3+	3+	3+	3+	–	–

[a] ND = not done.

Adapted from Kanerva et al.[9]

TABLE 6 Patch Test Results of Positive "Own" Dental Composite Resins (DCR) and Other Positive Relevant Allergies[a]

Patient no.	1	2	3	4	5	6	7	8
"Own" DCR	Concise Resin A and B 3+	Concise Resin A and B 2+	Miradapt Universal Paste 2+	Silar Paste A and B 3+	Silar Paste A and B 2+	Silar Paste A and B 3+	Silar Paste A and B 2+ Paste 2+	Delton Pit & Fissure Sealant, Universal, Catalyst and Light Curing 2+
	Concise Paste A and B 3+/2+	Silar Paste A and B 2+	Miradapt Catalyst Paste 2+	Silux Universal Opaque Paste 3+	Silux Universal Opaque Paste 2+	Delton Pit & Fissure Sealant Universal and Catalyst 3+	Aurafill 2+	
			Bonding Agent Universal Resin and Catalyst Resin 2+	Aurafill 3+			Delton Pit & Fissure Sealant Curing 3+	
Other relevant positive patch tests	TMTD 2+	Desimex® 0.5% 2+	Ampholyte® 103 G 1% 3+ 0.33% 2+ (0.1% neg)	Formaldehyde 2% and 1% 2+; 0.32% 1+	Glutaraldehyde 3+	Ampholyte® 103 G 1% 3+	Thiuram mix 2+	Fragrance mix 2+
	TMTM 2+		Desimex® 1% 2+; 0.5% 2+	Grotan BK 2+		Desimex® 10% 2+; 5% 1+	TMTD 2+	
	ZDC 2+			Black rubber mix 2+ IPPD 2+		Balsam of Peru 2+	TMTM 3+	
	Own rubber gloves 2+						Palavit G® 1% 3+	

[a] See also Table 4.

Adapted from Kanerva et al.[9]

TABLE 7   **List of Trade Names of Dental Composite Resins Handled by Eight Sensitized Patients**

Composite materials	Polymerization activated	DCR[a]	Manufacturer	Patient no.
Concise	By chemicals	BIS-GMA 22% TREGDMA 25%	3M Company, MN, U.S.	1, 2, 4, 5, 6, 8
Silar	By chemicals	Dimethacrylates 40–50%	3M Company, MN, U.S.	2, 4, 5, 6, 7, 8
Miradapt	By chemicals	BIS-GMA TREGDMA	Johnson & Johnson Dental Products Co., NJ, U.S.	3
Delton	By chemicals By light	BIS-GMA TREGDMA	Johnson & Johnson Dental Products Co., NJ, U.S.	6, 7, 8
Silux	By light	Dimethacrylates 40–50%	3M Company, MN, U.S.	5, 6, 8
Aurafill	By light	BIS-GMA TREGDMA	Johnson & Johnson Dental Products Co., NJ, U.S.	4, 7

[a]   DCRs included in composite materials according to material safety cards or other information given by the manufacturer.

Adapted from Kanerva et al.[9]

The commercial names of the DCR causing ACD are given in Table 7. Patients 1 and 2 were tested with MMA and their own DCR only (in 1979 and 1982, respectively). MMA was negative but the DCR (Concise and Silar) gave an allergic patch test reaction.

Epoxy resin was negative with these two patients, but the next four (i.e., Patients 3 to 6) had a positive patch test reaction caused by epoxy resin and some epoxy acrylates, e.g., BIS-GMA.

To summarize: all the patients were women; seven dental nurses and one dentist. Half of the patients were atopics. In addition to hand and finger dermatitis, three of the patients (two of them atopics) also had face dermatitis. The reason was probably a combination of atopy, air-borne allergic contact dermatitis, and ACD caused by dental resins from contamination via the hands. All patients, except Patient 8, also had occupational ACD caused by agents other than the DCR — from rubber chemicals, disinfectants and preservatives (Table 8). Patients 1 to 6 did not continue in their previous jobs as dental nurses; Patient 1 partly because of her relatively high age, and Patients 2 and 3 because of their young age. We often encourage young subjects who have relapsing ACD to consider retraining for another line of work.

COMMENT: dental composite resins (DCR) based on bisphenol A and (meth)acrylates, e.g., BIS-GMA, have been used since 1962.[18] Although BIS-GMA monomer is synthesized from glycidyl ethers containing epoxy groups, it does not itself contain epoxy groups. DCRs are interesting substances from the allergological point of view, since they contain several contact allergens: firstly, chemically reactive prepolymers, usually acrylated epoxies or acrylated urethanes;[19] secondly, monofunctional, and especially multifunctional aliphatic acrylates, i.e., acrylates, methacrylates, diacrylates, and dimethacrylates;[3,19,20] and thirdly, additives that trigger the polymerization at an appropriate time such as initiators (e.g., benzoyl peroxide), activators (e.g., tertiary aromatic amines), and inhibitors (e.g., hydroquinone).[3,20] DCRs also contain additional components that usually are probably not allergens: pigments, inorganic fillers, nonreactive inert polymers, and polymeric waxes.[20]

DCRs contain many sensitizing acrylates.[9,19] Epoxy acrylates are also used in many other compounds, but only a few reports on contact allergy have been published. The sensitized workers have mainly been in the ultraviolet (UV) light printing industry.[21-23] A dentist and a few dental patients wearing acrylic materials have been reported to be sensitized to their DCR, but the allergen has not been clarified.[24-27] DCRs also contain monoacrylates. Ruyter and Sjovik[19] identified acrylic monomers in 13 resin coating materials and 22 resin filling materials. They found monomers of low viscosity such as MAA (methacrylic acid), MMA, HEMA, EGDMA, DEGDMA (diethylene glycol dimethacrylate), TREGDMA, TEGDMA (tetraethylene glycol dimethacrylate), and PEGDMA (pentaethylene glycol dimethacrylate) as well as dimethacrylate derivatives of bisphenol-A, such as BIS-MA, linear and branched BIS-GMA, BIS-EMA, and BIS-PMA [2,2-bis(4-(3-methacrylox-ypropoxy)phenyl)propane], and dimethacrylate monomers containing urethane groups such as UEDMA. Because of this complexity of the acrylates present in DCR, it is difficult to know whether the patch test allergic reactions are due to concomitant sensitization or to cross-allergy.[28] Commercial DCR products vary in composition.[19] Most DCR studied contained BIS-GMA and TREGDMA, but other monomers were found in several of the DCR investigated.[19] Delton Fiss & Sealant was found to contain TREGDMA, BIS-GMA, and BIS-MA, but not MMA or EGDMA. Concise contained BIS-GMA and TREGDMA, but not BIS-MA, MMA, or EGDMA.[19] It is probable that the patients sensitized to epoxy acrylates and dimethacrylates were concomitantly sensitized to these two different allergens present in the same DCR. A concomitant sensitization probably also occurred from an impurity present in some compounds. This would explain why the patients reacted positively to both standard patch test epoxy resin and epoxy diacrylate. It is believed that epoxy resin MW 340 and epoxy acrylates do not cross-react.[29] Two patients showed allergic patch tests to several monoacrylates. This could be explained by cross-sensitivity,[28] but sensitization from several DCR containing different monoacrylates cannot be ruled out. The patients have probably been exposed to several DCRs during their years of work, and not only to those that they now are using and which we tested. It is clear that, in our patients, independent sensitization to other occupational allergens (rubber gloves, antimicrobials) had taken place.

The reason for the sensitization of the patients to standard epoxy resin is not known, but might be one of the following:

TABLE 8   Characteristics of Nine Patients Sensitized to Components of the Dentin Bonding System

Patient no.	1	2	3	4	5	6	7	8	9
Occupation	Dental nurse	Dental nurse	Dental nurse	Dentist	Dentist	Dentist	Dental nurse	Dentist	Dentist
Sex	Female	Female	Male	Female	Female	Female	Female	Female	Female
Age (when dx made)	49	36	40	48	45	47	36	50	56
Symptoms since	1987	1988	1989	1989	1990	1990	1975	1989	1990
Year of diagnosis	1988	1989	1990	1990	1990	1990	(1975)	1990	1991
Localization of dermatitis	Fingers, hands	Eyelids	Fingertips (left, 1–3)	Fingertips (left 1–3, right 1–4)	—	Finger (left 2,3)	Fingertips (left 1–3)	Fingertips (left 1,2)	Fingertips (left 1–3)
Own/family atopy	–/–	–/+	–/–	–/–	–/–	–/–	+/–	–/–	–/+
Use and type of protective gloves	PVC	PVC	PVC	PVC and rubber	Various occasionally	No	PVC	PVC	No
Paresthesiae	No	No	Yes	Yes	No	Yes	No	Yes	Yes

Adapted from Kanerva et al.[9]

1. DCR contains epoxy resin MW 340 as an impurity. Traces of epoxy resin MW 340 in Concise products have been demonstrated,[30] although we did not find oligomer MW 340 in Miradapt, Delton, or Bonding Agent Universal Resin,[8] but did find about 0.001% of oligomer MW 340 in one Concise patch.
2. Epoxy resin MW 340 and epoxy acrylates could cross-react, but Nethercott[23] reported lack of cross-reactivity between these compounds.
3. DCR is contaminated with (other) materials that cross-react with bisphenol A epoxy resin oligomers.
4. The standard patch test epoxy resin may contain impurities that react with substances in DCR.

Purity is a problem in the investigation of acrylate allergy. Van der Walle[5] found 45% contaminants in a sample of acrylic acid that the manufacturer claimed to be 98% pure. Thus, the impurities in "pure" chemicals can cause a substance to be erroneously labeled as a sensitizer.[20]

The acrylated urethanes are used in dental composite and sealant applications, playing the same role as BIS-GMA,[19] and they are allergens.[29] The aliphatic urethane acrylates are the most common ones,[6] but none of the urethane acrylates tested (i.e., aliphatic or aromatic urethane diacrylates or urethane dimethacrylates) gave positive patch tests in any of our patients.

VI. OCCUPATIONAL ALLERGIC CONTACT DERMATITIS CAUSED BY DENTIN PRIMERS

Altogether, ten sensitized patients are presented. Data on nine patients are given in Tables 8 and 9. The tenth patient (data on whom were kindly supplied by Dr. Tuula Nissi, Turku, Finland) is also reviewed briefly. Patients 1 to 6 have been described in a recent article.[10]

Patient 7 had earlier worked as a hairdresser, but developed occupational asthma in 1975. The patient was retrained to become a dental nurse, although she continuously had hand dermatitis. Later, allergy from protective gloves was suspected, but all skin tests in 1987 were negative. Dental resins were not tested before 1990, and then the dental primer allergy was detected (Table 9). The patient also had rubber chemical allergy, tetramethylthiuramdisulfide giving an allergic patch test reaction. This was considered occupational, caused by protective rubber gloves and/or polishing disks.[9]

Patient 8 had worked for 24 years as a dentist before she started to get dermatitis on her left forefinger and thumb. Later, dermatitis also developed on the other fingertips, accompanied by paresthesia. As with several other of the patients allergic to the primer, the start of dermatitis coincided with the start of using SB-2-DAS, indicating that this was the sensitizer. Later she has used the Tripton Primer and the Tripton Universal Bonding Agent (ICI). On patch testing, several acrylics gave a positive reaction (Table 9), the strongest being caused by MMA, EMA, 2-EHA, 2-HEMA, 2-HPMA, EGDMA, and TREGDMA. SDP (1% pet) gave only a 1+ reaction and SB-2 was negative (1% pet). Tripton Dentine Primer (2% pet) and several other DCR which she had used (Espe Ketac Bond, 1% pet; P-50 3M Gray with APC, 1% pet; Silux Universal Paste 1% pet; Paladur powder 100%; and Espe Ketac Bond 100%) gave negative patch test reactions. On the other hand, Paladur (2% pet) gave a 2+ allergic patch test reaction and Tripton Universal Bonding Agent (containing TREGDA, urethane dimethacrylate, and camphoroquinone) gave a 3+ allergic reaction. It can be concluded that she was allergic to SB-2-DAS containing 2-HEMA, Paladur containing MMA, and Tripton Universal Bonding Agent containing TREGDA. The other acrylic reactions may represent cross-reactions.

Patient 9 had worked as a dentist for 29 years before she started to get fingertip dermatitis. Having heard a lecture given by one of us (LK) on acrylics allergy she contacted a dermatologist, and ACD caused by SB-2-DAS was verified by patch testing. One year later she also started to get respiratory symptoms suspected to be caused by acrylics, and as a result was referred to our Institute for detailed investigations. Her ACD caused by acrylics was verified. In addition, neomycin and bacitracin allergy was revealed by patch testing. On patch testing, Silux Plus (3M) (1% pet) gave a negative reaction although it contains dimethacrylates (Table 7) and EGDMA was positive

TABLE 9 Results of Patients Sensitized to Dentin Primers

(Meth)acrylates		%(w/w)	1	2	3	4	5	6	7	8	9
Ethyl acrylate	(EA)	0.1	—	—	ND[a]	ND	ND	ND	ND	+	ND
Butyl acrylate	(BA)	0.1	—	—	ND	ND	ND	ND	ND	—	—
2-Ethylhexyl acrylate	(2-EHA)	0.1	—	—	ND	ND	ND	ND	ND	—	ND
2-Hydroxyethyl acrylate	(2-HEA)	0.1	2+	3+	ND	ND	ND	ND2	ND	3+	ND
2-Hydroxypropyl acrylate	(HPA)	0.1	—	—	ND	ND	ND	ND	—	?+	—
Methyl methacrylate	(MMA)	2	+?	—	+	+	—	+	—	3+	—
Ethyl methacrylate	(EMA)	2	—	—	ND	ND	ND	ND	ND	2+	—
n-Butyl methacrylate	(BMA)	2	—	—	ND	ND	ND	ND	ND	?+	—
2-Hydroxyethyl methacrylate	(2-HEMA)	2	3+	3+	3+	3+	3+	3+	3+	3+	—
2-Hydroxypropyl methacrylate	(2-HPMA)	2	3+	3+	ND	ND	ND	ND3	ND	3+	—
Ethylene glycol dimethacrylate	(EGDMA)	2	3+	3+	2+	3+	—	3+	3+	3+	2+
Triethylene glycol dimethacrylate	(TREGDMA)	2	3+	3+	+	2+	—	2+	—	2+	—
1,4-Butanediol dimethacrylate	(BUDMA)	2	+?	—	ND	ND	ND	ND	—	+	—
Urethane dimethacrylate	(UEDMA)	2	—	—	—	—	—	—	—	—	—
2,2-Bis[4-(2-methacryloxyethoxy)phenyl]propane	(BIS-EMA)	1	—	—	ND	ND	ND	ND	ND	—	—
2,2-Bis[4-(methacryloxy)phenyl]propane	(BIS-MA)	2	—	—	—	—	—	—	—	—	—
2,2-Bis[4-(2-hydroxy-3-methacryloyloxypropoxy)phenyl]propane	(BIS-GMA)	2	—	—	—	—	—	—	—	—	—
1,4-Butanediol diacrylate	(BUDA)	0.1	—	—	ND	ND	ND	ND	—	—	—
1,6-Hexanediol diacrylate	(HDDA)	0.1	—	—	ND	ND	ND	ND	—	—	—
Diethylene glycol diacrylate	(DEGDA)	0.1	—	—	ND	ND	ND	ND	—	—	—
Tripropylene glycol diacrylate	(TPGDA)	0.1	—	—	ND	ND	ND	ND	—	—	—
Trimethylolpropane triacrylate	(TMPTA)	0.1	—	—	ND	ND	ND	ND	—	—	—

Patient

Material		%								
Pentaerythritol triacrylate	(PETA)	0.1	—	—	—	ND	ND	ND	—	—
Oligotriacrylate 480	(OTA 480)	0.1	—	—	—	ND	ND	ND	—	—
Epoxy diacrylate	(BIS-GA)	0.5	—	—	—	ND	ND	ND	—	—
Urethane diacrylate (aliphatic)		0.1	—	—	—	ND	ND	ND	—	—
Urethane diacrylate (aromatic)		0.1	—	—	—	ND	ND	ND	—	—
Triethylene glycol diacrylate	(TREGDA)	0.1	3+	—	—	ND	ND	ND	—	—
N,N-Methylenebisacrylamid		1	—	ND	ND	ND	ND	ND	ND	ND
Tetrahydrofurfuryl methacrylate		2	ND	ND	ND	ND	ND	ND	ND	ND
N,N-Demethylaminoethyl methacrylate		2	ND	ND	ND	ND	ND	ND	—	+
Scotchbond-2-Dental Adhesive System										
Scotchprep Dentin Primer		1	3+	3+	3+	3+	3+	3+	2+	2+
Scotchbond-2-Light Cure Dental Adhesive		1	ND	3+	2+	3+	3+	3+	2+	2+
Other positive patch test reactions			Silux Universal®, Opaque Paste®, Eugenol, Nickel sulfate	—	—	Palladium Nickel	Servibond®	Servibond®	Thiuram (TMTD)	Paladur® 2%; 2+; Universal Bond®; Tripton 2%; 3+ Neomycin Bacitracin

a ND = not done.

Adapted from Kanerva et al.[10]

on patch testing. This is explained by the data given by the manufacturer: Silux Plus Restorative Material contains 15 to 20% TREGDMA, 15 to 20% BIS-GMA, and less than 7% acrylic acid, but no EGDMA. Provocation chamber tests to detect asthma caused by acrylics[31] were negative, but the patient is on follow-up with regard to her respiratory symptoms.

Patient 10 was a 53-year-old dentist who had been working as a dentist for 21 years. She started to get dermatitis on fingertips 2 and 3 of both hands, and on patch testing (dental series) was positive with EGDMA (3 +). MMA gave a weak (1 +) reaction. She was not tested with 2-HEMA. She related her symptoms to the use of the SB-2-DAS system, but further patch testings have not been performed. She also complained of fingertip paresthesia.

COMMENT: increased use of composite resins as dental restorative materials[32] has made it necessary to develop substances that induce firm adhesion of the dental composite resins (DCR) to the tooth. It has been difficult to obtain strong bonding to the dentin, and for this reason many adhesive agents, some of which require pretreatment of the dentin prior to application and polymerization of the adhesive material, have been introduced recently (Table 10). In 1988, Aasen and Oxman[33] of the 3M Corporation (St. Paul, MN, U.S.) patented a system based on maleic acid and 2-HEMA called the Scotchbond 2 Dental Adhesive System (SB-2-DAS), which has been commercially available in Finland since 1987, having been introduced some months earlier in the U.S. We diagnosed our first case of allergy to SB-2-DAS in 1988 (Patient 1).[34,35] Since then we have seen nine more patients who probably have been sensitized by components of SB-2-DAS. These findings indicate that SB-2-DAS is an important sensitizer, and stress the importance of using no-touch techniques when handling this adhesion promoter. Recently reports of allergy caused by SB-2-DAS have also been reported from Denmark.[36]

Most primers are di- or multifunctional molecules that contain groups capable of reacting with the calcium or protein in the tooth, and methacrylate groups for bonding to the resin restorative.[32] SB-2-DAS bonds anterior and posterior DCR to tooth structure and features two no-mix formulas (Table 10). The dentin is first handled by Scotchprep Dentin Primer (SDP), followed by Scotchbond 2 Light Cure Dental Adhesive (SB-2). This is then polymerized with a visible-light curing unit. Finally, the restorative material is applied to the tooth and cured chemically or with light. Thus, a "sandwich" is formed where the dentin is at the bottom, followed by layers of SDP, SB-2, and the restorative material.

TABLE 10   Dentin Bonding System Descriptions

System/manufacturer	Components	Precautions
All-Bond/Bisco Dental Products	Etchant: 10% phosphoric acid (All-Etch Technique) Conditioner: 20% SAMA in water Primers: (A) 2% NTG-GMA in ethanol and acetone, (B) 16% BPDM in acetone Bonding resin: BIS-GMA, UDMA, HEMA	1. May require as many as five coats of primer 2. Shelf life = 24 months
Clearfil Photo-Bond/J. Morita, Inc., U.S.	Etchant: 40% phosphoric acid, colloidal silica Catalyst: BIS-GMA, 10-MDP, HEMA, camphoroquinone, benzoyl peroxide Universal: aromatic sodium sulfinate, tertiary aromatic amine in ethanol	1. 1:1 Mix of catalyst and universal must be fresh 2. Refrigeration required 3. Shelf life (not released by manufacturer)
Gluma/Miles Inc., Dental Products	Cleanser: 16% EDTA Primer: 35% HEMA, 5% glutaraldehyde in water Sealer: BIS-GMA resin	1. Shelf life = 30 months at least 2. Sealing resin may require separate light curing

TABLE 10 Dentin Bonding System Descriptions (continued)

System/manufacturer	Components	Precautions
Mirage-Bond/Mirage Dental Systems	Conditioner: 4% NPG in 2.5% nitric acid in aqueous solution Adhesive: 10% PMDM in acetone	1. Conditioner cartridge requires careful handling to prevent air contamination 2. Adhesive must be allowed to evaporate 3. Refrigeration recommended 4. Shelf life = 24 months
Pertac Universal Bond/ ESPE Premier Sales Corp	(No conditioner or primer required) Adhesive: methacrylated carboxylic acid, hydrophilic and hydrophobic dimethacrylates, camphoroquinone, activator	1. Refrigeration recommended 2. Shelf life = 12 months
Prisma Universal Bond-3/ Caulk/Dentsply	Primer: 30% HEMA + 6% PENTA in ethanol Adhesive: 5% PENTA, 55% urethane resin, 39% polymerizable monomers (TEG-DMA, HEMA, etc.), <1% glutaraldehyde, <1% photoinitiators	1. Shelf life = 12 months
Restobond-3/Lee Pharmaceuticals	Conditioner: 4% NPG in 2.5% nitric acid in aqueous solution Sealant: 10% PMDM in acetone Resin: (Unfilled resin not identified)	1. Sealant must be allowed to evaporate 2. Refrigeration recommended 3. Shelf life = 12 months
Scotchbond 2/3M	Primer: 2.5% maleic acid, 58.5% HEMA in water Adhesive: 62.5% BIS-GMA, 37.5% HEMA, photoinitiators	1. Adhesive must not be air-thinned to less than 75 μm 2. Refrigeration recommended 3. Shelf life not released by manufacturer
Syntac/Ivoclar North-America, Inc.	Primer: 25% TEG-DMA + 4% maleic acid in acetone and water Adhesive: 35% PEG-DMA, 5% glutaraldehyde in water Resin: (Heliobond) 60% BIS-GMA, 40% TEG-DMA	1. Newly introduced to the U.S. 2. Cool storage recommended 3. Shelf life = 24 months
Tenure Solution/Den-mat, Inc.	Conditioner: 3.5% aluminum oxalate in 2.5% nitric acid in aqueous solution Bonding agent: (2 solutions) Soin A-5% NTG-GMA in acetone, Soin B-10% PMDM in acetone	1. Solutions A & B must be freshly mixed (1:1); allow to evaporate after applying 2. Shelf life = 18 months
XR-Bond/Kerr Manufacturing Co.,	Primer: 3.75% phosphonated dimethacrylate ester, 50% ethanol, 46% water, camphoroquinone Resin: 10% phosphonated dimethacrylate ester, UDMA, aliphatic dimethacrylate, camphoroquinone	1. Shelf life = 24 months

Adapted from Johnson et al.[57]

SB-2-DAS contains two known allergens, 2-HEMA and BIS-GMA. Our patients' allergy to SB-2-DAS was caused by 2-HEMA, and none of the patients had allergic reactions from BIS-GMA. Initially, when SDP is manufactured it does not contain methacrylic acid (MA). However, up to 18% of MA is formed during storage, especially at room temperature. MA makes the primer highly irritant, and contact between the mucosal tissue of the (dental) patient and the primer should strictly be avoided. The irritant action may also promote penetration of the allergens and thus contribute to sensitization. Therefore, it is important to store the SB-2-AS at ice box (4°C) temperature to prevent the formation of MA.

2-HEMA has caused sensitization in anaerobic acrylic sealants,[37,38] printing plates,[39-41] and during the manufacture of soft disposable contact lenses.[42] Six of our patients (Table 8 and Patient 10 complained of paresthesiae of the fingertips, which has earlier been reported from MMA[43] and 2-HEMA.[44] In the guinea pig maximization test 60 to 100% reacted to high concentrations of 2-HEMA, but there was no or only slight response to sensitization with low concentrations of 2-HEMA.[45] 2-HEMA may cross-react with other acrylates, e.g., 2-hydroxypropyl methacrylate.[6]

DCR may contain 2-HEMA,[19] and therefore dental personnel may have been exposed to 2-HEMA before exposure to SB-2-DAS. It could thus be argued that the patients were sensitized from products other than SB-2-DAS; this possibility cannot be excluded. In fact, Patient 1 was allergic to Silux universal paste (3M, St. Paul, MN, U.S.) which contains at least dimethacrylates (Table 7), and Patients 5 and 6 were allergic to Servibond (Ortho Enterprises, Ltd., Sheffield, U.K.) which, according to the manufacturer, contains TREGDMA and isobutyl methacrylate. Patient 7 was allergic to Paladur (containing MMA) and Tripton (containing TREGDMA). On the other hand, within a relatively short period, we have seen these new allergy patients, some of whom suspected that SB-2-DAS was the cause of their eczema. It is therefore plausible that SB-2-DAS was the (major) cause of their sensitization. One contributing factor could be that SB-2 is a very sticky substance, and thus it may contaminate instruments and the dentist's office. Furthermore, when opening and closing the bottle, the fingers are easily contaminated with SB-2 because of its stickiness. The 3M Corporation has recently informed us that a new bottle for SB-2 has been manufactured and this hopefully will reduce skin exposure to SB-2.

Many acrylates quickly penetrate practically all surgical rubber and PVC gloves. A commercial laminated disposable glove (4H-glove, Safety 4 A/S, Denmark) has been introduced on the market recently, but it is expensive and not of a good anatomical fit. We have recommended the use of a fingertip-piece of the 4H-glove under a disposable latex or PVC glove (Figure 3).

Dental patients treated with SB-2-DAS are probably at a much smaller risk of contracting allergy than are dental personnel, because they are exposed to uncured monomers for only a short time. Very few dental patients have been reported to have become sensitized to DCR.[24-26] However, uncured acrylics, e.g., those in the SB-2-DAS, are theoretically capable of sensitizing the patient even after a single exposure,[13] for which reason mucosal exposure should be avoided. Even though some of the acrylics from SB-2-DAS may remain uncured, they probably do not sensitize via the oral mucosa once the restoration has been finalized, because they are covered with DCR.

MMA previously was in widespread use as a standard allergen for patch testing screening for acrylate allergy.[28] However, both our and other studies[5,46,47] indicate that MMA is a poor screening substance for allergy to acrylates. No single (meth)acrylate has been able to screen all of our cases of allergy to DCR or SB-2-DAS, but patch testing with 2-HEMA, EGDMA and BIS-GMA would have detected all the cases.

In occupational dermatology we consider it important to use the patients' own substances for patch testing, since this is the only way to detect new allergens. However, possible sensitization when testing with their own substances, especially acrylates, has to be taken into consideration. Recently we have seen one patient who was sensitized from patch testing (elsewhere) with 100% SDP and SB-2.[48] Also, others have recently reported occupational acrylics allergy in dental personnel.[49-51]

Patient 5 had only respiratory symptoms, although in patch testing she had allergic reactions to SB-2-DAS, HEMA, and 15 other acrylics of the (meth) acrylate series.[52] In addition, she was patch-test positive to the new acrylate substance of the Chemotechnique (meth)acrylate series, i.e., tetrahydrofurfurylmethacrylate (3 + , 2% pet). We do not consider her positive (meth)acrylate reactions as an insignificant "false" positive response, but rather believe that they are connected

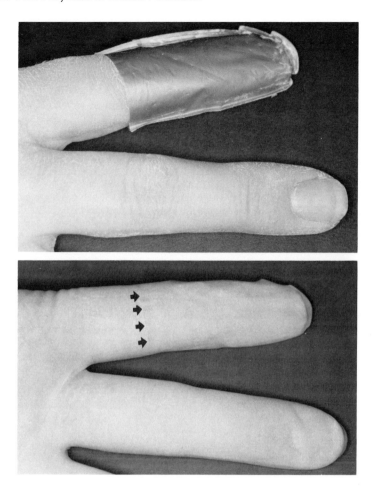

FIGURE 3. Because the 4-H glove is thick and not of good anatomical fit, we recommend the cutting of a fingertip from the 4-H glove (top) and using it under a latex or PVC glove (bottom). Arrows indicate the margin of the 4-H glove piece.

with her symptoms. Immediate hypersensitivity and/or bronchial asthma from cyanoacrylates, methyl methacrylate,[31,53] acrylic acid,[54] and unspecified acrylics[55] has been reported. The reason for the positive patch test reactions (Type IV allergy) in our patient with respiratory symptoms (Type I allergy?) is currently not understood.

Most DCR contain the same (partly cross-reacting) acrylics,[19,32] and currently there are probably no nonallergenic alternatives which can be used by the affected dental personnel. The 3M Corporation has done a good job in supplying new instructions regarding the precautions for dental personnel using acrylate resins (Table 11). Because of the difficulty in avoiding exposure to the various allergens present in everyday dental work, six out of seven patients allergic to DCR could not continue in their occupation.[9] Two of the ten patients with ACD from dentin primers have, so far, changed jobs. As private dentists in Finland are not automatically covered by insurance against occupational diseases, we strongly recommend all workers in dentistry to take private insurance against occupational disease.

VII. SUMMARY

All cases of occupational skin diseases caused by acrylics and detected at the Section of Dermatology, Institute of Occupational Health, Helsinki, during 1974 to 1992 have been reviewed. There

TABLE 11   Precautions for Dental Personnel and Patients Using the Scotchbond 2 Dental Adhesive System According to the 3M Company, St. Paul, MN, U.S.

1. ETCHING PRECAUTION: Avoid Etching Gel contact with oral soft tissue, eyes and skin. If accidental contact occurs, flush immediately with large amounts of water. Contains 35% phosphoric acid.
2. DENTIN PRIMER AND ADHESIVE CONTAIN HEMA. HEMA IS A KNOWN CONTACT ALLERGEN. USE OF PROTECTIVE GLOVES AND A NO-TOUCH TECHNIQUE IS RECOMMENDED. If adhesive contacts skin, wash immediately with soap and water. Acrylates may penetrate commonly used gloves. If adhesive contacts glove, remove and discard glove, wash hands immediately with soap and water and then reglove.
3. DENTIN PRIMER PRECAUTIONS: Scotchprep Dentin Primer is a severe eye irritant. Avoid contact with eyes. If contact occurs, flush immediately with large amounts of water and consult a physician. Scotchprep dentin primer should be refrigerated. Failure to refrigerate can increase the possibility of mucosal tissue irritation if the primer contacts the tissue. May cause irritation to mucosal membranes with whitening and/or swelling followed by tissue sloughing in some individuals. Avoid mucosal tissue contact. Isolation with rubber dam is the best means to avoid mucosal tissue contact and is highly recommended. If contact occurs, flush with large amounts of water. A small percentage of the population is known to have an allergic response to acrylate resins. To reduce the risk of allergic response, minimize exposure to these materials. If skin contact occurs, wash immediately with soap and water. Contains maleic acid, methacrylic acid, and 2-hydroxyethylmethacrylate (HEMA).
4. ADHESIVE PRECAUTION: A small percentage of the population is known to have an allergic response to acrylate resins. To reduce the risk of allergic response, minimize exposure to these materials. In particular, exposure to uncured resins should be avoided. If accidental contact with eyes or prolonged contact with oral soft tissue occurs, flush with large amounts of water. If skin contact occurs, wash immediately with soap and water. Contains bisGMA and 2-hydroxyethylmethacrylate (HEMA).

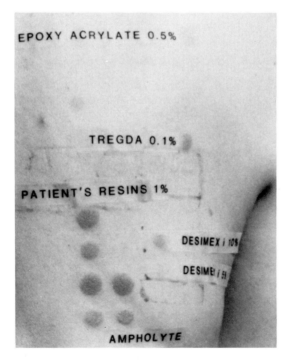

FIGURE 4.   Allergic patch-test reactions caused by the patient's own resins, TREGDA and epoxy acrylate, in a patient allergic to dental composite resins. The patient was also allergic to a disinfectant, Desimex.®

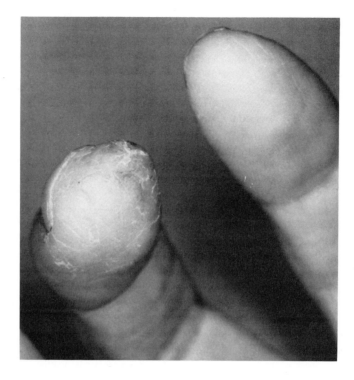

FIGURE 5.　Fingertip dermatitis (pulpitis) in a patient allergic to dentin primer.

were 6 cases of irritant and 22 cases of allergic contact dermatitis reported. The irritant contact dermatitis developed in dental technicians. A contributing factor was the numerous daily hand washings. Allergic contact dermatitis was caused by acrylics from work with dental prostheses (four cases), dental composite resins (eight cases), and dentin primers (ten cases). The patch test reactions are given in detail. Both cross and concomitant sensitization to different acrylics were detected. The newer, light-cured acrylic resins seem to be much more potent sensitizers than methyl methacrylate. The characteristic clinical feature is fingertip dermatitis (pulpitis) (Figures 4 and 5), which is sore, heals slowly, and causes many of the patients to change jobs. In fact, eight of the allergic patients have changed their occupation. Because acrylics are strong sensitizers and quickly penetrate most gloves, no-touch techniques should be used.

ABBREVIATIONS

Allergic contact dermatitis, ACD. Irritant contact dermatitis, ICD. (Meth)acrylates: abbreviations are given in Tables 2, 5, and 9. Dental composite resin, DCR. Polyvinyl chloride, PVC. Scotchbond 2 Dental Adhesive System, SB-2-DAS. Scotchprep Dentin Primer, SDP. Scotchbond 2 Light Cure Dental Adhesive, SB-2.

ACKNOWLEDGMENT

This work is part of the Allergy and Work program of the Finnish Institute of Occupational Health. The Allergy and Work program is headed by one of the authors (LK).

REFERENCES

1. Bradford, E. W., Case of allergy to methyl-methacrylate, *Br. Dent. J.*, 84, 195, 1948.
2. Fisher, A. A., Allergic sensitisation of the skin and oral mucosa to acrylic denture materials, *J. Am. Med. Assoc.*, 156, 238, 1954.
3. Calnan, C. D. and Stevenson, C. J., Studies in contact dermatitis. XV. Dental materials, *Trans. St John's Hosp. Dermatol. Soc.*, 49, 9, 1963.
4. Cronin, E., *Contact Dermatitis*, Churchill Livingstone, Edinburgh, 1980.
5. Van der Walle, H. B., Sensitizing Potential of Acrylic Monomers in Guinea Pigs, thesis, Katholieke Universiteit te Nijmegen, Krips Repro Meppel, 1982.
6. Björkner, B., Sensitizing Capacity of Ultraviolet Curable Acrylic Compounds, M.D. thesis, University of Lund, Lund, Sweden, 1984.
7. Estlander, T., Rajaniemi, R., and Jolanki, R., Hand dermatitis in dental technicians, *Contact Dermatitis*, 10, 201, 1984.
8. Kanerva, L., Jolanki, R., and Estlander, T., Occupational dermatitis due to an epoxy acrylate, *Contact Dermatitis*, 14, 80, 1986.
9. Kanerva, L., Estlander, T., and Jolanki, R., Allergic contact dermatitis from dental composite resins due to aromatic epoxy acrylates and aliphatic acrylates, *Contact Dermatitis*, 20, 201, 1989.
10. Kanerva, L., Turjanmaa, K., Estlander, T., and Jolanki, R., Occupational allergic contact dermatitis from 2-hydroxyethyl methacrylate (2-HEMA) in a new dentin adhesive, *Am. J. Contact Dermatitis*, 2, 24, 1991.
11. Estlander, T., Occupational skin disease in Finland. Observations made during 1974–1988 at the Institute of Occupational Health, Helsinki, *Acta Derm. Venereol.*, Suppl. 155, 1990.
12. Jolanki, R., Occupational skin diseases from epoxy compounds. Epoxy resin compounds, epoxy acrylates and 2,3-epoxypropyl trimethyl ammonium chloride, *Acta Derm. Venereol.*, Suppl. 159, 1, 1991.
13. Kanerva, L., Estlander, T., and Jolanki, R., Sensitization to patch test acrylates, *Contact Dermatitis*, 18, 10, 1988.
14. Kanerva, L., Estlander, T., and Jolanki, R., Double active sensitization caused by acrylics, *Am. J. Contact Dermatitis*, 3, 23, 1992.
15. Kanerva, L., Jolanki, R., and Estlander, T., Allergic contact dermatitis from epoxy resin hardeners, *Am. J. Contact Dermatitis*, 2, 89, 1991.
16. Kanerva, L., Estlander, T., and Jolanki, R., Active sensitization caused by 2-hydroxyethyl methacrylate, 2-hydroxypropyl methacrylate, ethyleneglycol dimethacrylate and N,N-dimethylaminoethyl methacrylate, *J. Eur. Acad. Derm. Venereol.*, 1, 165, 1992.
17. Kanerva, L., Jolanki, R., and Estlander, T., Organic pigment as a cause of plastic glove dermatitis, *Contact Dermatitis*, 13, 41, 1985.
18. Bowen, R. L., Dermatitis Filling Material Comprising Vinyl Silane Treated Fused Silica and a Binder Consisting of the Reaction Product of Bis Phenol and Glycidyl Acrylate, U.S. Patent 3,066, 112, 1962.
19. Ruyter, I. E. and Sjövik, I. J., Composition of dental resin and composite materials, *Acta Odontol. Scand.*, 39, 133, 1981.
20. Rietschel, R. L., Contact allergens in ultraviolet-cured acrylic resin systems, *Occup. Med. State of the Art Rev.*, 1(2), 301, 1986.
21. Emmett, E. A. and Kominsky, J. R., Allergic contact dermatitis from ultraviolet cured inks, *J. Occup. Med.*, 19, 2, 113–115, 1977.
22. Björkner, B., Allergic contact dermatitis from acrylates in ultraviolet curing inks, *Contact Dermatitis*, 6, 405, 1980.
23. Nethercott, J. R., Allergic contact dermatitis due to an epoxy acrylate, *Br. J. Dermatol.*, 104, 697, 1981.
24. Nathanson, P. and Lochart, P., Delayed extraoral hypersensitivity to dental composite material, *Oral Surg. Oral Med. Oral Pathol.*, 47, 329, 1979.
25. Niinimäki, A., Rosberg, J., and Saari, S., Allergic stomatitis from acrylic compounds. Report of a case, *Contact Dermatitis*, 9, 148, 1983.

26. Malten, K. E., Dermatological problems with synthetic resins and plastics in glues. Part II, *Derm. Beruf Umwelt*, 32, 118, 1984.
27. Riva, F., Pigatto, P. D., Altomare, G. F., and Riboldi, A., Sensitization to dental acrylic compounds, *Contact Dermatitis*, 10, 245, 1984.
28. Jordan, W. P., Jr., Cross-sensitization patterns in acrylate allergies, *Contact Dermatitis*, 1, 13, 1975.
29. Nethercott, J. R., Jakubovic, H. R., Pilger, C., and Smith, J. W., Allergic contact dermatitis due to urethane acrylate in ultraviolet cured inks, *Br. J. Ind. Med.*, 40, 241, 1983.
30. Niinimäki, A., Rosberg, J., and Saari, S., Traces of epoxy resin in acrylic dental filling materials, *Contact Dermatitis*, 9, 532, 1983.
31. Savonius, B., Keskinen, H., Tuppurainen, M., and Kanerva, I., Occupational respiratory disease caused by acrylics, *Clin. Exp. Allergy*, in press.
32. Vanherle, G. and Smith, D. C., *Posterior Composite Resin Dental Restorative Materials*, Peter Szule, Holland, 1985.
33. Aasen, S. M. and Oxman, J. D., Method For Priming Hand Tissue, U.S. Patent 4,719, 149, 1988.
34. Kanerva, L., Estlander, T., and Jolanki, R., Kosketusallergiaa akrylaateista hammashoitoalalla (Contact dermatitis from acrylates in dental personnel) (in Finnish with English summary), *Suomen Hammaslääkärilehti* (Finnish Dent. J.), 37, 164, 1990.
35. Kanerva, L., Estlander, T., and Jolanki, R., Allergic occupational dermatoses from epoxy resins and acrylates, in Occupational Health and Industrial Toxicology: State of the Art. Kahn, H. and Hernberg, S., Eds., Tallinn 92–98, 1989.
36. Munksgaard, E. C., Knudsen, B., and Thomsen, K., Kontaktallergisk håndeksem blandt tandplejepersonale af (di)metakrylater, (in Danish), *Tandlaegbladet*, 94, 270, 1990.
37. Conde-Salazar, L., Guimaraens, D., and Romero, L. V., Occupational allergic contact dermatitis from anaerobic acrylic sealants, *Contact Dermatitis*, 18, 129, 1988.
38. Kanerva, L., Estlander, T., and Jolanki, R., Occupational allergic contact dermatitis from acrylates: observations concerning anaerobic sealants and dental composite resins, in Current Topics in Contact Dermatitis, Frosch, P. J., Dooms-Goossens, A., Lachapelle, J.-M., Rycroft, R. J. G., and Scheper, R. J., Eds., Springer-Verlag, New York, 1989, 352.
39. Malten, K. E. and Bende, W. J. M., 2-Hydroxy-ethyl-methacrylate and di- and tetraethylene glycol dimethacrylate: contact sensitizers in a photoprepolymer printing plate procedure, *Contact Dermatitis*, 5, 214, 1979.
40. Pedersen, N. B., Senning, A., and Nielsen, A. O., Different sensitising acrylic monomers in napp printing plate, *Contact Dermatitis*, 9, 459, 1983.
41. Wahlberg, J. E., Contact sensitivity to NAPP printing plates secondary to a relapsing hand dermatitis, *Contact Dermatitis*, 9, 239, 1983.
42. Peters, K. and Andersen, K. E., Allergic hand dermatitis from 2-hydroxyethyl-acrylate in contact lenses, *Contact Dermatitis*, 15, 188, 1986.
43. Fisher, A. A., *Contact Dermatitis*, 3rd ed., Lea & Febiger, Philadelphia, 1986.
44. Mathias, C. G. T., Turner, M. C., and Maibach, H. I., Contact dermatitis and gastrointestinal symptoms from hydroxyethyl methacrylate, *Br. J. Dermatol.*, 110, 447, 1979.
45. Clemmensen, S., Sensitizing potential of 2-hydroxyethylmethacrylate, *Contact Dermatitis*, 12, 203, 1985.
46. Nethercott, J. R., Skin problems associated with multifunctional acrylic monomers in ultraviolet curing inks, *Br. J. Dermatol.*, 98, 541, 1978.
47. Fisher, A. A., Cross-reactions between methyl methacrylate monomers and acrylic monomers presently used in acrylic nail preparations, *Contact Dermatitis*, 6, 345, 1980.
48. Kanerva, L., Turjanmaa, K., Jolanki, R., and Estlander, T., Occupational allergic contact dermatitis from iatrogenic sensitization by a new acrylate dentin adhesive, *Eur. J. Dermatol.*, 1, 25, 1991.
49. Jacobsen, N. and Hensten-Pettersen, A., Occupational health problems and adverse patient reactions in periodontics, *J. Clin. Periodontol.*, 16, 428, 1989.
50. Tosti, A., Rapacchiale, S., Piraccini, B. M., and Peluso, A. M., Occupational airborne contact dermatitis due to ethylene glycol dimethacrylate, *Contact Dermatitis*, 24, 152, 1991.

51. Blichmann, C. W. and Roed-Petersen, J., Occupational skin problems in dental technicians, *Ugeskr. Laeg.*, 148, 1370, 1986.
52. Kanerva. L., Estlander, T., Jolanki, R., and Pekkarinen, E., Occupational pharyngitis associated with allergic patch test reactions from acrylics, *Allergy*, 47, 571, 1992.
53. Lozewicz, S., Davison, A. G., Hopkirk, A. et al., Occupational asthma due to methyl methacrylate and cyanoacrylates, *Thorax*, 40, 836, 1985.
54. Fowler, J. F., Jr., Immediate contact hypersensitivity to acrylic acid, *Derm. Clin.*, 8, 193, 1990.
55. Taylor, J. S., Acrylic reactions — ten years' experience, in *Current Topics in Contact Dermatitis*, Frosch, P. J., Dooms-Goossens, A., Lachapelle, J.-M., Rycroft, R. J. G., and Scheper, R. J., Eds., Springer-Verlag, New York, 1989, 346.
56. Kanerva, L., Estlander, T., Jolanki, R., and Tarvainen, K., Occupational allergic contact dermatitis caused by exposure to acrylates during work with dental prostheses, *Contact Dermatitis*, in press.
57. Johnson, G. H., Powell, L. V., and Gordon, G. E., Dentin bonding systems. A review of current products and techniques, *J.A.D.A*, 122, 34, 1991.

23

Hand Eczema from Rubber Gloves

Kristiina Turjanmaa

CONTENTS

0-8493-7355-7/94/$0.00 + $.50

I. INTRODUCTION

Rubber gloves have been protecting hands against different kinds of chemicals and infectious agents for over a hundred years.[1] The use of gloves has increased continually, the biggest increase being in recent years because of HIV. Besides their benefits, gloves can also elicit unfavorable effects like eczema. The chemicals added to natural rubber in the glove manufacturing process have long been known to cause allergic contact dermatitis (delayed Type IV allergy), but it is only in the last 13 years that it has been realized that proteins in natural rubber, which are still present in the finished gloves, can cause contact urticaria, and even eczema in sensitized persons (immediate Type I allergy).[2-4] Apart from immunological reactions to natural rubber and compounds added to it, it must be emphasized that irritant dermatitis from gloves is the most common symptom among glove users.[5] Since the clinical picture is not predictive of the eliciting agent, all glove users with hand eczema should be examined for delayed and immediate rubber allergy.[6]

II. MANUFACTURE OF LATEX GLOVES

Surgical and cleaning gloves are manufactured by dipping them in natural rubber latex; 99% of the world's rubber consumption is supplied by liquid latex tapped from the rubber tree, *Hevea brasiliensis,* which contains 34% rubber (polyisoprene), 2% proteins, 0.4% fatty acids, 1.6% resins, 0.6% ash, 1.4% sugar, and 60% water. The latex is first stabilized in the field by adding ammonia, and then further treated at the collection station with zinc oxide or tetramethylthiuram disulfide or more ammonia to make it stable for transport. For optimum product performance and manufacturing efficiency the latex requires the addition of several chemicals. The most important additive is sulfur, which produces the rubber polymer cross-linking (known as vulcanization) essential for good tensile properties. The assimilation of sulfur into the rubber polymer is aided by the addition of activators, which increase the reaction speed, thus reducing the time required for polymerization to take place. Other additives include antioxidants, which help to reduce the decline in physical properties as the product ages, and surfactants, which ensure film uniformity during dipping, and pigments or dyes if a colored product is required. In principle, all dipped products are manufactured by coating a former or mold in the shape of the ultimately desired product with latex and drying it to a continuous film which can then be stripped from the mold. Thin latex products are made by dipping the former directly into latex two or three times, depending on the thickness required. For thicker articles like cleaning gloves, multiple dipping of the former is possible, but efficiency can be improved by using a coagulant or heat-sensitization process, which gives a relatively thick film in a few seconds. Irrespective of the dipping method, the rest of the process is roughly the same.

Typically, latex dipping is followed by leaching (which removes excess chemicals, especially coagulant, from the film), drying, and curing (vulcanization). The final stages may include further leaching, chlorination, and powdering before the finished product is stripped from the mold. Most rubber products are quite tacky, so powdering is essential to prevent surfaces sticking together. Powders are often included in the coagulant solution as "mold-release agents" to ease stripping and prevent unwanted adhesion.[7,8] Surgical and examination gloves are now generally powdered with corn starch. The finished surgical gloves are packed in sealed paper envelopes and sterilized using ethylene oxide, or generally, today, by gamma irradiation.

III. SYMPTOMS

Cronin studied the clinical patterns of hand eczema in 263 women and found that allergens, irritants, and endogenous factors produce similar, indistinguishable patterns.[6] However, a very typical feature of delayed-type rubber contact allergy is localization of the eczema on the dorsal side of the fingers and hands, and on the flexor or extensor surfaces of the forearms, not extending to the area outside glove contact.[9]

The main symptoms of Type I allergy to rubber proteins include contact urticaria, rhinitis, conjunctivitis, angioedema, generalized urticaria, and anaphylaxis.[10,11] Information on the frequency of eczema caused by rubber proteins, the so-called protein contact dermatitis, in these patients is rather limited. In 27 subjects with latex glove contact urticaria, 9 had hand eczema. Only 3 of them complained of redness, itchiness, or exacerbation of hand eczema as the only symptoms of using gloves, while the other 24 patients showed all the symptoms typical of contact urticaria syndrome.[4] In another study consisting of 42 patients with latex glove contact urticaria, 28 presented with hand eczema, and in 9 (32%) the hand eczema disappeared or improved markedly with avoidance of latex gloves, which suggests that the gloves were the main cause of the dermatitis.[4] Irritant dermatitis on the hands often begins as simple dryness of the dorsal aspects of the hands, later leading to eczema.

IV. FREQUENCY OF ECZEMA

Chemicals, especially the accelerators, are frequently responsible for delayed-type sensitization to rubber that elicits eczema on the contact area. Thiurams, and to a lesser extent mercaptobenzo-thiazole (MBT), used to be the most common allergens in gloves. Carbamates are thought to sensitize less frequently than thiurams and MBT, and have consequently replaced them in many glove brands.[9]

In the U.K., at St John's Hospital, London, the incidence of rubber glove dermatitis increased between 1965 and 1976 from 2 to 3.5% for women and from 0.4 to 2.1% for men, as diagnosed by patch testing. During the same period the annual incidence of thiuram allergy varied between 3.4 and 7.0% in women and between 0.5 and 4.3% in men. The corresponding figures for MBT and the mercapto group were 1.6 to 5.2% for women and 1.1 to 2.7% for men. Sensitivity to carba mix alone was less frequent, but it was clearly associated with thiuram allergy, probably because of their chemical similarity.[9] In Singapore, Goh found only 7 (1%) subjects allergic to thiuram mix among 721 hand eczema patients, 32% had irritant dermatitis, and 23% allergic contact dermatitis.[12] In Finland, Lammintausta and Kalimo[13] patch-tested 3332 eczema patients over a 3-year period and found rubber allergy in 158 (4.7%) of them; 59 (2.5%) out of 2337 female patients were allergic to thiurams and most of them were sensitized by using gloves.[13] Estlander et al.[14] analyzed 542 patients with occupational skin diseases and found that in 63 (12%) cases the disorder was caused by rubber gloves; 52 (83%) of the patients were women, 18 were cleaners, 17 worked in kitchens or in the food industry, and 17 in other nonmedical jobs. In the Finnish National Register for Occupational Diseases the frequency of allergy to rubber chemicals was 19.9% in data collected from 1974 to 1983.[15] About 60% of the rubber allergies were caused by rubber gloves. Lammintausta et al.[16] in Finland examined 536 hospital wet-workers; 9 (1.7%) were allergic to thiurams and 7 had relevant hand eczema symptoms from gloves.

Immediate Type I allergy from gloves seems infrequent in the literature, as compared with the frequency of delayed allergy. In Finland, Lammintausta and Kalimo[13] patch-tested 3332 patients with eczema and found that 46 (1.4%) patients had a history of immediate skin reactions to various rubber materials, but only 3 patients out of 46 (7%) were elicited by gloves.[13] In Sweden, Nilsson studied 142 hospital wet-workers and found that only 4 (2.8%) exhibited contact urticaria symptoms caused by rubber cleaning gloves.[17] Estlander et al.[14] found 2 patients in an occupational outpatient clinic with immediate allergy from cleaning gloves, and 63 with delayed allergy to rubber gloves; i.e., the ratio of immediate to delayed rubber glove allergy was 1:32. The patients in this study were not routinely examined for protein-contact dermatitis. Wrangsjö et al.[18] studied 15 patients with discomfort and itching produced by rubber gloves within 1 h of working in thin latex gloves; 13 of them had hand dermatitis. They found a positive provocation test result with wheal reactions in 40%. In 1990 Turjanmaa diagnosed 15 cases of positive skin test reactions to thiuram mix out of 609 patch-tested patients.[19] During the same period, 28 new cases of immediate allergy to rubber proteins were diagnosed at the same clinic; 16 of them presented with hand eczema. This result shows that by testing all patients with hand eczema with both patch tests and prick tests, even more Type I allergy to rubber proteins can be found than contact allergy to rubber additives.

Turjanmaa and Reunala[20] studied the simultaneous occurrence of Type I allergy to rubber proteins and Type IV allergy to rubber additives. Out of 18 patients (89% with existing or previous hand eczema) with previously diagnosed rubber-glove contact dermatitis, 1 (6%) was verified by RAST, prick, and use tests as also having immediate allergy to rubber proteins. Out of 35 glove-using patients (97% with existing or previous hand eczema) with previously diagnosed Type I allergy to gloves, 5 (14%) produced positive patch tests to thiurams and 1 (3%) to naphthyl mix. Simultaneously, sensitization to dibenzothiazyl disulfide was found in one patient, to carba mix in another, and to cyclohexylparaphenylenediamine in a third. Altogether, 7 out of 53 patients allergic to rubber gloves had, at the same time, immediate and delayed type allergy to gloves.

Nilsson studied a selected group of 142 hospital wet-workers with hand eczema. In 92%, water, cleaning agents, hand disinfectants, wearing of gloves, and other trivial irritants were claimed to have caused the hand eczema.[17] Turjanmaa studied 512 hospital employees using gloves;[21] 26% of them complained of irritation from the gloves, especially blaming the glove powder, while 2.9% were found to have immediate allergy to rubber gloves. Irritation from using rubber gloves seems to be much more frequent than sensitization to rubber components or additives, but the exact numbers have not been studied. Ruutu et al.[22] investigated seven brands of latex catheters for cellular toxicity after an epidemic of severe urethral strictures in cardiac surgery patients. Four of the seven brands showed marked cytotoxicity and inhibited almost all cell growth in various human cell cultures. Identical results have been found in some brands of latex surgical gloves.[23] The significance of this finding in relationship to irritant properties of gloves has to be studied more carefully.

V. DIAGNOSIS

A. Allergic Contact Eczema

Cell-mediated, Type IV allergic contact dermatitis from rubber gloves can be diagnosed by patch tests using different rubber mixes, individual rubber chemicals, and pieces of gloves as allergens. The guidelines for testing are laid down by the International Contact Dermatitis Research Group (ICDRG) or local research groups. At the moment, the standard patch test series recommended by the European group includes thiuram mix, black-rubber mix, mercapto mix, and mercaptobenzothiazole as rubber allergens. Carba mix has been abandoned because it has been shown to elicit too many irritant reactions. Individual rubber chemicals are tested by using special screening series.[9,13]

Storrs et al.[24] studied the relevance of allergic patch test reactions in North America during 1984 and 1985. Thiuram mix 1% pet was tested on 1137 persons, 68% of 44 positive patch test reactions were relevant; 38 out of 1135 tested persons were allergic to carba mix 3% pet, with a relevance of 71%, and 30 out of 1132 tested persons were allergic to mercapto mix 1% pet, with a relevance of 80%. Carba mix elicited suspect reactions in 14 cases and irritant reactions in 6 cases, while thiuram mix elicited 8 and mercapto mix 3 doubtful reactions, and no irritant reactions were recorded. Between 1985 and 1990 von Hintzenstern et al.[25] analyzed 145 patients with rubber allergy and found that 67 had occupational rubber glove allergies — 72% of them had positive patch test reactions to thiuram mix, 25% to carba mix, and 3% to mercapto mix. Estlander et al.[14] analyzed 63 rubber glove eczema patients: 38 had positive reactions to rubber chemicals and glove materials, 14 to glove material only, and 11 to rubber chemicals (the glove material was not available).

The importance of testing with pieces of the patients' own gloves is also evident from two patients of Rich et al.[26] Both of them had clear symptoms from latex gloves but did not react to the usual rubber allergens. Patch testing with different latex gloves elicited some positive reactions, and the allergens responsible could be traced: 4,4'-thiobis(6-*tert*-butyl-*m*-cresol) Lowinox 44S36) and butylhydroxyanisole (BHA), both antioxidants used in glove manufacture. In the same way, other rubber additives, such as dyes, may prove to be responsible for the allergic reaction. Heese et al.[27] recently pointed out the possibility of allergic contact eczema from rarely used corn starch ingredients such as epichlorhydrin, sorbic acid, and an isothiazolin-3-one derivative.

B. Protein Contact Dermatitis

For a clinical diagnosis of protein contact dermatitis there must be eczema following contact with the suspect proteinaceous material.[28] The mechanism is still obscure: an IgE-mediated late-phase hypersensitivity or a reaction via IgE-receptors on Langerhans cells, leading to same kind of reaction as occurs in delayed type contact allergy, have been suggested.[29,30] Scratch tests have been recommended by several authors for diagnosing protein contact dermatitis in cases of Type I allergy with dermatitis from fish and shellfish, fruit and vegetables, and, in the case of veterinary surgeons, from cows.[31-33] In a recent study, Susitaival et al.[34] used prick and patch test methods to study about 100 farmers with hand dermatosis. Allergy to cow dander was diagnosed in 46% of work-related eczema. Of the cow allergies, one in three was only detected in the skin prick test or in a 30-min patch test, one in three only in 24-h patch tests, and one in three in both immediate and delayed skin tests. A similar test result distribution might occur in protein contact dermatitis caused by rubber gloves, but so far there has been only one publication on successful, delayed-type latex patch test results.[35]

Testing with rubber proteins has been problematic so far, since there is no reliable commercially available allergen for skin testing. Excessively effective test material can cause systemic reactions, while skin test material containing small amounts of allergens may produce false negative reactions.[10,36,37] Various methods also have been used: from the rub test to the open patch test, and from testing with undiluted ammoniated latex to the use of diluted glove extracts.[38] Turjanmaa used the latex glove scratch chamber test on 512 hospital employees using gloves;[21] 23 were found to be positive by this method but 8 of the 23 were negative in prick testing with latex glove eluates. In accordance with the prick test result, these eight patients all had negative 15-min use tests, and afterwards they were able to use the gloves in their daily work without any symptoms. Of the 15 prick-test-positive persons, 14 had a positive 15-min use test with latex gloves, while 1 developed wheal and flare reactions after 4 h. Glove eluates have been compared by the skin prick test method with the sap and leaf of the rubber tree and found to give concordant results.[39] They have never caused harmful side effects, even when several allergenic glove brands have been tested at the same time in highly sensitive patients.

The glove powder in glove eluates seems not to disturb the skin testing, as so far there is little evidence of allergenicity in glove powders.[40] The powder taken from gloves has been studied by immunoblotting and found to contain the same allergenic proteins as the gloves.[41] In contrast, two glove powders (Biosorb, Johnson & Johnson, Arlington, TX and Elastyren glove powder, Remy Industries, Wijgmaal-Leuven, Belgium) supplied by glove manufacturers produced no positive skin reactions when tested on 42 and 32 patients, respectively, with immediate rubber allergy.[4] Marked differences have been found in the allergenicity of different gloves, and it is thus advisable to use two or three different glove brand eluates at the same time to avoid false negative results.[37] The use test, initially with one finger, and in negative cases with the whole glove, is important for verifying doubtful skin prick test results. An anaphylactic reaction has been reported in the whole-hand use test, therefore the test must be performed under emergency-care conditions.[38] Latex RAST (k82, Pharmacia Diagnostics, Uppsala, Sweden) is not suitable for screening because it gives positive reactions in only 60 to 65% of the cases with immediate allergy to rubber proteins.[4]

C. Irritant Dermatitis

So far, there is no reliable method for diagnosing irritant dermatitis; it only remains to exclude the different types of allergic reaction. Irritant dermatitis is more common among atopic persons, and in working conditions where hands are frequently washed and exposed to chemicals.[42] Some allergens, like acrylates and epoxy resin, can penetrate the glove and thus replicate glove allergy. In such cases, irritant dermatitis can be falsely diagnosed if other chemicals are not tested at the same time.[43]

VI. ALLERGENICITY OF DIFFERENT LATEX GLOVES

Thiurams, and to a lesser extent MBT, used to be the most common delayed-type allergens in gloves. Certain gloves are now marketed as "hypoallergenic" because known sensitizers are avoided, used in lower concentrations, or washed away during the manufacturing process. Carbamates are thought to sensitize less frequently, and have therefore replaced thiurams and MBT in many glove brands. Fisher called gloves manufactured using carbamates "hypoallergenic".[44]

The immediately allergenicity of different latex surgical and household gloves has been studied by prick testing of people with Type I allergy to rubber gloves with eluates of 19 different glove brands;[37] 6 out of 17 surgical gloves and 1 in 2 household gloves caused positive reactions in over

87% of the allergic subjects; 4 less-allergenic latex surgical gloves caused positive reactions in 8 to 21%, confirming that not all rubber gloves are equally allergenic. The term "hypoallergenic" does not refer to rubber proteins and can thus be misleading.

VII.   PROPHYLAXIS

Household gloves are often used for personnel protection in cleaning and industrial work. Their use is promoted by preexisting hand eczema, which is known to be a predisposing factor for both Type I and Type IV allergies to rubber gloves. Thus, people with hand eczema preferably should use household gloves made from non-rubber materials to avoid rubber sensitization.[14]

Many brands of latex gloves are known to contain proteins which have caused sensitization in atopic people, especially in medical workers. The physical properties of surgical latex gloves are not easily replaced by gloves made from non-rubber materials, which are also many times more expensive than latex gloves. People already sensitized to rubber proteins should use non-latex surgical gloves, such as: Dermaprene (Ansell America, Eatontown, NJ), Elastyren (Allerderm Laboratories, Mill Valley, CA and Hermal Pharmaceutical Laboratories, NY), Neolon (Deseret Medical Inc., Sandy, UT), or Tactylon (SmartPractice, Phoenix, AZ).[27] In the future, if it is not possible to totally eliminate the proteins, levels of allergenic proteins should be minimized to a point where they do not sensitize people.

VIII.   CONCLUSIONS

Eczema from rubber gloves is a common problem today, both generally and in occupational praxis. The clinical picture of rubber allergy has been expanded since immediate allergy was detected. Immediate rubber protein allergy is even known to cause lethal anaphylactic reactions.[45] In addition to contact urticaria from gloves, hand eczema may also be the first sign of a sensitization ending in life-threatening symptoms, e.g., during medical examinations or operations.[46] All patients with hand eczema therefore should always be examined for the two modalities of rubber allergy.

To allow suitable gloves to be chosen for rubber-allergic patients, manufacturers should indicate on their packages the rubber chemicals used and also, for example, the amounts of protein allergens in the finished gloves. The misleading term "hypoallergenic" should be abandoned.

REFERENCES

1. Geelhoed, G. W., 'Hand in Glove': a centennial observation on the surgical use of rubber gloves, *South. Med. J.,* 84, 1012, 1991.
2. Downing, J. G., Dermatitis from rubber gloves, *N. Engl. J. Med.,* 208, 196, 1933.
3. Nutter, A. F., Contact urticaria to rubber, *Br. J. Dermatol.,* 101, 597, 1979.
4. Turjanmaa, K., Latex Glove Contact Urticaria, thesis, Acta Univ. Tamperensis, Ser. A, Vol. 254, University of Tampere, 1988.
5. Singgih, S. I. R., Lantinga, H., Nater, J. P., Woest, T. E., and Kruyt-Gaspersz, J. A., Occupational hand dermatoses in hospital cleaning personnel, *Contact Dermatitis,* 14, 14, 1986.
6. Cronin, E., Clinical patterns of hand eczema in women, *Contact Dermatitis,* 13, 153, 1985.
7. Blackley, D. C., *High Polymer Latices,* Vols. 1 and 2, Applied Science Publishers, London, 1966.
8. Hofman, W., *Kautschuk-Technologie,* Gentner Verlag, Stuttgart, 1980.
9. Cronin, E., *Contact Dermatitis,* Churchill Livingstone, Edinburgh, 1980, 714.
10. Frosch, P. J., Wahl, R., Bahmer, F. A., and Maasch, H. J., Contact urticaria to rubber gloves is IgE-mediated, *Contact Dermatitis,* 14, 241, 1986.
11. Turjanmaa, K. and Reunala, T., Contact urticaria from rubber gloves, Occupational dermatoses, in *Dermatologic Clinics,* Vol. 6, Taylor, J. S., Ed., W. B. Saunders, Philadelphia, 1988, 47.

12. Goh, C. L., An epidemiological comparison between hand eczema and non-hand eczema, *Br. J. Dermatol.*, 118, 797, 1988.

13. Lammintausta, K. and Kalimo, K., Sensitivity to rubber, study with rubber mixes and individual rubber chemicals, *Dermatosen*, 33, 204, 1985.

14. Estlander, T., Jolanki, R., and Kanerva, L., Dermatitis and urticaria from rubber and plastic gloves, *Contact Dermatitis*, 14, 20, 1986.

15. Kanerva, L., Estlander, T., and Jolanki, R., Occupational skin disease in Finland, An analysis of 10 years of statistics from an occupational dermatology clinic, *Int. Arch. Occup. Environ. Health*, 60, 89, 1988.

16. Lammintausta, K., Kalimo, K., and Havu, V. K., Occurrence of contact allergy and hand eczemas in hospital wet work, *Contact Dermatitis*, 8, 84, 1982.

17. Nilsson, E., Contact sensitivity and urticaria in "wet" work, *Contact Dermatitis*, 13, 321, 1985.

18. Wrangsjö, K., Mellström, G., and Axelsson, G., Discomfort from rubber gloves indicating contact urticaria, *Contact Dermatitis*, 15, 79, 1986.

19. Turjanmaa, K., unpublished data.

20. Turjanmaa, K. and Reunala, T., Latex contact urticaria associated with delayed allergy to rubber chemicals, in *Current Topics in Contact Dermatitis*, Frosch, P. J., Dooms-Goossens, A., Lachapelle, J.-M., Rycroft, R. J. G., and Scheper, R. J., Eds., Springer-Verlag, Heidelberg, 1989, 460.

21. Turjanmaa, K., Incidence of immediate allergy to latex gloves in hospital personnel, *Contact Dermatitis*, 17, 270, 1987.

22. Ruutu, M., Alfthan, O., Talja, M., and Andersson, L. C., Cytotoxicity of latex urinary catheters, *Br. J. Urol.*, 57, 82, 1985.

23. Cormio, L., Ruutu, M., Talja, M., Turjanmaa, K., and Andersson, L. C., *Clin. Exp. Allergy*, in press.

24. Storrs, F. J., Rosenthal, L. E., Adams, R. M., Clendenning, W., Emmett, E. A., Fisher, A. A., Larsen, W. G., Maibach, H. I., Rietschel, R. L., Schorr, W. F., and Taylor, J. S., Prevalence and relevance of allergic reactions in patients patch tested in North America — 1984 to 1985, *J. Am. Acad. Derm.*, 20, 1038, 1989.

25. von Hintzenstern, J., Heese, A., Koch, H. U., Peters, K.-P., and Hornstein, O. P., Frequency, spectrum and occupational relevance of type IV allergies to rubber chemicals, *Contact Dermatitis*, 24, 244, 1991.

26. Rich, P., Belozer, M. L., Norris, P., and Storrs, F. J., Allergic contact dermatitis to two antioxidants in latex gloves: 4,4′-thiobis(6-*tert*-butyl-*meta*-cresol) (Lowinox 44S36) and butylhydroxyanisole, *J. Am. Acad. Derm.*, 24, 37, 1991.

27. Heese, A., von Hintzenstern, J., Peters, K.-P., Koch, H. U., and Hornstein, O. P., Allergic and irritant reactions to rubber gloves in medical health services, *J. Am. Acad. Derm.*, 25, 831, 1992.

28. Veien, N. K., Hattel, T., Justesen, O., and Norholm, A., Causes of eczema in the food industry, *Dermatosen*, 31, 84, 1983.

29. Bruynzeel-Koomen, C., van Wichen, D. F., Toonstra, J., Berrens, L., and Bruynzeel, P. L. B., The presence of IgE molecules on epidermal Langerhans cells in patients with atopic dermatitis, *Arch. Dermatol. Res.*, 278, 199, 1986.

30. Clark, R. A. F., Cell-mediated and IgE-mediated immune responses in atopic dermatitis, *Arch. Dermatol.*, 125, 413, 1989.

31. Hjorth, N. and Roed-Petersen, J., Occupational protein contact dermatitis in food handlers, *Contact Dermatitis*, 2, 28, 1976.

32. Prahl, P. and Roed-Petersen, J., Type I allergy from cows in veterinary surgeons, *Contact Dermatitis*, 5, 33, 1979.

33. Hannuksela, M., Atopic contact dermatitis, *Contact Dermatitis*, 6, 30, 1980.

34. Susitaival, P., Husman, K., Husman, L., Hollmén, A., Horsmanheimo, M., Hannuksela, M., Vohlonen, I., and Notkola, V., Prevalence, cause and prognosis of hand dermatoses in Finnish dairy farmers, in *Abstr. Third Int. Course Occup. Dermatoses*, Åland, Finland, June 3 to 7, 1991.

35. Goertz, J. and Goos, M., Immediate and late type allergy to latex: contact urticaria, asthma and contact dermatitis, Poster 4, *Eur. Symp. Contact Dermatitis,* Heidelberg, May 27 to 29, 1988.

36. Spaner, D., Dolovich, J., Tarlo, S., Sussman, G., and Buttoo, K., Hypersensitivity to natural latex, *J. Allergy Clin. Immunol.,* 83, 1135, 1989.

37. Turjanmaa, K., Laurila, K., Mäkinen-Kiljunen, S., and Reunala, T., Rubber contact urticaria, allergenic properties of 19 brands of latex gloves, *Contact Dermatitis,* 19, 362, 1988.

38. Turjanmaa, K. and Reunala, T., Contact urticaria to surgical and household rubber gloves, in *Exogenous Dermatoses: Environmental Dermatitis,* Menné, T. and Maibach, H. I., Eds., CRC Press, Boca Raton, FL, 1991, 317.

39. Turjanmaa, K., Reunala, T., and Räsänen, L., Comparison of diagnostic methods in latex surgical glove contact urticaria, *Contact Dermatitis,* 19, 241, 1988.

40. Fisher, A. A., Contact urticaria and anaphylactoid reaction due to corn starch surgical glove powder, *Contact Dermatitis,* 16, 224, 1987.

41. Turjanmaa, K., Reunala, T., Alenius, H., Brummer-Korvenkontio, H., and Palosuo, T., Allergens in latex surgical gloves and glove powder, *Lancet,* 336, 1588, 1990.

42. Rystedt, I., Hand eczema in patients with history of atopic manifestations in childhood, *Acta Derm. Venereol. Stockholm,* 65, 305, 1985.

43. Kanerva, L., Estlander, T., and Jolanki, R., Allergic contact dermatitis from dental composite resins due to aromatic epoxy acrylates and aliphatic acrylates, *Contact Dermatitis,* 20, 201, 1989.

44. Fisher, A. A., "Hypoallergenic" surgical gloves and gloves for special situations, *Cutis,* 15, 797, 1975.

45. Slater, J. E., Mostello, L. A., and Shaer, C., Rubber-specific IgE in children with spina bifida, *J. Urol.,* 146, 578, 1991.

46. Ownby, D. R., Tomlanovich, M., Sammons, N., and McCullough, J., Anaphylaxis associated with latex allergy during barium enema examinations, *A.R.J.,* 156, 903, 1991.

24

Hand Eczema in the Construction Industry

Chee-Leok Goh

CONTENTS

0-8493-7355-7/94/$0.00 + $.50

I. EPIDEMIOLOGY OF HAND ECZEMA IN THE CONSTRUCTION INDUSTRY

The construction industry is one of the major contributors of patients with occupational hand eczema in many countries. In Singapore, the largest number of patients attending its occupational skin disease clinic were construction workers.[1] There are few field studies on the prevalence and incidence of occupational skin disease in the construction industry;[2,3] this is because of the difficulties in conducting field studies under the conditions of construction work. Most workers with occupational eczema in the construction industry present with hand eczema.[3,4] Most construction workers with hand eczema also had contact eczema to cement. In the Netherlands, the prevalence of hand eczema among construction workers was 7.1% (of 112 construction workers surveyed in a population survey). In the Netherlands, workers from the construction industry were the third commonest occupational group presenting with hand eczema, after the chemical industry and metal industry.[6] In a field survey of occupational eczema in a construction factory in Singapore, 47% of 15 workers with allergic contact eczema presented with pure hand eczema, and 68% of 22 workers with irritant eczema presented with pure hand eczema.[4] Cement is the most common cause of hand eczema among construction workers.[1,4]

In Sweden, a 1-year-period prevalence survey of hand eczema in a population of hand eczema showed that hand eczema was prevalent in 3.6% of concrete workers.[5] The 1-year-period prevalence of hand eczema in relation to occupational exposure from cement was 7.1% in males and 30% in females (overall 9.2%) compared to other occupational exposures in 7810 people with hand eczema. Burrows and Calnan estimated that about 200,000 workdays were lost each year in the building industry through eczema.[7] In Singapore, it was estimated that about 14,000 workdays per year were lost through occupational eczema in the construction industry.[8]

Studies have also indicated that the most common cause of allergic dermatitis among construction workers is hexavalent chromate. Hexavalent chromate is present as an impurity in most cement.[1,4,6-9]

The prevalence of eczema among construction workers varies in different countries. In Singapore, 16.9% of 272 workers surveyed in a prefabrication construction factory were found to have an occupational contact eczema; 46% (7/15) of these workers with allergic contact eczema (from cement and/or rubber gloves) presented with pure hand eczema; and 68% (15/22) with irritant contact eczema presented with pure hand eczema.[4] Of 1071 construction workers surveyed, 8.2% had cement contact eczema;[12] 5.6% of 366 workers surveyed in Norway had cement contact eczema,[2] and 7.8% of 1691 workers surveyed had hand cement eczema compared to a prevalence of 4.6% in the general population in Groningen.[3] The most common cause of hand eczema was contact allergy to chromate.

II. IRRITANT AND ALLERGIC HAND ECZEMA IN CONSTRUCTION WORKERS

Construction workers presenting to a skin clinic in Singapore more often suffer from allergic contact eczema than irritant contact eczema, unlike workers from industries where irritant contact eczema is a more common presentation.[1] Among 155 construction workers with occupational contact eczema attending an occupational skin disease clinic in Singapore, 68% had allergic contact eczema compared to only 25% of 208 metal and engineering workers with allergic contact eczema and 40% of 86 electrical and electronic workers.[1] The rest had irritant contact eczema, predominantly. This is probably the observation in most other countries. This is probably because cement allergic contact eczema tends to be more severe than irritant contact eczema and therefore workers with cement allergic contact eczema are more likely to seek treatment.

However, the actual prevalence of irritant contact eczema in the construction industry exceeds allergic contact hand eczema among construction workers.[3,4] This is because most construction workers with mild irritant eczema usually do not seek treatment as they often regard eczema as an accepted risk in their occupation. The ratio of allergic contact eczema to irritant contact eczema was 1:1.4 in Singapore and 1:3.3 in the Netherlands. In the survey in the Netherlands, the prevalence of hand eczema in construction workers (7.8%) was significantly higher in comparison with a sample from the general population, in which the crude prevalence was 4%.[6] Irritant eczema represented a substantial portion of all cases of eczema in the construction industry and accounted for most of the difference from the general population.[6]

Avnstorp, in his survey among construction workers in Denmark, reported that most construction workers with cement irritant hand eczema tend to have mild eczema. Workers with allergic hand eczema from chromate were distributed more equally between the mild to severe eczema groups.[17] This confirmed the observation that there is a higher proportion of allergic contact eczema than irritant contact eczema among construction workers attending skin clinics. That is, workers with allergic cement eczema tend to have more severe eczema.

Coenraads et al.,[3] in the Netherlands, reported that positive patch tests (to one or more allergens including dichromate, cobalt, thiuram mix, and epoxy resin) were found in 15% of the workers with hand eczema (among 1700 construction workers surveyed), compared to a rate of 5.5% in the control group without eczema. In carpenters, there was very little difference between the proportion of positive patch tests in workers with hand eczema (6.1%) and that in controls (4.3%); in bricklayers and plasterers, these percentages were 27.5 and 7.6%, respectively.[3] The prevalence of irritant eczema was 4.0% compared to 1.9% (irritant eczema alone or in combination with other forms of eczema was 4.8%) in the general population, and of allergic contact eczema, 1.4% compared to 0.9% in the general population.

III. HAND ECZEMA AMONG DIFFERENT TYPES OF WORKERS IN THE CONSTRUCTION INDUSTRY

Contact eczema in construction workers usually affects the hands. In a report from Singapore, 46.7% of construction workers with allergic contact eczema presented with pure hand eczema and 68.2% of the construction workers with irritant contact eczema presented with pure hand eczema.[3]

In the U.K., half of 134 patients with cement eczema presented with hand and/or arm eczema, and of these 57% had chromate allergy; 9% had involvement of the palms only (of which 58% had chromate allergy).[32]

In Groningen, contact allergy could be established in 15% of 126 construction workers with hand eczema and in 5.5% of 307 workers without eczema. Of bricklayers and plasterers with hand eczema in the construction industry, 24% had contact allergy (manifesting as having one or more positive patch test reactions) compared to a rate of 7% of workers in the control group. In carpenters, however, no significant difference between the proportions of persons with positive patch tests was noted.[3] In the job category of persons handling cement and plaster, 12.6% of 357 workers were found to have hand eczema, and was the most affected group compared to carpenters (6.1% of 840 workers), unskilled workers (8.7% of 184 workers), technicians/plumbers (5.9% of 119 workers), and administration/supervisors (7.3% of 191 workers).[3]

In Singapore, chromate allergy among construction workers was most prevalent in occupations that require workers to be exposed to cement most frequently. For example, it was found that chromate allergy was most prevalent among workers employed in the concrete bay (10.9%) where workers' contact with cement was most frequent and intense, and was less prevalent in other areas, e.g., the repair/maintenance section (7.7%), repair/storage section (8.3%), or steel yards (3.2%), and the concrete laboratory (0%).

IV. CONTACT ALLERGENS IN THE CONSTRUCTION INDUSTRY

A. Chromate

Jaegar and Pelloni, in 1950, were the first to associate cement eczema with the chromates in cement.[22] The role of chromates in cement as a direct cause of allergic contact eczema in construction workers has been confirmed in several studies.[23-25] The water-soluble hexavalent chromates in cement are the causative allergen. Chromate is present in cement as an impurity. It is not added into cement during the manufacturing process. Several studies in different countries have shown that hexavalent chromates are present in cement in varying concentrations, ranging from 1 to 40 μg/g.[25-27]

Cement does not have a constant composition. Rather, it is made from chalk (or limestone), clay (or shale), and gypsum (calcium sulfate); coal, used as fuel in the kiln, is often incorporated during the manufacturing process. The chromate in cement comes from the chrome steel grinders and ash. Johnston and Calnan found chromates in clay, coal ash, and chalk.[23] Most of these chromates exist in an insoluble trivalent form, but are converted into water-soluble hexavalent chromates in the kiln.[28]

A survey in Groningen showed that 11% of 126 construction workers with hand eczema had chromate allergy compared to a rate of 2.6% in 307 workers without eczema. Burrows and Calnan reported a prevalence of 78% (of 171 patients) of chromate allergy in construction workers with cement eczema.[32] In Singapore, 15 (of 272 workers) in a prefabrication factory had contact allergy to chromates. These findings further support the role of chromates as a cause of hand eczema among construction workers.

B.   Cobalt and Nickel

Although the total cobalt content (ranging from 8.1 to 14.2 $\mu g/g$), nickel content (ranging from 14.9 to 28.5 $\mu g/g$), and chromium content of cement are almost identical, isolated contact sensitivity to cobalt or nickel from cement is uncommon.[21,24,29,30] This is explained by the low concentration of water-soluble cobalt and nickel salts. Cobalt and nickel exist in cement mainly as insoluble salts not readily absorbed into the skin, and hence do not sensitize.

In Groningen, the prevalence of cobalt allergy among construction workers with hand eczema was 2.3% (among 126 persons) compared to a rate of 0.7% among 307 workers without eczema. In Singapore, the prevalence of cobalt and nickel sensitivity in a prefabrication construction factory was low (4 of 272 workers); these workers had concomitant chromate allergy. Of the 5 (out of 272) construction workers with nickel allergy, 2 were nonoccupational (from watches), 2 had asymptomatic nickel allergy, and 1 worker with nickel and cobalt allergies also had allergic contact eczema to chromate in cement.[30]

The absence of isolated nickel allergy among these construction workers with cement eczema indicated that nickel in cement does not appear to sensitize normal skin. Fregert demonstrated that, unlike cobalt salts, insoluble nickel salts in cement could not be dissolved by water or by cysteine, an amino acid constituent of body fluid. He theorized that insoluble cobalt oxides in cement can form complexes with other constituents of body fluid on eczematous skin, and sensitize the skin.

It would appear that cobalt sensitivity can occur simultaneously and aggravate the eczema in persons with allergic contact eczema to chromate in cement. Since cement contains minute amounts of cobalt, contact allergy to cobalt is not unexpected.

C.   Rubber Chemicals

Rubber chemical allergy in construction workers is not uncommon. Many construction workers wear rubber gloves and boots during work and become sensitized to rubber chemicals in their protective gear. In Groningen, the prevalence of thiuram-mix allergy in workers with hand eczema was 3.2% (out of 126 workers) compared to a rate of 1% (of 307) workers without eczema. In Singapore, 2.9% (8/272) of construction workers in a prefabrication factory had contact allergy to one or more rubber chemicals. These workers were allergic to carba mix and/or PPD mix and/or mercapto mix. None of their workers was allergic to thiuram mix.[19]

D.   Rubber Gloves/Boots Allergy

Construction workers frequently wear gloves to protect themselves against contact eczema. A population survey of occupational hand eczema in Goetenborg, Sweden, revealed that 43% of 109 workers handling cement used gloves regularly or frequently during work, compared to a rate of 21.6% in the total population of 12,750 people surveyed. The study revealed that regular or frequent use of gloves was significantly more common among people with hand eczema.[5] The motivation for protecting the hands is probably increased when hand eczema is present. Frequent use of protective gloves was seen in the groups with high figures for irritant contact eczema.[5]

Avnstorp[17] reported that individual preventive measures, including the use of gloves, creams, and handwashing, were not found to influence the development of irritant contact eczema among construction workers with hand eczema. In his survey of various risk factor profiles, including the use of protective gloves, among construction workers in Denmark, he found them to be equal among those workers who had cement eczema and those who did not. He explained that the absence of influence of individual preventive measures was because the construction work process is so hazardous that it overwhelmed the protective effect of the gloves.

In a field survey in Singapore, 30.5% (of 272 construction workers) in a prefabrication construction factory used rubber gloves and/or boots as protective clothing and 8 workers had rubber chemical allergies; i.e., 9.5% of all workers who used rubber gloves/boots had rubber chemical allergies. The prevalence of rubber chemical allergy in the construction industry will depend on the prevalence of occupational contact eczema among the workers, as there is evidence to suggest that sensitization to rubber chemicals in gloves often occurs secondary to an existing dermatitis.[19-21] In the report, three of the four workers with relevant positive reactions to rubber chemicals (from rubber gloves) also had allergic contact eczema from chromate in cement.[19]

E. Epoxy Resin

Contact allergy to epoxy resin among construction workers has seldom been reported. Epoxy resin is mixed with cement and used as a grouting agent. Allergic contact eczema to epoxy resin among construction workers has been uncommon until recently. Epoxy resin cement is now more widely used in repair and maintenance work in the construction industry. Contact allergy from epoxy resin in cement in construction workers is seldom present with pure hand eczema. Eczema is often present on the arms, face, and other parts of the body.

None of the construction workers in Groningen with hand eczema had allergy to epoxy resin compared to a rate of 1.3% of 307 workers without eczema.

I. Effect of Elimination of Chromate in Cement on Allergic Contact Eczema in the Construction Industry

Over the past decade there were indications that the incidence and prevalence of chromate allergy (in particular, from cement) had declined.[14-16] Cited reasons for the decline included improvement in work processes, increased awareness of cement eczema, and an increased use of individual preventive measures. Avnstorp believed that allergic cement eczema in Denmark was associated with the concomitant lowering of the content of water-soluble chromate in Danish cement.[16] Under Danish law, cement used in the country must not contain more than 2 μg/g of water-soluble chromate.

Recently, Avnstorp studied the prevalence of cement eczema and chromate allergy in two groups of construction workers who were exposed to different concentrations of chromate in cement. There was a significant decrease in the number of workers with cement hand eczema found in the group that was exposed to cement with a lower, water-soluble chromate concentration (<2 ppm) than workers exposed to cement containing a high concentration of water-soluble chromate (>10 ppm). The rates were 12% (27/227) and 25% (47/190), respectively. In the group exposed to low chromate concentration cement, the prevalence of chromate allergy among workers with hand eczema was 11% (3/28) compared to 36% (17/47) in the other group.

The study also revealed that the prevalence of irritant cement hand eczema did not differ significantly among workers who were exposed to either low or high concentrations of water-soluble chromate in cement: 64% (30/47) of the workers exposed to high chromate concentration cement had irritant cement eczema compared to 89% (25/28) exposed to low chromate concentration cement.[17]

V. PROGNOSIS OF HAND ECZEMA FROM CEMENT

Several reports have indicated that occupational contact eczema from cement gradually has a poor prognosis.[32-34] Others have reported a better prognosis.[35] Allergic contact eczema from cement tends to be more severe than irritant contact eczema.[17] This is also an observation for other causes of allergic contact eczema in comparison to irritant contact eczema.[5] Several reports have indicated that workers with allergic contact eczema from chromate in cement tend to have a poor medical prognosis. They continued to develop frequent episodes of hand eczema and frequently require topical steroid treatment.[18] The eczema tends to occur even after years of avoidance of contact with cement and a job change.

Hovding[2] found that bricklayers and bricklayers' assistants who developed cement hand eczema without chromate allergy tend to suffer from eczema for a short duration, whereas those with concomitant chromate allergy tend to suffer from long-lasting symptoms.

Burrows and Calnan[32] did not find any significant difference in prognosis in patients with chromate-sensitive and nonchromate-sensitive cement eczema whose eczema had persisted for more than 5 months.[32] The authors found that 57% (26/46) of workers with cement eczema were not cleared of their eczema after a 5-month follow-up, even after they have avoided contact with cement. Only five workers had improved considerably, and six were entirely clear after a change of jobs. The prognosis of cement eczema appeared to be poor.

Chia and Goh[35] reported a better prognosis in their construction workers with cement eczema. Five patients with irritant cement eczema had complete clearance of eczema[1] after ceasing exposure to cement and four others improved even with continuation of exposure to cement. In five of the six workers with chromate allergy from cement, the eczema cleared upon ceasing contact with cement; one worker had persistent dermatitis when he continued to work with cement.[35]

VI. REHABILITATION AND PREVENTIVE MEASURES

Many patient with cement eczema failed to improve significantly after apparent removal of contact with cement. Burrows reiterated that advice about a change of occupation, particularly in the more profitable occupations, should not be given without careful thought, even in those cases with a positive chromate patch test.[32] Chromate is difficult to avoid in daily life. Minute quantities are certainly present in many commonplace articles. This may partly explain the chronicity of eczema in these patients.

It has been stated that a job change should only be recommended when absolutely necessary. Many dermatologists probably underestimate the effects of a change of occupation on earnings and job satisfaction.[36] Hovding reported that 50% of workers with cement eczema had never been off work because of eczema, and those who had been off work only stayed away on an average of 3 to 4 days/year.[2] The important conclusion from Hovding's work was that the medical prognosis should be kept strictly apart from the social prognosis. The medical prognoses of many cases of occupational eczema may be poor, but in spite of this, the social prognosis may be excellent.[36]

Fregert et al. demonstrated that the addition of ferrous sulfate into cement converts the soluble hexavalent chromate in cement into insoluble trivalent chromate, which is "less sensitizing."[31] It appears to be an effective preventive measure against allergic chromate dermatitis from cement.[17] Swedish and Danish cement manufacturers have added ferrous sulfate into their cement to prevent allergic cement eczema. The prevalence of chromate allergy and cement eczema in Denmark appears to have declined. However, the decline in the prevalence of chromate allergy is also seen in countries which did not introduce similar measures to reduce water-soluble chromates in cement. The cost effectiveness of such measures must be considered against the background of generally lower labor costs and poor workmen's compensation laws in some developing countries.

REFERENCES

1. Goh, C. L., Occupational skin disease in Singapore: epidemiology and causative agents, *Ann. Acad. Med. Singapore*, 16, 303, 1987.
2. Hovding, G., Cement Eczema and Chromium Allergy. An Epidemiological Investigation, thesis, University of Bergen, Norway, 1970.
3. Coenraads, P. J. et al., Prevalence of eczema and other dermatoses of the hands and forearms in construction workers in the Netherlands, *Clin. Exp. Dermatol.*, 9, 149, 1984.
4. Goh, C. L., Gan, S. L., and Ngui, S. J., Occupational dermatitis in a prefabrication construction factory, *Contact Dermatitis*, 15, 235, 1986.

5. Meding, B. and Swanbeck, G., Occupational hand eczema in an industrial city, *Contact Dermatitis*, 22, 13, 1990.

6. Coenraads, P. J., Prevalence of eczema and other dermatoses of the hands and forearms in the Netherlands. Association with age and occupation, *Clin. Exp. Dermatol.*, 8, 495, 1983.

7. Burrows, D. and Calnan, C. D., Cement dermatitis. II. Clinical aspects, *Trans. St. John's Hosp. Dermatol. Soc.*, 51, 27, 1965.

8. Goh, C. L., Sickness absence due to occupational dermatitis in a prefabrication construction factory, *Contact Dermatitis*, 15, 28, 1986.

9. Pirila, V., On the role of chrome and other trace elements in cement eczema, *Acta Derm. Venereol.*, 34, 136, 1954.

10. Skog, E. and Tottie, M., Occupational eczema causing disablement, *Acta Derm. Venereol.*, 41, 205, 1961.

11. Goh, C. L., Chromate sensitivity in Singapore, *Int. J. Derm.*, 24, 514, 1985.

12. Wahlberg, J. E., Health screening for occupational skin diseases in building workers, *Berufs-Dermatosan*, 17, 184, 1969.

13. Rystedt, I., Work-related hand eczema in atopics, *Contact Dermatitis*, 12, 164, 1985.

14. Farm, G., Changing patterns in chromate allergy, *Contact Dermatitis*, 15, 298, 1986.

15. Van Ketal, W. G., Low incidence of occupational dermatitis from chromate, *Contact Dermatitis*, 10, 249, 1984.

16. Avnstorp, C., Prevalence of cement eczema in Denmark before and since addition of ferrous sulfate to Danish cement, *Acta Derm. Venereol.*, 69, 151, 1989.

17. Avnstorp, C., Risk factors for cement eczema, *Contact Dermatitis*, 25, 81, 1991.

18. Avnstorp, C., Follow-up of workers from the pre-fabricated concrete industry after the addition of ferrous sulphate to Danish cement, *Contact Dermatitis*, 20, 365, 1989.

19. Goh, C. L. and Gan, S. L., Rubber allergy among construction workers in a prefabrication construction factory, *Clin. Exp. Dermatol.*, 12, 332, 1987.

20. Goh, C. L., Kwok, S. F., and Gan, S. L., Cobalt and nickel content of Asian cements, *Contact Dermatitis*, 16, 169, 1986.

21. Fregert, S. and Gruvberger, B., Solubility of cobalt in cement, *Contact Dermatitis*, 4, 14, 1978.

22. Jaeger, H. and Pelloni, E., Test epicutanees aux bichromates, positifs dans l'eczema au ciment, *Dermatologica*, 100, 200, 1950.

23. Johnston, A. J. M. and Calnan, C. D., Cement dermatitis. I. Chemical aspects, *Trans. St. John's Hosp. Dermatol. Soc.*, 41, 11, 1958.

24. Fregert, S. and Gruvberger, B., Chemical properties of cement, *Berufs-Dermatosen*, 20, 238, 1972.

25. Goh, C. L. and Kwok, S. F., Chromate allergy: chromate content of Asian cement, *J. Derm.*, 13, 393, 1986.

26. Meneghini, C. L., Rantuccio, F., and Pertruzzelis, V., Cr VI content in cements, *Contact Dermatitis Newsl.*, 5, 108, 1969.

27. Wahlberg, J. E., Lindstedt, G., and Einarsson, O., Chromium, cobalt and nickel in Swedish cement, detergents mould and cutting oils, *Berufs-Dermatosen*, 25, 220, 1977.

28. Cronin, E., *Contact Dermatitis*, Churchill Livingstone, Edinburgh, 1980, 297.

29. Gimenez-Camarasa, J. M. G., Cobalt contact dermatitis, *Acta Derm. Venereol.*, 47, 287, 1967.

30. Goh, C. L., Kwok, S. F., and Gan, S. L., Cobalt and nickel content of Asian cement, *Contact Dermatitis*, 15, 169, 1986.

31. Fregert, S., Gruvberger, B., and Sandahl, E., Reduction of chromate in cement by iron sulphate, *Contact Dermatitis*, 5, 39, 1979.

32. Burrows, D. and Calnan, C. D., Cement dermatitis. II. Clinical aspect, *Trans. St. John's Hosp. Dermatol. Soc.*, 51, 27, 1965.

33. Fregert, S., Occupational dermatitis in a 10-year material, *Contact Dermatitis*, 1, 96, 1975.

34. Burrows, D., Prognosis in industrial dermatitis, *Br. J. Dermatol.*, 87, 145, 1972.

35. Chia, S. E. and Goh, C. L., Prognosis of occupational dermatitis in Singapore workers, *Am. J. Contact Dermatitis*, 2, 105, 1991.

36. Hjorth, N. and Avnstorp, C., Rehabilitation in hand eczema, *Dermatosen*, 34, 74, 1986.

25

Hand Eczema in Caterers: Social and Medical Prognosis

Jytte Roed-Petersen

CONTENTS

I. INTRODUCTION

Sandwich-makers have a high prevalence of occupational hand dermatitis. Both immediate and delayed contact allergy as well as irritant reactions to foods are considered the main causes.[1-4]

In 1976, Hjorth and Roed-Petersen[1] reported an analysis of 33 cases of occupational hand dermatitis among food handlers — 9 male chefs and 24 female sandwich-makers. At that time the majority had not changed occupation — and common to all of them was a high motivation for their work.

The aim of this chapter is to evaluate the medical and social prognosis in sandwich-makers with occupational hand dermatitis.

II. POPULATION

From the 24 female sandwich-makers discussed in the original report[1] we succeeded in contacting 14 for a follow-up. A further 26 female sandwich-makers who were referred to us and tested in our department between 1976 and 1980 also could be traced for a follow-up. The study thus comprised a total of 40 female sandwich-makers (we have never seen a male sandwich-maker in our department). All except three were seen in the department in the period 1981 to 1986 in a personal interview and, if necessary, further testing (patch test, prick test, scratch chamber test[2]) was performed in connection with the interview. Within 2 to 4 years after this visit the patients were interviewed again by telephone. Three were interviewed by telephone only.

III. PROGNOSIS

Of the 40 female sandwich-makers, 28 had given up their work. Among the 28 who ceased to handle food professionally, hand dermatitis cleared in 3, and among the 12 still working as sandwich-makers the dermatitis cleared in 1 (Table 1).

Hand dermatitis usually starts within the first 4 years of employment (Table 2). A subsequent change of work mostly follows after more than 5 years in the occupation, and an early cessation of work is associated with a better chance for the clearing or improvement of hand eczema.

The social prognosis appears to be more favorable for patients who attended school for 9 to 10 years compared to those who attended school for 7 to 8 years (Table 3). Years in the occupation and age at change of work did not influence the social prognosis except for the four who had a disablement pension. From Table 4, it appears that those who had changed to a skilled profession generally were satisfied in their new occupation, while the rest were not.

The results of the patch tests, scratch chamber tests, and prick tests among the 28 who had given up professional food handling and among the 12 who continued to work as sandwich-makers appears in Tables 5 and 6.

Among those with positive patch tests in the standard series, eight were allergic to nickel; all eight belonged to the group that had changed occupation. Positive patch-test reactions to onions were seen in ten, nine of them in the group of patients who had changed occupation. All patients

TABLE 1   Medical Prognosis in 40 Female Sandwich-Makers with Hand Eczema

	Hand eczema	
	Cleared	Not cleared
Change of occupation	2	17
Unemployed	0	5
Disablement pension	1	3
Continued work	1	11
Total	4	36

TABLE 2   Work History of 40 Female Sandwich-Makers with Hand Eczema

No. of sandwich-makers	Years in occupation before onset of eczema
24	0–2
10	2–4
6	>5

TABLE 3   Social Prognosis of 28 Female Sandwich-Makers after Change of Occupation in Relation to Years in School

Years in school	No. of patients			
	Skilled work	Unskilled work	Unemployed	Disablement pension
7	1	6	3	4
8	0	1	1	0
9	4	2	1	0
10	3	2	0	0

TABLE 4   Social Prognosis of 28 Female Sandwich-Makers after Change of Occupation

	Decline in income	Satisfied with social state of affairs	
		Yes	No
Skilled work	2/8	6	2
Unskilled work	8/11	5	6
Unemployed	4/5	0	5
Disablement pension	4/4	1	3
Total	18/28	12/28	16/28

TABLE 5   Results of Patch, Scratch Chamber, and Prick Tests on 40 Female Sandwich-Makers

	Change of occupation (n = 28)	No change of occupation (n = 12)
Only patch test positive	4	3
Scratch chamber and prick test positive	9	6
Patch, scratch chamber, and prick test positive	13	0
All tests negative	2	3

allergic to nickel and/or onions had eczema constantly or intermittently. There were 28 patients in the group of 40 who had positive scratch chamber and/or prick test reactions to food allergens — in 2 the eczema cleared after a change of occupation, while those who continued to handle food had eczema intermittently.

Among the 40 female sandwich-makers, 5 had a personal history of atopic disease (4/28 who had changed occupation and 1/12 who continued the work). In one of the atopics, the hand dermatitis cleared after a change of occupation.

IV.   DISCUSSION

Cronin[3] investigated 47 caterers with dermatitis of the hands. A diagnosis of atopy was found in 30/47. She succeeded in following 32/47 for about 2 years after the primary investigation. The

TABLE 6   Results of Patch, Scratch Chamber, and Prick Tests on 40 Female Sandwich-Makers

	Change of occupation (n = 28)	No change of occupation (n = 12)
Positive patch test		
Standard series	13[a]	1
Onions	9	1
Others[b]	2	1
Positive scratch chamber and prick test		
Food allergens	22	6
Others[c]	1	1

All tests negative
[a]Nickel: 8
[b]Curry: 1, cayenne pepper: 1, carrot: 1
[c]Pollen: 1, house dust: 1

hand dermatitis persisted in 15/19 who continued cooking and in 9/13 who changed their job. Among those who continued cooking, 12/19 were atopics and the hands returned to normal in 3 of those 12. Among those who had changed their job, 8/13 were atopics and the dermatitis healed in 3 of those 8. Cronin thus had a majority of atopics among the caterers investigated and followed.

Among the 40 patients presented in this chapter, only 5 had a personal history of atopic disease and a further 2 had a family history of atopic disease only. But, nevertheless, the medical prognosis was equally poor in atopic and nonatopic patients from England and Denmark, suggesting that once a hand dermatitis has developed in a caterer, the medical prognosis is independent of possible atopic disease.

It is, however, not possible from this study to conclude whether atopics have a greater risk than others for developing hand dermatitis if they work in the catering industry as sandwich-makers.

Evaluation of the data from the 40 patients in this survey especially points to two important factors regarding medical and social prognosis: the number of years of school attendance and the results of skin tests. The most important factor regarding the social prognosis was related to years in school. All eight patients with a positive patch test to nickel and nine of the ten with a positive patch test to onions had to give up catering because of hand eczema. Among the 28 who had changed their occupations, 22 had positive Type I reactions to food allergens, while 6/12 who continued to work had positive Type I reactions to food allergens.

REFERENCES

1. Hjorth, N. and Roed-Petersen, J., Occupational contact dermatitis in food handlers, *Contact Dermatitis*, 2, 28, 1976.
2. Niinimäki, A., Scratch-chamber tests in food handler dermatitis, *Contact Dermatitis*, 16, 11, 1987.
3. Cronin, E., Dermatitis of the hands in caterers, *Contact Dermatitis*, 17, 265, 1987.
4. Hannuksela, M. and Lahti, A., Immediate reactions to fruits and vegetables, *Contact Dermatitis*, 3, 79, 1977.

26

Hand Eczema in Farmers

Niels K. Veien

CONTENTS

I. INTRODUCTION

Persons employed in agriculture are exposed to a wide range of substances which are potentially harmful to the skin.

Recent years have seen the small, family farm give way to highly specialized industries in which exposure to agricultural chemicals has intensified. More than 4000 chemical compounds are registered for sale to farmers in Japan.[1] Burrows[2] has provided an extensive list of chemicals used as feed additives, and Adams,[3] in his book, reviews the substances most likely to cause contact dermatitis in farmers.

Few epidemiological studies have been made of the skin diseases affecting farmers. Difficult to carry out under the best of circumstances for such a diversified occupation, such studies are further complicated by variations in farming tradition, climate, and individually preferred crops in various parts of the world.

II. EPIDEMIOLOGY

Mathias and Morrison[4] reported data from the Annual Survey of Occupational Injuries and Illnesses in the U.S. from 1973 through 1988. The data were gathered from a representative sample of 280,000 employers throughout the country. Self-employed individuals were excluded, as were employees in industries employing fewer than 11 persons.

The overall incidence of occupational skin disease was shown to decrease from 16.2/10,000 full-time workers in 1973 to 6.2/10,00 full-time workers in 1983. In agriculture, the incidence of occupational skin disease decreased from 40.2/10,000 full-time workers in 1973 to 28.5/10,000 in 1984, and the total number of reported cases of occupational skin disease among agricultural workers decreased from 3200 in 1973 to 2200 in 1984. There was, however, an increase in the relative rate of occupational skin disease in agriculture, from a low of 2.4 in 1974 to 5.6 in 1983. During this same period, the relative rate of skin disease in manufacturing industries decreased from 4.1 to 3.0. Of 15 occupations listed, agricultural production had the highest incidence of occupational skin disease in the U.S. In 1984, followed by forestry. The occupation listed as ''agricultural services'' had the fifth highest incidence. Among 15 manufacturing industries, ''poultry and egg processing'' was in 12th place, with an incidence of 49.1/10,000 full-time workers.

The high frequency of occupational skin disease among agricultural workers seen in this study may have been the result of a large number of sensitizations to various members of the Toxicodendron family.

In his study of a group of 1282 patients treated at a clinic specializing in occupational dermatology, Fregert[5] ranked agriculture 9th among 17 occupations predominantly held by males which can cause occupational dermatoses.

Of the 424 patients with occupational dermatoses seen in an occupational disease clinic in Great Britain, 9 were employed in agriculture or horticulture.[6]

Wall and Gebauer[7] reexamined 954 Australian patients with occupational dermatoses, and found that 30 were crop-growing farmers, florists, or gardeners, while 18 handled animals or feedstuffs on a daily basis.

The prevalence of hand dermatoses among Finnish farmers was determined on the basis of questionnaires sent to 10,847 farmers — 4% of the men and 11% of the women who responded to the questionnaire had hand dermatoses. An additional 3% of the men and 5% of the women had suffered from hand dermatoses within the year prior to their response. Risk factors included an increasing workload, milking, and the handling of chemicals such as disinfectants and silage preservatives. Atopy was also a risk factor, and there was an especially high prevalence of atopy among young women.[8]

Poultry workers are frequently seen to have work-related hand dermatoses caused by the wetness of the work itself, allergic contact dermatitis to rubber accelerators in gloves, and microorganisms which invade intertriginous areas and paronychia.[9]

In a study of occupational dermatoses in a well-defined area of Denmark with 1.2 million employed persons, 1039 of these had occupational dermatoses severe enough to warrant referral to a dermatologist.[10] The prevalence of occupational dermatoses among this group was found to be 89/100,000 employed persons. There were 80,657 farmers in the region, and 58 of these (72/100,000) were diagnosed as having occupational dermatosis. The majority of the patients examined had hand eczema.

The above figures indicate that farmers in Denmark do not run the same risk of occupational skin disease as do farmers in North America.

III. PREDISPOSING FACTORS

Atopic dermatitis in childhood is the most important predictor of possible occupational hand eczema in whatever occupation is chosen later in life.[11] Other studies have shown a clear relationship between hand eczema and wet-work occupations.[12]

Cutaneous reactions to mechanical trauma from, for example, grain fibers are often more severe among atopic persons. In a study involving 1954 grain elevator operators and 689 control persons not employed in grain elevators, Hogan et al.[13] found that 67% of the operators who had had eczema in infancy developed pruritus upon exposure to grain dust, compared with 51% of those who had not had eczema in infancy. Only 1 of 689 controls complained of pruritus following grain dust exposure. A history of asthma or hay fever was not associated with an increased risk of pruritus following exposure to grain dust.

Sweat retention problems are also more common among atopics. *Miliaria rubra,* or ''prickly heat'', is more common in atopic persons who carry out demanding physical labor in a hot working environment. Sweat retention can also aggravate existing atopic dermatitis of the skin folds.

Psoriasis of the hands may flare if a patient is exposed to strenuous physical labor — a typical phenomenon in many agricultural jobs.

The etiology of hyperkeratotic palmar eczema remains unknown. It is known, however, that mechanical trauma aggravates this dermatitis and causes fissures and hyperkeratosis.[14]

IV. CONTACT DERMATITIS

Today, farming is so specialized that the risk of contact dermatitis of the hands very much depends on the type of farming done. In temperate climates, most farmers plant field crops, raise pigs or cattle (cows or sheep), or produce milk. A few farmers have even more specialized operations and raise deer or cultivate apple, pear, peach, or cherry orchards or raise other types of fruits or vegetables.

A. Irritants

Regardless of the type of farming done, a farmer is exposed to a wide range of irritants. Farm work often also includes the repair of buildings and machinery and, therefore, contact with oils and hydraulic fluids, cement, wood preservatives, and paint. Other possible irritants include plants and wet soil. In one study, 11 of 57 farmers with occupational dermatoses had irritant dermatitis.[15]

B. Dairy Farming

Dairy farmers usually do not wear gloves as they carry out their work, and many have wet hands for much of the working day. Their hands are in contact with disinfectants such as the hypochlorite solutions used to clean the udder, and other solutions used for cleaning milking equipment. These may include sodium hydroxide solutions used to saponify lipids in milk and a nitric acid solution used to neutralize alkalinity and remove protein and calcium residues. In a study of occupational dermatoses among farmers, carried out in the former DDR from 1981 to 1985, milkers were among the workers with the highest risk of developing occupational dermatoses, with an incidence of 6.4%.[15]

Milkers are also in contact with animal hair and the saliva of cows and calves, which may act as mechanical and chemical irritants, respectively. Amniotic fluid, as well as the bodily excretions of the animals, may also irritate the skin.

C. Animal Feed

The components of animal feed can also be skin irritants. In an epidemiological study of 204 employees in an animal feed manufacturing company, 28 (13.7%) had occupational contact dermatitis on the hands and 16 had irritant dermatitis.[16] Finely cut straw in animal feed may cause mechanical irritation. Dust from various grains, notably barley and oats, may also contain fibers which can cause irritation.[13]

Chemical irritation from ammonia used to treat straw used for animal feed is not uncommon, and numerous feed additives may also act as irritants.

D. Pesticides

Many pesticides contain irritants in either the active substances or in solvents such as kerosene. Most farmers in industrialized countries are aware of the dangers associated with the use of pesticides and wear protective clothing when handling these compounds. Cutaneous eruptions or itching following the use of pesticides, or the actual absorption of pesticides through the skin, are usually the result of the accidental, uncontrolled release of the compounds. Lisi et al.[17] patch-tested 652 persons with various pesticides and reported that 274 of these patients had contact dermatitis of the hands; 92 of them were employed in agriculture, and 11 were ex-agricultural workers. Of 350 persons tested, 45 had irritant patch test reactions to 1% fentin hydroxide, while 5 of 109 reacted to a 0.5% solution of fentin hydroxide, and none of 109 reacted to a 0.25% solution. Captan 1% in petrolatum produced irritant reactions in 13 of 442 persons; 6 of 389 reacted to a 0.5% solution, and none of 279 reacted to a 0.25% or to a 0.1% solution. Only a few irritant reactions were found when the same patients were patch-tested with several other pesticides. Although it is difficult to convert patch-test data involving irritant patch-test reactions to clinical situations, this study indicates that the irritant potential of pesticides is limited to a few active components. Reactions to ready-to-use products can be caused by solvents and additives.

E. Plants

At least 14 of 42 workers pulling weeds in a California sugar-beet field developed bullous contact dermatitis on exposed areas of the hands, arms, thighs, and abdomen. Pesticide dermatitis was suspected, but it was determined that the most likely cause of the eczema was Mayweed *(Anthemis cotula)*.[18]

In another study, employees in plant nurseries were seen to have a 23% prevalence of eczema. Most of the workers in this study had hand eczema.[19]

Of 111 Japanese okra *(Hibiscus esculentus* L.) farmers, 18 developed irritant dermatitis, largely on the fingertips, hands, and arms. It was felt that the irritation could have been mechanical, caused by the plant's prickly surface.[20] Mechanical dermatitis commonly occurs following contact with plants with thorns and spikes. Castelain and Ducombs[21] reported two patients with contact dermatitis on the hands caused by madder. The mechanical dermatitis of one of these patients was caused by the thorns of *Rubria peregrina* L., and the other patient had a mechanical reaction to the roots of *Rubria tinctorum* L., which contains a substance previously used to dye French military uniforms. Mechanical and chemical irritant reactions are also common following contact with various plants of the *Dieffenbachia* species, which contain calcium oxalate crystals that can penetrate the skin.[22] A chemical irritant reaction to tobacco may cause hand eczema in individuals who handle tobacco leaves.[23]

Persons employed in agriculture commonly suffer phototoxic reactions caused by the furocoumarins in the juice of plants of the *Umbilliferae* species. One large variety of this species, giant hogweed, is rapidly spreading throughout northern Europe. The use of rotary string bush cutters (strimmers) can spread the juice of this and other plants to exposed areas of the skin.[24] When raised in large amounts for human consumption, plants such as celery, parsley, and parsnip may cause phytophotodermatoses. The juice of citrus fruits can also cause phototoxic contact dermatitis.

V. ALLERGIC CONTACT DERMATITIS

Most cases of allergic contact dermatitis can be detected with the aid of a standard patch test series. When treating patients employed in certain occupations, however, it may be necessary to test with additional, job-specific substances. This is illustrated by the patch test results among 57 farmers with occupational dermatoses, most of whom raised pigs. In this study, 14 of the farmers had allergic contact dermatitis. The most common allergen for these patients was spiramycin (five positive reactions), while four patients reacted to the thiuram mixture, four to black-rubber mix, and two to animal feed.[10]

In another study, a group of 34 agricultural workers had a significantly greater number of positive patch tests to paraphenylene diamine, balsam of Peru, neomycin, carba mix, mercury, and cobalt, compared to a control group.[25]

A woman with hand eczema who worked with fertilizer containing between 22 and 45 ppm. of nickel reacted to both nickel and cobalt.[26]

A. Animal Feed and Feed Additives

Reactions to the grains which are often the basic ingredients of animal feeds are rarely reported. Cronin described one patient with delayed-type hypersensitivity to barley.[27]

A number of chemical compounds such as vitamins, minerals, and antioxidants are added to animal feedstuffs. Antibiotics may also be mixed with feed, both to prevent disease and to promote growth.[2]

Animal feed mill workers are exposed to higher concentrations of potentially sensitizing substances in feedstuffs than farmers, and most cases of allergic contact dermatitis to animal feed reported to date have involved mill workers. Mancuso et al.[16] reported allergic contact dermatitis among 12 of 204 animal feed mill workers patch-tested with 34 allergens commonly used as feed additives. All 12 had hand eczema.

Ethoxyquin, an antioxidant commonly used in pig feed, and previously also used to prevent apple scab, has been shown to sensitize in a few instances.[28-30]

Allergic contact dermatitis to vitamin K added to pig feed was seen in a man who presented with hand dermatitis which later spread to other exposed areas of his body.[31] Furazoline, used as a pig feed additive, caused fingertip dermatitis in a pig farmer who had a positive patch test to 2% furazoline in polyethylene glycol. This substances is also used to promote growth in poultry.[32]

A piglet dealer who used azaperone to sedate his animals prior to transport developed hand eczema and dermatitis on other exposed areas of the body. He had a positive patch test to 0.4% azaperone in water. A patch test site exposed to UV-A showed a stronger reaction than a nonexposed site.[33]

The photodistribution of dermatitis in pig farmers may be due to olaquindox in the feed they use.[34,35] This substance is chemically related to quindoxin, which was withdrawn from the market almost 20 years ago after it was shown to induce photosensitization.

An airborne pattern of contact dermatitis involving the hands, arms, neck, and face of a cattle breeder was caused by multiple sensitizations to antibiotics mixed with feed for calves. He had positive patch tests to oxytetracycline, tylosin, penicillin, and spiramycin.[36]

B. Medicaments Used to Treat Animals

Some feedstuffs contain antibiotics used as growth promoters. In certain circumstances, the same antibiotics are used by the farmers to treat sick animals or to prevent disease. One woman developed hand dermatitis and later an airborne pattern of dermatitis following the use of tylosin to inject chicks.[37] A similar procedure produced hand eczema in two women who used lincomycin and spectinomycin to vaccinate chickens.[38]

The contact dermatitis of 15 farmers primarily engaged in raising pigs was caused by antibiotics.[39] Eight of these farmers had positive patch tests to 5% spiramycin as well as to 5% tylosin in petrolatum. Four reacted only to spiramycin, two reacted only to tylosin, two reacted to benethamate, and one reacted to a sulfonamide. Most of the 15 patients had chronic hand eczema, and several also had an airborne pattern of dermatitis. The addition of tylosin to feed as a growth promoter is permitted in Denmark. Although one would expect to see an increasing number of sensitizations to tylosin because of its use in feed, no such increase has as yet been seen. This may be because the concentration of the substance in feedstuffs is lower than the sensitization threshold.

C. Pesticides

A wide range of chemical compounds are used as fungicides, herbicides, insecticides, rodenticides, and soil fumigants. In spite of their widespread use, sensitization to pesticides is rarely reported. A study of 62 workers in a mushroom production facility where the carbamate, benomyl, was used regularly over a period of 10 years, showed no instance of sensitization.[40] Lisi et al.[17] carried out extensive testing of 36 pesticides in 652 persons, 103 of whom were agricultural workers or had previously been employed in agriculture; 125 persons (38 of them agricultural workers) were considered to have allergic contact dermatitis. Allergic contact dermatitis to pesticides was seen in 27 persons, 14 of whom were agricultural workers. Fungicides, in particular thiophthalimide, captan, and captafol, and the dithiocarbamates, maneb, zineb, and ziram, were the most common allergens. Of the insecticides, parathion produced a positive patch test in one person, as did the fumigant, dazonet. Based on their experience, the authors suggested the use of a pesticide patch test tray.[17]

Thirty Indian farmers who suspected pesticides to be the cause of their dermatitis were patch tested with a series of pesticides. While most of these patients had dermatitis on exposed parts of the body, only seven had dermatitis of the hands and feet. Eleven of the farmers reacted to at least one pesticide, most frequently to one of the dithiocarbamates, to which there were seven positive reactions. Four patients reacted to organophosphorus compounds.[41]

Six of seven workers on a strawberry farm who had contact dermatitis, and were available for patch testing, had positive patch tests to the fungicide anilazine (2,4-dichloro-6-(*o*-chloroanilino)-s-trizine). Most of these workers had hand eczema as well as eczema at other sites.[42] There have been several reports from Italy of allergic contact dermatitis caused by dithiocarbamate fungicides.[43-45]

It is important to bear in mind that many pesticides are able to penetrate the skin and cause systemic toxicity with no recognizable skin lesions. This emphasizes the significance of the skin as an organ of absorption as well as the importance of wearing gloves and other protective clothing when working with pesticides and other chemical compounds which readily penetrate the skin. The problems associated with systemic toxicity following percutaneous absorption of industrial chemicals has recently been reviewed in detail.[3]

D. Plants

Allergic contact dermatitis in farmers caused by plants is likely to involve the hands as well as other exposed areas of the body. Although most allergic contact dermatitis to plants is caused by weeds, in today's specialized farming, the produce itself may sensitize.

The urushiols in some *Toxicodendron* species are strong sensitizers, and poison oak dermatitis is a common cause of occupational disability due to skin disease among agricultural workers in California. While poison oak is prevalent in the western U.S., poison ivy is a more widespread *Toxicodendron* in the midwestern U.S. Contact dermatitis from these weeds has been only sporadically reported outside the U.S., but several other plants containing chemically related substances may cross-react with urushiols. Such cross-reactors include the shells of cashew nuts, the Indian marking nut tree, the Japanese lacquer tree, the fruit of the ginkgo tree, and the rind of the mango fruit.[3]

The family of plants known as Composita includes common weeds regularly encountered by most crop-growing farmers. A number of these weeds contain strong sensitizers — sesquiterpene lactones — also found in liverworts (Frullania), a common sensitizer of wood cutters in humid climates.[46] One farmer who presented with hand dermatitis which had spread to his face and genitalia reacted to a number of Compositae plants as well as to lichens.[47]

One Composita, *parthenium hysterophorus,* or wild feverfew, was introduced into India in the late 1950s. The plant found very favorable conditions for growth there, and is today a very common weed in some parts of the country.[48] Many Indian farmers have developed incapacitating contact dermatitis on exposed areas of the body. Wild feverfew is also seen in Australia.[49] Ragweed (Ambrosia) is a frequent cause of contact dermatitis in the midwestern U.S. Compositae dermatitis is most commonly seen on the face and neck, but most of those affected also have dorsal hand eczema and eczema of the forearms.[44]

Farmers who specialize in the growing of certain plants may develop hand eczema from contact with their produce. A Japanese woman developed hand eczema from contact with a vegetable, *Cryptotaemia Japonica,* cultivated in the family business.[51] Fisher reviewed the cutaneous problems associated with edible plants.[52] He pointed out the potential of contact urticaria to plants or plant components to evolve into hand eczema following repeated exposures. Protein contact dermatitis, a term coined by Hjorth and Roed-Petersen,[53] is most common among persons employed in the catering industry. Farmers are exposed to the same food items as cooks, and vegetable farmers may also develop hand eczema from exposure to the same plants as cooks.[54-57] The risk associated with contact with plants has been emphasized in studies of plant-related occupations such as work with ornamental flowers: 56 of 675 persons who grew and sold ornamental flowers were tested with the flowers, and half were shown to have allergic contact dermatitis to one or more plants. The most common allergens were chrysanthemums, tulips, and Alstromeria. Of the 56 persons with allergic contact dermatitis, 51 had hand eczema.[58]

E.   Dairy Farming

Dairy farming is associated with a risk of contact sensitization to the rubber used in milking equipment or in gloves.[15] In one study, 28 of 51 milkers with allergic contact dermatitis to rubber products had positive patch tests to isopropylaminodiphenylamine (IPPD).[59] Among 57 farmers with occupational dermatoses, Veien et al.[10] found 11 farmers with allergic contact dermatitis. Four had positive patch tests to the thiuram mixture and four to the black-rubber mix. Allergic contact dermatitis to rubber gloves may be detected by battery testing, but a surprising number of cases of rubber allergy can be detected only by testing with the gloves themselves.[60]

One farmer with hand eczema who milked regularly had a weakly positive patch test to the black-rubber mix, an elevated total serum IgE, and a positive RAST (class 3) to whole milk.[61] Three men who worked as ewe milkers developed hand eczema. All these patients had positive patch tests to the ewe's wool, and two of them also had weakly positive patch tests to wool alcohols.[62,63]

Determination of the percentage of butterfat in cows' milk has traditionally been carried out in laboratories following the collection of samples of the milk. A classic example of sensitization to dichromates, previously used to preserve the milk until the time of analysis, was seen among the laboratory technicians who carried out this work.[64] Of 16 women employed as milk testers, 8 had a history of hand dermatitis, and 3 had dermatitis at the time of the study. Two of those with current dermatitis were allergic to potassium dichromate. Grattan et al.[65] reported allergic contact dermatitis of the hands to the modern milk preservatives, Bronopol® (2-bromo-L-nitropropane-1,3 diol) and Kathon CG (5-chloro-2-methyl-4-isothiazolin-3-one and 2-methyl-4-isothiazon-3-one), in three milk testers in the U.K.

VI.   NAIL LESIONS IN FARMERS

The wet work associated with dairy farming, in particular, may cause chronic paronychia with infection and inflammation of the nail folds. Periungual telangiectases were seen in 19 of 34 coffee plantation workers,[66] and wet work in irrigation canals in India caused koilonychia in 25 of 226 persons.[67]

REFERENCES

1. Matsushita, T., Nomura, S., and Wakatsuki, T., Epidemiology of contact dermatitis from pesticides in Japan, *Contact Dermatitis,* 6, 255, 1980.
2. Burrows, D., Contact dermatitis in animal feed mill workers, *Br. J. Dermatol.,* 92, 167, 1975.
3. Adams, R. M., *Occupational Skin Disease,* 2nd ed., W. B. Saunders, Philadelphia, 1990.
4. Mathias, C. G. T. and Morrison, J. H., Occupational skin diseases, United States, *Arch. Dermatol.,* 124, 1519, 1988.
5. Fregert, S., Occupational dermatitis in a 10-year material, *Contact Dermatitis,* 1, 96, 1975.
6. Wilkinson, D. S., Budden, M. G., and Hambly, E. M., A 10-year review of an industrial dermatitis clinic, *Contact Dermatitis,* 6, 11, 1980.
7. Wall, L. M. and Gebauer, K. A., Occupational skin disease in Western Australia, *Contact Dermatitis,* 24, 101, 1991.
8. Sustaival, P., Husman, K., Vohlonen, I., Husman, L., and Horsmanheimo, M., The prevalence of hand dermatoses among Finnish farmers: a questionnaire study, *Contact Dermatitis,* 23, 303, 1990.
9. Marks, J. G., Jr., Rainey, C. M., Rainey, M. A., and Andreozzi, F. J., Dermatoses among poultry workers: "chicken poison disease", *J. Am. Acad. Dermatol.,* 9, 852, 1983.
10. Veien, N. K., Heydenreich, G., Kaaber, K., and Willumsen, P., Hudsygdomme. Arbejdsbetingede Hudsygdomme Diagnosticeret af Hudlæger i Jylland, Industrial Environment Fund, Copenhagen, Denmark, 1986.
11. Rystedt, I., Hand Eczema and Long-term Prognosis in Atopic Dermatitis, Ph.D. Thesis, Karolinska Institute, Stockholm, 1985.
12. Nilsson, E., Individual and Environmental Risk Factors for Hand Eczema in Hospital Workers, Ph.D. thesis, *Acta Derm. Venereol. Stockholm,* Suppl. 128, 1986.
13. Hogan, D. J., Dosman, J. A., Li, K. Y. R., Graham, B., Johnson, D., Walker, R., and Lane, P. R., Questionnaire survey of pruritus and rash in grain elevator workers, *Contact Dermatitis,* 14, 170, 1986.
14. Hersle, K. and Mobacken, H., Hyperkeratotic dermatitis of the palms, *Br. J. Dermatol.,* 107, 195, 1982.
15. Laubstein, H., Monnick, H. T., and Hofmann, S., Epidemiology of occupational dermatoses in the Potsdam district, *Dermatol. Monatsschr.,* 175, 425, 1989.
16. Mancuso, G., Staffa, M., Errani, A., Berdondini, R. M., and Fabbri, P., Occupational dermatitis in animal feed mill workers, *Contact Dermatitis,* 22, 37, 1990.
17. Lisi, P., Caraffini, S., and Assalve, D., Irritation and sensitization potential of pesticides, *Contact Dermatitis,* 17, 212, 1987.
18. O'Malley, M. A. and Barba, R., Bullous dermatitis in field workers associated with exposure to Mayweed, *Am. J. Contact Dermatitis,* 1, 34, 1990.
19. Lander, F., Jeune, B., and Skytthe, A., Prævalensen af allergiske og irritative symptomer blandt gartneriarbejdere, *Ugeskr. Laeger,* 149, 44, 1986.
20. Matsushita, T., Aoyama, K., Manda, F., Ueda, A., Yoshida, M., and Okamura, J., Occupational dermatoses in farmers growing okra (*Hibiscus esculentus* L.), *Contact Dermatitis,* 21, 321, 1989.
21. Castelain, M. and Ducombs, G., Contact dermatitis from madder, *Contact Dermatitis,* 19, 228, 1988.
22. Ippen, H., Wereta-Kubek, M., and Rose, U., Haut- und Schleimhautreaktionen durch Zimmerpflanzen der Gattung Dieffenbachia, *Dermatosen,* 34, 93, 1986.
23. Rycroft, R. J. G., Tobacco dermatitis, *Br. J. Dermatol.,* 103, 225, 1980.
24. Freeman, K., Hubbard, H. C., and Warin, A. P., Strimmer rash, *Contact Dermatitis,* 10, 117, 1984.
25. Garcia-Perez, A., Garcia-Bravo, B., and Beneit, J. V., Standard patch tests in agricultural workers, *Contact Dermatitis,* 10, 151, 1984.
26. Pecegueiro, M., Contact dermatitis due to nickel in fertilizers, *Contact Dermatitis,* 22, 114, 1990.

27. Cronin, E., *Contact Dermatitis,* Churchill Livingstone, Edinburgh, 1980.
28. Zachariae, H., Ethoxyquin dermatitis, *Contact Dermatitis,* 4, 117, 1978.
29. Van Hecke, E., Contact dermatitis to ethoxyquin in animal feeds, *Contact Dermatitis,* 3, 341, 1977.
30. Savini, C., Morelli, R., Piancastelli, E., and Restani, S., Contact dermatitis due to ethoxyquin, *Contact Dermatitis,* 21, 342, 1989.
31. Dinis, A., Brandao, M., and Faria, A., Occupational contact dermatitis from vitamin K3 sodium bisulphite, *Contact Dermatitis,* 18, 170, 1988.
32. De Groot, A. C. and Conemans, J. M. H., Contact allergy to furazolidone, *Contact Dermatitis,* 22, 202, 1990.
33. Brasch, J., Hessler, H.-J., and Christophers, E., Occupational (photo)allergic contact dermatitis from azaperone in a piglet dealer, *Contact Dermatitis,* 25, 258, 1991.
34. Dunkel, F. G., Elsner, P., Pevny, I., and Burg, G., Olaquindox-induced photoallergic contact dermatitis and persistent light reaction in a pig breeder, *Contact Dermatitis,* 23, 301, 1990.
35. Schauder, S., Gefahren durch Olaquindox, *Dermatosen,* 37, 183, 1989.
36. Guerra, L., Venturo, N., Tardio, M., and Tosti, A., Airborne contact dermatitis from animal feed antibiotics, *Contact Dermatitis,* 25, 333, 1991.
37. Barbera, E. and De La Cuadra, J., Occupational airborne allergic contact dermatitis from tylosin, *Contact Dermatitis,* 20, 308, 1989.
38. Vilaplana, J., Romaguera, C., and Grimalt, F., Contact dermatitis from lincomycin and spectinomycin in chicken vaccinators, *Contact Dermatitis,* 24, 225, 1991.
39. Veien, N. K., Hattel, T., Justesen, O., and Nørholm, A., Patch testing with substances not included in the standard series, *Contact Dermatitis,* 9, 304, 1983.
40. Larsen, A. I., Larsen, A., Jepsen, J. R., and Jørgensen, R., Contact allergy to the fungicide benomyl?, *Contact Dermatitis,* 22, 278, 1990.
41. Sharma, V. K. and Kaur, S., Contact sensitization by pesticides in farmers, *Contact Dermatitis,* 23, 77, 1990.
42. Schuman, S. H. and Dobson, R. L., An outbreak of contact dermatitis in farm workers, *J. Am. Acad. Dermatol.,* 13, 220, 1985.
43. Manuzzi, P., Borrello, P., Misciali, C., and Guerra, L., Contact dermatitis due to Ziram and Maneb, *Contact Dermatitis,* 19, 148, 1988.
44. Piraccini, B. M., Cameli, N., Peluso, A. M., and Tardio, M., A case of allergic contact dermatitis due to the pesticide maneb, *Contact Dermatitis,* 24, 381, 1991.
45. Peluso, A. M., Tardio, M., Adamo, F., and Venturo, N., Multiple sensitization due to bis-dithiocarbamate and thiophthalimide pesticides, *Contact Dermatitis,* 25, 327, 1991.
46. Mitchell, J. and Rook, A., *Botanical Dermatology,* Greengrass, Vancouver, 1979.
47. De Corrés, L. F., Leanizbarrutia, I., Muñoz, D., Bernaola, G., Fernández, E., and Audícana, M. T., Multiple sensitizations to plants in a farmer, *Contact Dermatitis,* 17, 315, 1987.
48. Lonkar, A., Nagasampagi, B. A., Narayanan, C. R., Landge, A. B., and Sawaikar, D. D., An antigen from *Parthenium hysterophorus* Linn., *Contact Dermatitis,* 2, 151, 1976.
49. Burry, J. N. and Kloot, P. M., The spread of composite (compositae) weeds in Australia, *Contact Dermatitis,* 8, 410, 1982.
50. Paulsen, E., Compositae dermatitis: a survey, *Contact Dermatitis,* 26, 76, 1992.
51. Kanzaki, T., Contact dermatitis due to *Cryptotaemia japonica* Makino, *Contact Dermatitis,* 20, 60, 1989.
52. Fisher, A. A., Allergic eczematous contact dermatitis due to foods, *Cutis,* 16, 603, 1975.
53. Hjorth, N. and Roed-Petersen, J., Occupational protein contact dermatitis in food handlers, *Contact Dermatitis,* 2, 28, 1976.
54. Tosti, A. and Guerra, L., Protein contact dermatitis in food handlers, *Contact Dermatitis,* 19, 149, 1988.
55. Odom, T. B. and Maibach, H. I., Contact urticaria: a different contact dermatitis, *Cutis,* 18, 672, 1976.

56. Valdivieso, R., Moneo, I., Pola, J., Muñoz, T., Zapata, C., Hinojosa, M., and Losada, E., Occupational asthma and contact urticaria caused by buckwheat flour, *Ann. Allergy*, 63, 149, 1989.

57. Veien, N. K., Hattel, T., Justesen, O., and Nørholm, A., Causes of eczema in the food industry, *Derm. Beruf Umwelt*, 31, 84, 1983.

58. Hausen, B. M. and Oestmann, G., Untersuchungen über die Häufigkeit berufsbedingter allergischer Hauterkrankungen auf einem Blumengrossmarkt, *Dermatosen*, 36, 117, 1988.

59. Jung, H.-D. and Wolff, F., Das Melkerekszem im Industrie-Agrarbezirk Neubrandenburg, *Dermatol. Monatsschr.*, 166, 523, 1980.

60. Veien, N. K., Hattel, T., and Laurberg, G., Patch testing with non-standard substances, *Derm. Beruf Umwelt*, 40, 217, 1992.

61. Crippa, M., Misquith, L., and Pasolini, G., Contact dermatitis from animal proteins in a milker, *Contact Dermatitis*, 22, 240, 1990.

62. Quirce, S., Olaguibel, J. M., Muro, M. D., and Tabar, A. I., Occupational dermatitis in a ewe milker, *Contact Dermatitis*, 27, 56, 1992.

63. Zemtsov, A., A case of contact allergy to Kathon® CG in the United States, *Contact Dermatitis*, 25, 135, 1991.

64. Herzog, J., Dunne, J., Aber, R., Claver, M., and Marks, J. G., Jr., Milk tester's dermatitis, *J. Am. Acad. Dermatol.*, 19, 503, 1988.

65. Grattan, C. E. H., Harman, R. R. M., and Tan, R. S. H., Milk recorder dermatitis, *Contact Dermatitis*, 14, 217, 1986.

66. Narahari, S. R., Srinivas, C. R., and Kelkar, S. K., LE-like erythema and periungual telangiectasia among coffee plantation workers, *Contact Dermatitis*, 22, 296, 1990.

67. Dolma, T., Norboo, T., Yayha, M., Hobson, R., and Ball, K., Seasonal koilonychia in Ladakh, *Contact Dermatitis*, 22, 78, 1990.

27

The Prognosis of Hand Eczema

Daniel J. Hogan

CONTENTS

0-8493-7355-7/94/$0.00 + $.50

I. INTRODUCTION

It is unusual for dermatologic texts to specifically address prognosis even though this is a very important topic and is usually one of the chief concerns of the patient, the employer, and of the workers' compensation authority.[1] Despite the introduction of corticosteroids, immunosuppressives, and ultraviolet light treatment, (including PUVA), and improvement in the science of patch testing, the prognosis for those with hand eczema, especially disabling hand eczema, remains poor in terms of a complete and permanent recovery.

A small proportion of workers with occupational contact dermatitis develop disabling dermatitis.[2] The number of workdays lost because of occupational dermatitis has declined in England and in the U.S.[3] Occupational dermatitis is now the second leading occupational disease in the U.S., rather than the main occupational disease that it had been for many years. This appears to reflect improvements in working conditions, rather than a change in the natural history of contact dermatitis once clinical dermatitis has occurred. Workers disabled by contact dermatitis do benefit more from intense investigation and rehabilitation than patients disabled by other chronic skin diseases, such as severe congenital ichthyosis or refractory psoriasis.[4] Workers with contact hand dermatitis are usually younger than workers with other occupational diseases. This facilitates reeducation and retraining of the affected worker, but makes early retirement of a worker because of occupational dermatitis impractical.

Most studies of the prognosis of hand eczema are retrospective and are based on workers' compensation records or on patients referred to specialized clinics because of severe dermatitis.[1] Occupational and nonoccupational hand eczema have a similar prognosis.[5] Hand eczema, particularly occupational contact dermatitis of the hands, affects younger workers more than those affected by other occupational illnesses.[3]

Studies on the prognosis of hand dermatitis tend to select individuals with persistent or severe dermatitis. In a large survey of the Swedish population, Agrup noted that individuals with hand dermatitis who attended a follow-up examination were more likely than those declining a follow-up examination to complain of nonhealing dermatitis.[6] Persistent and more severe cases also show up in studies of workers' compensation cases. Conversely, individuals with mild hand dermatitis generally do not consult physicians for this problem. In some occupations, such as nursing, large numbers of workers accept varying degrees of irritant contact dermatitis as the price they pay for their chosen profession.[7-9]

Most hand dermatitis does not originate from the workplace. Agrup found that only 22% of the hand dermatitis cases she examined in an industrial area of Sweden were occupational in origin.[6] One-third of her hand eczema cases were housewife's eczema.

Most studies have not found that a job change improves the prognosis of workers with chronic hand dermatitis. One exception may be workers with soluble oil dermatitis from cutting fluids. Workers who may require a job change include those with a severe allergy to a workplace allergen where indirect and direct contact with the allergen cannot be curtailed. Workers with atopic hand dermatitis exacerbated by cutaneous irritants will do better if they can switch to work where there is no exposure to cutaneous irritants such as water, soaps, and solvents.

Most workers do best if they continue to work for their current employer, recognizing that they may miss brief periods of work for severe flares of their dermatitis. It is preferable for a worker to continue to work at a worksite where he/she knows the irritants and allergens that exacerbate his/her dermatitis and can follow measures to avoid contact with them.

Many workers are able to continue to work despite hand dermatitis. Many workers recognize the need to continue working at their present occupation despite their hand dermatitis. For example, very few surgeons, at least in North America, will switch careers if they develop hand dermatitis. Similarly, a skilled trades person who is allergic to chromate can usually continue to work with mortar and cement despite allergic contact dermatitis to chromate.[10]

II. TIME OFF WORK

Some workers with mild hand dermatitis of occupational origin may not require time off work. Other workers may require up to 3 weeks off work to allow their dermatitis to respond to treatment and to heal. Workers with moderate hand dermatitis often require up to 1 month of time off work. Workers with severe hand dermatitis usually require 2 to 10 weeks of time off work and some never fully recover. Experts in European countries, particularly Scandinavian countries, recommend a longer period of time off work for occupational hand dermatitis than is customary in North America.[11] This may reflect differences in workers' compensation and social welfare laws. It is clear, both in clinical experience and basic immunologic investigations, that both irritant and allergic contact dermatitis may precipitate a self-perpetuating cycle of dermatitis.

This book clearly documents the importance of hand eczema. In addition to the morbidity caused by hand eczema, it is a major occupational disease and patients, particularly older workers, may suffer significant financial losses from their hand eczema[12] if they are forced to stop working because of hand dermatitis. The high cost of hand eczema is further increased by the loss of productive workers, the cost of workers' compensation, and the cost of treatment and rehabilitation of these workers. This article will focus on the crucial topic of prognosis so that we can advise our patients about the prognosis of hand eczema, using the most complete data currently available.

III. ALLERGIC CONTACT DERMATITIS

Nickel and chromate contact allergies have been associated with a poor prognosis for complete healing of dermatitis, particularly in Europe.[13]

Healthcare workers who develop occupational allergic contact hand dermatitis to glutaraldehyde have a poor prognosis for healing of hand dermatitis, even with a change of occupation or careful avoidance of glutaraldehyde.

Allergic contact dermatitis to rubber chemicals may have a good prognosis if accurately diagnosed and appropriate substitutions made by the patient.[14] However, it is known that individuals may begin wearing rubber gloves because of the development of hand dermatitis, and allergy to rubber gloves may be only one component of multifactorial hand eczema.

IV. IRRITANT CONTACT DERMATITIS

Irritant contact dermatitis is the most common form of hand eczema. In the general population, this is typically a multifactorial process with interaction between workplace cutaneous irritants, household irritants, and a propensity to hand dermatitis, particularly among those with underlying atopic dermatitis.[9] Not surprisingly, occupational irritant contact dermatitis has been found to have a worse prognosis than occupational allergic contact dermatitis in some studies.[15,16] A major limitation is our lack of diagnostic tests for irritant dermatitis and the need to rely on clinical examination, careful history, and exclusion of allergic contact dermatitis by patch testing.

V. PROGNOSTIC FACTORS

As one would suspect, the likelihood for clearing of hand eczema diminishes with the duration of the eczema.[5] Accurate diagnosis and therapeutic intervention in the late stages of hand eczema may be unable to alter an eczematous process which appears to enter a self-perpetuating stage in some individuals.

A. Dermatitis Artefacta

Occupational dermatitis artefacta has been reported rarely.[17] It has been suggested that some workers, particularly lowly paid, unskilled workers with young children at home, may be better off economically if they can receive workers' compensation for hand eczema rather than continuing to work despite hand eczema.[18] However, in general, workers suffer financial loss if they are disabled by hand eczema and this is a positive motivating factor for workers to follow medical advice and treatment and to make workplace modifications to allow them to be employed. Older workers, in particular, suffer severe financial losses if they terminate their normal work because of occupational hand eczema.[12]

B. Morphology

Vesicular hand dermatitis is associated with a worse prognosis than milder forms of hand dermatitis.[19] It is important to remember that even the most expert dermatologist can not reliably distinguish irritant from allergic from endogenous dermatitis of the hands.[20]

C. Inappropriate Treatment

Inappropriate treatment is an important remedial cause of hand eczema. The use of topical medications containing well-known sensitizers such as benzocaine, or neomycin, as self-medications or supplied by the workplace, or recommended by a physician, may provoke allergic contact dermatitis and contribute to the persistence of hand eczema. Rubber gloves are frequently used by those with hand dermatitis, but these individuals may develop allergic contact dermatitis to chemicals added to rubber gloves or contact urticaria to rubber. Individuals with a history of atopy and healthcare workers with hand dermatitis are at an elevated risk to develop contact urticaria to rubber.[21]

D. Atopic Dermatitis

As discussed in other chapters of this book, patients with a history of atopic dermatitis, particularly atopic dermatitis of the hands, tolerate cutaneous irritants poorly and are more susceptible to irritant contact dermatitis. Those with a history of atopic hand dermatitis who develop irritant hand dermatitis have a poorer prognosis for healing of hand dermatitis than nonatopic workers.[7-9]

Domestic exposures to cutaneous irritants is an important additional aggravating factor for women with hand eczema who often work in occupations, such as hairdressing and nursing, which put workers at an elevated risk to develop irritant contact dermatitis. Those with atopic hand dermatitis frequently have persistent dermatitis even if they change jobs.[22]

E. Allergen Avoidance

The accurate diagnosis of allergic contact dermatitis of the hand requires detailed and complete patch testing, as discussed elsewhere in this book. Hand dermatitis may be mixed in etiology with varying components of allergic contact dermatitis, irritant contact dermatitis, and endogenous hand eczema.

Contact allergies are not static. Contact allergies may diminish with time, but new contact allergies to old and new contactants may develop. The more knowledgeable a patient is of sources of exposure to relevant contact allergen(s) the better the prognosis.[23,24] Consideration of possible cross-reactions to contact allergens is important. Individuals allergic to neomycin are likely to develop allergic contact dermatitis if they are treated with gentamicin or tobramycin. Unfortunately, the same allergen may be known by various names. For example, Quaternium 15 is also known as Dowicil 200, and a worker could be exposed to Quaternium 15 in a moisturizer at home and, under a different name, in a cutting fluid at work.

F. Improper Hand Washing

It has been suggested that a dirty workplace induces workers to practice poor hygiene and increases their risk of occupational contact dermatitis.[25] An apparently more frequent problem is inappropriate cleansing of the skin with harsh cleansers and solvents at work.[26] No inspection of a worksite is complete until the worksite washing facilities are examined. Irritant hand cleansers may be the primary cause of occupational contact dermatitis or an important contributory factor for occupational contact dermatitis previously initiated by an allergen or occupational irritant. Occasionally, irritant contact dermatitis of the hands occurs in those who obsessively wash their hands frequently.[27]

Certain workers, such as farm workers, may work in areas distant from adequate washing facilities and may not be able to remove occupational irritants and allergens, particularly pesticides and plant products, rapidly from their skin following exposure to these materials. Appropriate legislation may help protect these often-disadvantaged workers.

G. Barrier Creams

Some studies indicate that barrier creams are not helpful and may even increase the severity of irritant contact dermatitis.[28] Some barrier creams are irritant when patch-tested as is under Finn chambers.[29] The irritant effect of such barrier creams is exacerbated on dermatitic skin. Barrier creams also contain potential allergens, particularly preservatives and fragrances.[29]

H. Rubber Gloves

Occupational allergens such as nickel and methyl methacrylate may penetrate intact rubber glove. Methyl methacrylate, in particular, can penetrate several pairs of rubber gloves and product paresthesias and allergic contact dermatitis of the hands in exposed surgeons.

I. Misdiagnosis

It is important to consider tinea manuum in those presenting with hand eczema, particularly if the eruption is unilateral and is predominantly erythematous and scaly. Given the high quality of dermatologic care in western countries, it is infrequent for tinea to be missed by a dermatologist and to be diagnosed only in a referral clinic. Psoriasis of the hands may be very difficult to distinguish from hand eczema, but the therapy of both disorders is generally similar, i.e., topical corticosteroids or PUVA, and there are cases of hand dermatitis where the morphology clearly varies between psoriasiform and vesicular. The author has seen porphyria cutanea tarda misdiagnosed as hand eczema and other dermatologists have had the same experience.[35]

J. Photoeruptions

Polymorphous light eruption may present as a hand dermatitis, but this condition usually involves other sun-exposed areas and is most severe in early spring and summer. Photoallergic and photoirritant contact dermatitis are uncommon causes of eruptions on the hands and would not be identified via standard patch testing.

K. Alcoholism

Alcoholism is frequent in Western countries, but very rarely mentioned as an adverse factor on the prognosis for recovery from dermatitis or psoriasis. A busy dermatologist will see several patients a day who suffer from alcoholism and it is important to consider this condition in patients whose dermatitis does not respond to treatment, who do not follow treatment or instructions, and who do not keep appointments. It is frequently difficult for physicians to arrange appropriate referral for treatment for a patient with alcoholism.

L. Lichen Simplex Chronicus

Lichen simplex chronicus may complicate hand dermatitis. The American Medical Association Guidelines in the Assessment of Impairment accepts lichen simplex chronicus as a compensable complication of occupational contact dermatitis (Table 1).[31] This self-perpetuating cycle of scratching and dermatitis can play a major role in allowing hand dermatitis to persist in some individuals.

The dermatologist should question patients about their hobbies and part-time jobs. Exposure to allergens and irritants from these sources may be more important than occupational exposures in the persistence of hand dermatitis.[32]

M. Sex

Irritant contact dermatitis is more common in women than men. For example, Coenraads found in his survey of a general population that 8% of women and 5% of men have hand dermatitis.[33] His follow-up study found that most of these individuals still had hand dermatitis 3 years later. Women

TABLE 1   American Guidelines to Impairment Ratings of
Occupational Skin Diseases

Class (% impairment)		Limitations in activities in daily living with treatment
American Medical Association	Minnesota	
I (0–5)	I (2)	0–minimal
II (10–20)	II (10)	Some
III (25–50)	III (20)	Many
IV (55–80)	IV (45)	Many
V (85–95)	V (70)	Severe

usually have greater exposure to cutaneous irritants used in household cleaning and in the care of children. The adverse effects of exposure to irritants at home are additive to occupational exposures.[9] Many high-risk occupations for hand eczema, i.e., hairdressing, nursing, and catering, typically employ more women than men. It is unknown if women with contact dermatitis have a worse prognosis than men with similar dermatitis and similar exposure to domestic and occupational allergens and irritants.

Menne and Bachman[13] found that, in Denmark, twice as many women as men had permanent disability pensions because of allergic contact dermatitis. Almost one-half of cases with permanent disability pensions because of allergic contact dermatitis were due to nickel, and 91 of these 96 cases were women. It is well known that a much higher percentage of women than men in the general population in Western countries are allergic to nickel.

N. Age

For any occupational disease there is the possibility of the healthy worker effect. An occupation may have more healthy individuals than average for a population as those workers who poorly tolerate workplace exposures tend to discontinue such work. It has been suggested that older workers are more susceptible to irritant contact dermatitis, particularly irritant contact dermatitis due to solvents. Burrows found that age had no effect on prognosis but that older workers had the greatest difficulty in finding new employment and suffered the greatest financial loss.[12] Early retirement may be considered for older manual workers who develop severe hand eczema.

O. Self-Perpetuating Dermatitis

It is the opinion of many experts in the field of occupational contact dermatitis of the hands that induction of a chronic, self-perpetuating cycle of dermatitis is a major cause of persistence of occupational dermatitis of the hands. There appears to be immunologic clues as to why dermatitis might persist once it occurs. It is of interest that more and more similarities in the immunology of the irritant and the allergic contact dermatitis are being discovered, and this may partially explain why the prognosis is so similar for both disorders once they are initiated.[34] It is hoped that further research into the pathogenesis and treatment of hand dermatitis will lead to a real change in the prognosis of hand dermatitis.

REFERENCES

1. Hogan, D. J., Dannaker, C. J., and Maibach, H. I., The prognosis of contact dermatitis, *J. Am. Acad. Dermatol.,* 23, 300, 1990.
2. Skog, E. and Tottie, M., Occupational eczema causing disablement, *Acta Derm. Venereol.,* 41, 205, 1961.
3. Griffiths, W. A. D., Industrial dermatitis, a national problem, in *Essentials of Industrial Dermatology,* Griffiths, W. A. D. and Wilkinson, D. S., Eds., Blackwell Scientific, Oxford, 1985, 1.

4. O'Quinn, S. E., Cole, J., and Many, H., Problems of disability and rehabilitation in patients with chronic skin diseases, *Arch. Dermatol.*, 105, 35, 1972.

5. Gallant, C. J., A long-term follow-up study of patients with hand dermatitis evaluated at St. Michael's Occupational Health Clinic in 1981 and 1982, Toronto, Canada, Masters thesis, University of Toronto, 1986.

6. Agrup, G., Hand eczema and other hand dermatoses in South Sweden, *Acta Derm. Venereol.*, 49 (Suppl. 61), 1, 1969.

7. Lammintausta, K., Kalimo, K., and Aantaa, S., Course of hand dermatitis in hospital workers, *Contact Dermatitis*, 8, 327, 1982.

8. Nilsson, E. and Back, O., The importance of anamnestic information of atopy, metal dermatitis and earlier hand eczema, *Acta Derm. Venereol.*, 66, 45, 1986.

9. Nilsson, E., Mikaelsson, B., and Anderson, S., Atopy, occupation and domestic work as risk factors for hand eczema in hospital workers, *Contact Dermatitis*, 13, 216, 1985.

10. Hunziker, N. and Musso, E., A propos de l' eczema au ciment, *Dermatology*, 21, 204, 1960.

11. Hogan, D. J., Dannaker, C. J., Lal, S., and Maibach, H. I., An international survey of expert opinion on the prognosis of contact dermatitis, *Dermatosen*, 38, 143, 1990.

12. Burrows, D., Prognosis in industrial dermatitis, *Br. J. Dermatol.*, 87, 145, 1972.

13. Menne, T. and Bachmann, E., Permanent disability from allergic contact dermatitis, *Contact Dermatitis*, 6, 59, 1980.

14. Cronin, E., *Contact Dermatitis*, Churchill Livingstone, Edinburgh, 1980.

15. Hellier, F. F., The prognosis in industrial dermatitis, *Br. Med. J.*, 1, 196, 1958.

16. Keczkes, K. and Bhate, S. M., The outcome of primary irritant hand dermatitis, *Br. J. Dermatol.*, 109, 665, 1983.

17. Meneghini, C. L. and Angelini, G., Occupational dermatitis artefacta, *Dermatosen*, 27, 163, 1979.

18. Morris, G. E., Why doesn't the worker's skin clear up?, *Arch. Ind. Hyg.*, 10, 43, 1954.

19. Christensen, O. B., Prognosis in nickel allergy and hand eczema, *Contact Dermatitis*, 8, 7, 1982.

20. Cronin, E., Clinical patterns of hand eczema in women, *Contact Dermatitis*, 13, 153, 1985.

21. Turjanma, K., Incidence of immediate allergy to latex gloves in hospital personnel, *Contact Dermatitis*, 17, 270, 1987.

22. Rystedt, I., Hand eczema and long-term prognosis in atopic dermatitis, *Acta Derm. Venereol.*, 65 (Suppl. 117), 1, 1985.

23. Edman, B., The usefulness of detailed information to patients with contact allergy, *Contact Dermatitis*, 19, 43, 1988.

24. Breit, R. and Turk, R. B., The medical and social fate of the dichromate allergic patient, *Br. J. Dermatol.*, 94, 349, 1976.

25. Phillips, B., Occupational dermatitis, *Practitioner*, 172, 531, 1954.

26. Mathias, C. G. T., Contact dermatitis from use or misuse of soaps, detergents, and cleansers in the workplace, *Occup. Med. State of the Art Rev.*, 1, 205, 1986.

27. Rasmussen, S. A., Obsessive compulsive disorder in dermatologic practice, *J. Am. Acad. Dermatol.*, 13, 965, 1985.

28. Fischer, T. and Rystedt, I., Skin protection against ionized cobalt and sodium lauryl sulphate with barrier creams, *Contact Dermatitis*, 9, 125, 1983.

29. Mellstron, G., Wrangjso, K., and Whalberg, J. E., Patch testing with barrier creams, *Contact Dermatitis*, 13, 40, 1985.

30. Savoie, J. M., Une porphyrie cutanee tardive simulant une dermatitie industrielle, *Nouv. Dermatol.*, 3, 205, 1984.

31. Anon., Impairment committee on rating of mental and physical: the skin, *J. Am. Med. Assoc.*, 211, 106, 1970.

32. Church, R., Hand eczema in industry and the home, in *Essentials of Industrial Dermatology*, Griffiths, W. A. D. and Wilkinson, D. S., Eds., Blackwell Scientific, Oxford, 1985, 85.

33. Coenraads, P. J., Prevalence of hand eczema: association with occupational exposure, especially in construction workers, Ph.D. thesis, University of Groningen, 1983.

34. Hogan, D. J., Dannaker, C. J., Lal, S., and Maibach, H. I., An international survey on the prognosis of occupational contact dermatitis of the hands, *Dermatosen Beruf Umwelt,* 38, 143, 1990.

35. Dannaker, C. J., personal communication.

28

UV-Light Treatment of Hand Eczema

Ole B. Christensen

CONTENTS

0-8493-7355-7/94/$0.00 + $.50

I. INTRODUCTION

Hand eczema occurs widely in the population. In a recent Swedish epidemiological study on 20,000 individuals between ages 20 and 65, the prevalence of hand eczema occasionally during the last year was found to be 11%.[1] In the same study, 2% of 1385 patients investigated had suffered from hand eczema continuously for the last year, indicating that chronic hand eczema also is a prevalent condition. Chronic hand eczema is often of multifactorial etiology (exogenous as well as endogenous). Especially, this mixed etiology exists in pompholyx patients with a combination of atopy and contact allergy.[2,3]

Managing patients with hand eczema, including a correct relevant medical history work-up with epicutaneous testing, prevention, information to the patient, and deciding on the proper treatment among the available possibilities, is a constant challenge for practicing dermatologists. Often, assistance by subspecialists with a knowledge of occupational dermatology, including epicutaneous testing as well as experience in special treatments like UV treatment, is required.

II. INDICATIONS FOR UV TREATMENT

Most patients with hand eczema can be controlled by topical corticosteroids and preventive measures. However, sometimes we are left with chronic recalcitrant cases that cannot be controlled either topically or by acceptable doses of systemic corticosteroids. Such cases are considered candidates for UV treatment. In the author's experience, often patients with eczema in the palmar region — the pompholyx type — belong to this category. Of course, duration of sick leave, workers compensation legislation, change of occupation, and the influence of the eczema on the quality of life should be taken into consideration when evaluating indications for UV treatment.

III. CONTRAINDICATIONS FOR UV TREATMENT

Patients with compromised liver and/or renal function should be monitored carefully during systemic PUVA therapy. In these cases, topical PUVA therapy or UV-B is an alternative. Skin diseases like lupus erythematosis and porphyria, which deteriorate from light therapy, should avoid this treatment. Actinic sun-damaged skin and an earlier or present history of malignant skin cancers represent a relative contraindication. Systemic PUVA therapy should not be carried out during pregnancy. Caution has to be taken in patients on phototoxic or photosensitizing drugs like phenothiazines, tetracycline, sulfones, etc. Treatment of patients abusing alcohol and with other signs indicating risk for bad compliance usually fails. If such suspicions exist, it is usually unwise to start a treatment which demands regularity to be successful.

IV. DIFFERENT TYPES OF UV TREATMENTS

A. PUVA

PUVA Treatment is usually carried out by ingestion of 8-methoxypsoralen (8-MOP), 0.6 mg/kg of body weight. In cases with severe side effects, 5-methoxypsoralen (5-MOP) in a dose of 1 mg/kg of body weight is usually a practical alternative. Also, 8-MOP or trioxsalen can be applied topically in a cream, organic solution, or bath before UV-A irradiation. Topical application of psoralens can have obvious advantages for the patient, but demands careful monitoring as a narrower spectrum between doses for improvement and burning exists under these conditions compared to oral PUVA treatment. Also, this type of treatment is usually more staff-consuming than the systemic PUVA treatment. When psoralen (8-MOP as well as 5-MOP) is taken orally, the starting dose of UV-A is usually 2 J/cm², whereas the UV-A dose has to be decreased four to ten times when the psoralens are applied topically. When treating only the hands, special considerations for different skin types is usually not necessary. Also, determination of the minimal phototoxic dose (MPD) is not required, except maybe when treating dorsal aspects of the hands in Type I skin or when administering topical PUVA treatment. PUVA treatment is carried out two to four times weekly and the UV-A dose should be increased according to the patient's report and objective findings following the last treatment. Experience teaches that one can be more aggressive with dose increments of systemic PUVA treatments when treating the hands than with other parts of the body, especially when treating the volar aspects of the hands. Increments of 1 to 2 J at each new treatment session, up to a maximum of 12 to 15 J, can be carried out in most cases.

B. UV-B

Treatment of chronic hand eczema can also be carried out with UV-B. Several units, home built or commercially produced, are on the market in different countries. When effective, UV-B treatment is very practical compared to PUVA, and with a suitable unit can be carried out by the patient at home. UV-B irradiation can be given to the hands only or combined with whole-body irradiation, with extra UV-B to the hands,[4] taking advantage of the proven downgrading effect of systemic UV-B on contact allergy.[5] In studies published so far[4,6,7] on the effect of UV-B on hand eczema, the same dose as was usually given in whole-body treatment for psoriasis and eczema patients has been administered to the hands. Such doses are probably not optimal for the hands where, at least in the palms, the thick stratum corneum results in a MED which is several times higher than that on the body skin. Taking this consideration into account, a new small and comfortable unit with a high output of UV-B has been constructed in Sweden.[8] For the moment, we are testing this unit in our clinic and patients are treated either in our day-care center or at home. From this study it is obvious that the hands tolerate considerably higher doses of UV-B (10 to 20 times) than tested before, without side effects.

V. CLINICAL EFFECT OF UV TREATMENT

A. PUVA

Most of the experience concerning PUVA treatment of refractory chronic hand eczema originates from 8-MOP given orally. In 1978, Morrison and co-workers[9] for the first time in a controlled study described five patients with symmetrical active endogenous hand eczema that cleared on the treated side only, after an average of 16 treatments.[9] In another controlled study of seven patients with dyshidrotic eczema of the palms, all patients cleared on the treated side.[10] Positive reports of PUVA treatment of allergic and irritant contact dermatitis and chronic hyperkeratotic dermatitis of the palms have been published.[11,12]

In 1985, Tegner and Thelin[13] treated 38 patients with chronic eczematous dermatitis — 26 with pompholyx, 10 with allergic contact dermatitis, and 2 with irritant contact dermatitis of the palms — with 8-MOP orally: 20 patients were completely free from lesions when treatment was stopped and 11 patients were improved. The initial PUVA course was followed by maintenance treatment with an average of 12 sessions in 13 patients, and this combination resulted in 9 patients healed and 3 patients improved.

B. UV-B

The first report of the effect of UV-B on hand eczema was by Mörk and Austad in 1982.[6] Ten patients with allergic contact dermatitis of the hands with an average duration of 9 years were treated with doses of UV-B from 0.2 to 1.2 J/cm^3, once or twice weekly for an average of 5.5 months. Seven patients cleared and the other three patients improved. The study was uncontrolled. Later on, Sjövall and Christensen[4] randomly allocated 18 patients with refractory hand eczema with an average duration of 9 years into 3 different groups. Group I was treated with UV-B on the hands only. Group II was given UV-B sham treatment to the hands. Group III was given whole-body UV-B + UV-B to the hands as in group I. All patients were treated 4 times weekly for 8 weeks, resulting in an accumulated dose of approximately 19 J/cm^2. One patient dropped out in each group. In group I, two patients cleared and three improved. In group II, one patient cleared and four patients remained unchanged. In group III all five patients cleared, indicating that the most effective treatment was the situation when whole-body UV-B irradiation was combined with UV-B irradiation of the hands.

At the moment, we are running a study[14] in our clinic to investigate the effect of a more aggressive UV-B treatment of chronic hand eczema with a new UV-B unit (Handylux).[8] The patients are randomly allocated to treatment, either in the clinic or at home. The dimensions and weight of the unit makes it easily transportable. The unit is equipped with 8×8 W Sankyo FL tubes with a continuous spectrum of 270 to 320 nm and a maximum at approximately 315 to 318 nm. The UV-B output is 3.23 mW/cm^2. The starting dose of UV-B for the volar and dorsal parts of the hands is 2 min $= 0.38$ J/cm^2 and 30 s $= 0.10$ J/cm^2, respectively. When possible, the treatment time is increased by 30 to 60 s in the palms and 10 to 20 s in the dorsal aspects of the hands, to a maximum of 15 min $= 2.9$ J/cm^2 and 6 min $= 1.16$ J/cm^2, respectively.

The treatment has been carried out 4 to 5 times weekly for 6 to 12 weeks. To date, we have treated 18 patients, 9 in the clinic and 9 at home; 1 patient in each group discontinued treatment after 5 to 6 weeks due to lack of effect. In total from both groups, 7 patients have cleared, 4 patients have almost cleared, and 3 patients have improved considerably, and the overall effect for the last 2 patients was estimated as an improvement. Side effects are few and minor and this treatment, especially the possibility of treatment at home, was highly evaluated by the patients. At the moment we see home treatment with UV-B as an effective and very practical possibility and a future treatment of choice in patients with chronic hand eczema. According to our present experience, the UV-B Handylux treatment is comparable to PUVA in efficacy and naturally much easier to perform, with no drawbacks as in PUVA treatment (visits to day-care centers, nausea, avoidance of sun exposure, wearing Polaroid sunglasses, effective anticonception, etc.).

C.   PUVA vs. UV-B

An extensive study comparing the effect of PUVA and UV-B in chronic hand eczema has been carried out by Rosén et al.[7] A group of 35 patients with symmetrical hand eczema were allocated to PUVA treatment (18 patients) or UV-B treatment (17 patients) on only one hand, whereas the other hand served as a control. Treatment was carried out three times weekly for a maximum of 3 months.

During the treatment, four patients dropped out of the PUVA group and one dropped out of the UV-B group. All 14 remaining patients in the PUVA group cleared on the treated hand; only 1 patient cleared on the untreated hand but 10 patients improved on this side. No patients cleared on the UV-B treated hand but 15 out of 16 improved. Also, in this group the control side improved somewhat, emphasizing that proper controls are necessary.

The number and duration of treatments were less in the PUVA than the UV-B group. The average UV-A dose was 100 J/cm^2 (range 21 to 329) compared with 11 J/cm^2 (2 to 27) of UV-B. Seven patients in the PUVA group developed more or less severe side effects (nausea, edema, pain, itching), whereas only two patients in the UV-B group developed side effects with bullouses in the treated palm.

In this rather extensive and well-monitored controlled study, PUVA is clearly superior in efficacy compared with UV-B. However, as mentioned above, the doses of UV-B that have been applied have not been optimal and can be increased several times, resulting in higher efficacy without major side effects.

D.   PUVA vs. Superficial Radiotherapy

Superficial radiotherapy is established as an effective treatment for chronic hand eczema resistant to conventional topical treatment.[15,16] In a double-blind study of 21 patients with chronic bilateral constitutional hand eczema, the therapeutic efficacy of conventional superficial radiotherapy and topical photochemotherapy (topical PUVA) was compared.[17] Significantly better clinical improvement was seen in superficial radiotherapy-treated hands over topical PUVA-treated hands after 6 weeks of treatment. At the time there was no significant difference in symptom severity between the two treatments, but superficial radiotherapy produced significantly more symptomatic improvement at 9 and 18 weeks. It is concluded that superficial radiotherapy is a less time-consuming procedure than topical PUVA and leads to more rapid improvements. However, it is not documented if any of the patients cleared from either radiotherapy or topical PUVA treatment. As pointed out in Chapter 29 in this book, Grenz-ray treatment of chronic hand eczema is most effective and practical to perform.

E.   PUVA vs. UV-A

The effect of PUVA on chronic hand eczema is generally accepted, though a controlled study vs. UV-A as placebo was not performed until the study by Gratten et al. in 1991.[19] In this study, topical PUVA was compared with UV-A in a double-blind randomized within-patient trial in 12 patients with chronic vesicular hand eczema. The mean dose of UV-A for the 8-week treatment period was 105.5 J/cm^2 (range 70 to 162). Both hands improved over the treatment period and remained substantially better objectively and subjectively at the 8-week follow-up. No statistical difference of assessments between the treated hands was found at any stage. On a visual analogue scale only the UV-A-treated hand showed significant improvement. Again, it has to be pointed out that none of the patients cleared during the treatment period, indicating that topical PUVA treatment is generally not as effective as systemic PUVA treatment. Also, as shown by Rosén et al.,[7] the untreated hand improved during PUVA as well as UV-B treatment, 49 and 37%, respectively. Therefore, the observed effect in the study by Gratten et al.[19] could correspond to a mainly placebo effect. However, in atopic eczema the effect of UV-A is documented,[20-22] indicating that the reported effect of UV-A in chronic hand eczema is due to a true biological effect which, however, needs to be confirmed in future trials.

F.   Follow-Up of UV Treatment

The longest follow-up period after discontinuation of systemic PUVA treatment of chronic hand eczema is from the study by Tegner and Thelin, who followed the patients for up to 5 years.[13] The mean remission time for 11 patients who cleared after an initial course was 8 months, whereas in 9 patients who cleared after the initial course, followed by maintenance treatment, the remission time was 14 months. Also, most patients reported that their eczema activity was reduced when recurring after rather than before PUVA treatment. Rosén et al.[7] report recurrence after a mean of 3 months (range 1 to 8 months) in 9 patients, whereas 5 patients were still cleared after a follow-up period of 3 weeks (2 patients) and 2, 8, and 16 months.

Only one report concerning the effect of UV-B in chronic hand eczema mention follow-up results.[4] Five patients, who cleared following local + systemic UV-B irradiation stayed clear for a mean of 6 weeks (3 to 10 weeks).

Obviously, follow-up data are relatively limited and no major conclusions can be drawn. However, phototherapy of recalcitrant chronic hand eczema is simply an effective symptomatic treatment, but unfortunately not a cure. Maintenance treatment seems to result in the longest eczema-free period and, therefore, this approach should be performed in most patients.

V.   SIDE EFFECTS OF UV TREATMENT

A.   PUVA

Unfortunately, PUVA treatment, systematically or topically, is not without side effects. Most patients who ingest 8-MOP complain about nausea, in some patients so extensively that vomiting occurs. Taking 8-MOP dissolved in water sometimes overcomes this side effect. If this problem is not eliminated 5-MOP is an alternative, as it usually is well tolerated by the patients. Naturally, topical PUVA treatment also is an alternative, but in the author's experience this treatment is not as effective as systemic PUVA treatment. The side effects of systemic PUVA treatment of psoriasis are extensively listed in a thesis by Tegner.[23] In this review only those side effects related to the treatment of chronic hand eczema will be mentioned.

Phototoxic blisters and localized edema can be observed when treating only the hands. These phenomena are usually related to an overly aggressive treatment regimen or skin atrophy from prolonged use of corticosteroids, but also the possibility of interaction with phototoxic or photosensitizing drugs or porphyria should be considered. Burning, pruritus, and seldomly, pain, are side effects of a minor degree probably also related to too frequent a treatment schedule and overly aggressive increments of the UV-A dose. Uncommon side effects like photoonycholyses and bleeding under the finger nails are also related to the circumstances mentioned above. When these side effects occur, treatment should be discontinued and proper etiologic investigations undertaken. When treatment is reinstituted, the UV-A dose given before the side effects appeared should be the new starting dose. Also, a decrease of the 8-MOP dose should be taken under consideration.

Contact and photocontact allergy to psoralens have been described in some cases.[24-28] The circumstances for sensitization are usually identical, namely, repeated painting with 8-MOP and exposure to UV-A on the same skin area. When sensitized on the hands, a severe flare-up can be elicited by systemic PUVA.[26] When severe acute vesicular eczema occurs during topical or systemic PUVA treatment, the possibility of contact and/or photocontact sensitization should be considered and investigated by relevant testing procedures.

In a few cases, liver damage following 8-MOP intake also has been reported.[29,30] Since the first report from our department,[29] we have had two more cases, as also described by Tegner.[23] This unusual complication, of course, is most serious and demands prompt discontinuation of treatment and future avoidance of systemic PUVA therapy. However, from a cost-benefit point of view this unusual side effect, in the author's opinion, dose not merit initial or regular control of liver enzymes.

PUVA lentigines is a well-known side effect of prolonged PUVA therapy.[31,32] This phenomenon can also occur in the palms and dorsal aspects of the hands and is related to a high cumulative dose of UV-A.

Several studies have dealt with the potential risk of cutaneous cancers in patients receiving PUVA therapy[33-37] for different skin disorders. By now, an increased risk of squamous cell cancer of the skin for patients on long-term PUVA treatment is agreed. Squamous cell cancer on the upper extremities including the hands, seems to be very uncommon,[37] and to the author's knowledge this skin cancer type has not been described as being located in the hands following long-term PUVA treatment. Therefore, the risk of developing squamous cell carcinoma in the hands, even at a very high cumulative UV-A dose, seems extremely low. However, we all know that actinic keratoses are very prevalent on the dorsal aspects of hands in elderly patients who have lived in heavily sun-exposed areas for a long time. With regard to the risk of developing cutaneous cancer, patients should always be carefully preselected before PUVA photochemotherapy. Patients with previous exposure to arsenic, methotrexate, ionizing irradiation, excessive exposure to tar and/or UV-B, and probably to azathioprine, run an increased risk of developing epidermal tumors. Obviously, these patients should be controlled at regular intervals during PUVA treatment.

Another potential side effect of concern during systemic PUVA therapy is the risk of developing cataracts. This risk has been known since the start of PUVA therapy and as a preventive measure Polaroid sunglasses are always worn. This seems to have been most protective, since no case of cataract development coarsely related to PUVA treatment has been reported.[38]

B. UV-B

In connection with a UV-B treatment overdose resulting in burning, painful erythema and superficial bullae formation sometimes occur. Topical corticosteroids, discontinuation of treatment for 3 to 5 days, and when restarting treatment applying the last dose which didn't induce any side effects, usually solves the problem. When applying high doses of UV-B in the future by patients at home,[14] the carcinogenic potential of UV-B must be considered. For this treatment, patients should be selected in relation to the risk factors mentioned above and controlled regularly.

VII. PRACTICAL ADVICE IN CONNECTION WITH UV TREATMENT OF HAND ECZEMA

Selection of patients with regard to indications, contraindications, risk factors, and compliance, as well as oral and written information by the doctor and a trained nurse, is obligate before start of treatment. Frequently, patients are frightened of PUVA therapy and ask many questions which have to be answered professionally, sometimes with some degree of persuasion. Several patients, after a successful treatment course, expressed thanks that they were convinced to start PUVA treatment. The patients should be informed that they have to attend at regular intervals, initially at least three times a week for several weeks, and that the effect comes slowly. When cleared or considerably improved, maintenance treatment twice weekly and then once weekly for 3 to 4 weeks, respectively, is recommended.

As mentioned earlier, not all patients clear or improve to an acceptable degree during PUVA therapy. In some cases the psoralens are not absorbed sufficiently, the dose is too low, patients do not take the tablets at recommended time intervals, or simply for different reasons avoid intake of tablets. Under such circumstances the serum level of psoralen should be controlled.[39] In the author's experience, an increased hyperpigmentation of the hands usually correlates very well with clinical improvement, meaning that the absence of hyperpigmentation when a reasonably high UV-A dose is achieved, is a circumstance indicating that the serum concentration of psoralens should be controlled. When lack of compliance is suspected, the patient shouldn't be informed about this control in advance.

During the initial phase of UV treatment of hand eczema, especially in pompholyx cases which sometimes flare aggressively, a flare can be interpreted as deterioration due to overtreatment. This is very seldom the case and except for contact or photo contact allergy or atrophy, treatment should be continued. The patient can be allowed to use potent corticosteroids for a few days or, if necessary, systemic corticosteroids to control the flare, whereas treatment is continued to reach optimal doses of UV-A. The same phenomenon and approach is also applicable during UV-B treatment of chronic hand eczema.

Patients with severe chronic hand eczema often have to be on sick leave. As the hand eczema improves during treatment, patients could return partly to their occupations while maintenance treatment is continued for some weeks, in order to test the influence of the occupation on the prognoses. Obviously, cases with relevant occupational allergic or irritant contact dermatitis need legal help to change their occupations.

VIII. PROSPECTS OF UV TREATMENT OF HAND ECZEMA

Today, 8-MOP is the most widely used psoralen. However, 5-MOP results in less side effects and allows better compliance. Therefore, 5-MOP probably to a large degree will replace 8-MOP in the future. At present, PUVA or whole-body UV-B with extra exposure of the hands are the most effective treatments in refractory cases of hand eczema. However, several drawbacks are involved in PUVA treatment. UV-B treatment can be optimized and, by the use of safe handheld units, turn out to be a future treatment carried out by the patients at home.

REFERENCES

1. Meding, B. and Swanbeck, G., Prevalence of hand eczema in an industrial city, *Br. J. Dermatol.*, 116, 627, 1987.
2. Christensen, O. B., Prognosis in nickel allergy and hand eczema, *Contact Dermatitis*, 8, 7, 1982.
3. Lodi, A., Betti, R., Chianetti, G., Urbané, C. E., and Crosti, C., Epidemiological, clinical and allergological observations on pompholyx, *Contact Dermatitis*, 26, 17, 1992.
4. Sjövall, P. and Christensen, O. B., Local and systemic effect of UVB irradiation in patients with chronic hand eczema, *Acta Derm. Venereol. Stockholm*, 67, 538, 1987.
5. Sjövall, P. and Christensen, O. B., Local and systemic effect of ultraviolet irradiation (UVB and UVA) on human allergic contact dermatitis, *Acta Derm. Venereol. Stockholm*, 66, 290, 1986.
6. Mörk, N. I. and Austad, J., Short-wave ultraviolet light (UVB) treatment of allergic contact dermatitis of the hands, *Acta Derm. Venereol. Stockholm*, 63, 87, 1983.
7. Rosén, K., Mobacken, H., and Swanbeck, G., Chronic eczematous dermatitis of the hands: a comparison of PUVA and UVB treatment, *Acta Derm. Venereol. Stockholm*, 67, 48, 1987.

8. Anon., Handylux, Esshå Dermatia AB, Box 528, S-331 25, Värnamo, Sweden.
9. Morrison, W. L., Parrish, I. A., and Fitzpatrick, T. B., Oral methoxalen photochemotherapy of recalcitrant dermatoses of the palms and soles, *Br. J. Dermatol.*, 99, 297, 1978.
10. Le Vine, M. I., Parrish, I. A., and Fitzpatrick, T. B., Oral methoxalen photochemotherapy (PUVA) of dyshidrotic eczema, *Acta Derm. Venereol. Stockholm*, 61, 570, 1981.
11. Bruynzell, D. P., Boouk, W. I., and van Keter, W. G., Oral psoralen photochemotherapy of allergic contact dermatitis of the hands, *Dermatosen*, 30, 16, 1982.
12. Mobacken, H., Rosén, K., and Swanbeck, G., Oral psoralen photochemotherapy (PUVA) of hyperkeratotic dermatitis of the palms, *Br. J. Dermatol.*, 109, 205, 1983.
13. Tegner, E. and Thelin, I., PUVA treatment of chronic eczematous dermatitis of the palms and soles, *Acta Derm. Venereol. Stockholm*, 65, 451, 1985.
14. Christensen, O. B. and Sjövall, P., unpublished observation, 1992.
15. Fairris, G. M., Mack, O. P., and Rowell, N. R., Superficial X-ray therapy in the treatment of constitutional eczema of the hands, *Br. J. Dermatol.*, 111, 445, 1984.
16. King, C. M. and Chalmers, R. I. G., A double blind study of superficial radiotherapy in chronic palmar eczema, *Br. J. Dermatol.*, 111, 451, 1984.
17. Sheehan-Dare, R. A., Goodfield, M. I., and Rowell, N. B., Topical psoralen photochemotherapy (PUVA) and superficial radiotherapy in the treatment of contact hand eczema, *Br. J. Dermatol.*, 121, 63, 1989.
18. Lindelöf, B., X-ray treatment of hand eczema, in *Hand Eczema*, Menne, T. and Maibach, H. I., Eds., CRC Press, Boca Raton, FL, 1993, chap. 29.
19. Gratten, C. E. H., Carmichard, A. I., Shottleuach, G. I., and Poolds, I. S., Comparison of topical PUVA with UVA for chronic vesicular hand eczema, *Acta Derm. Venereol. Stockholm*, 71, 118, 1991.
20. Middelfart, K., Shervald, S. E., and Volden, G., Combined UVB and UVA phototherapy of atopic eczema, *Dermatologica*, 171, 95, 1986.
21. Falk, S., UV-light therapies in atopic dermatitis, *Photodermatology*, 2, 241, 1985.
22. Jebler, J. and Larkö, O., Phototherapy of atopic dermatitis with ultraviolet A (UVA), low-dose UVB and combined UVA and UVB: two paired-comparison studies, *Photodermatol. Photoimmunol. Photomed.*, 8, 151, 1991.
23. Tegner, E., Observations of PUVA Treatment of Psoriasis and on 5-5-Cysteinyldopa After Exposure to UV Light, Doctoral dissertation, University of Lund, Sweden, 1983.
24. Saihan, E. M., Contact allergy to methoxalen, *Br. Med. J.*, II, 20, 1979.
25. Weissman, I., Wagner, G., and Plewig, G., Contact allergy to 8-methoxypsoralen, *Br. J. Dermatol.*, 102, 113, 1980.
26. Möller, H., Contact and photocontact allergy to psoralen, *Photodermatol. Photoimmunol. Photomed.*, 7, 43, 1990.
27. Fulton, I. E. and Willis, I., Photoallergy to methoxalen, *Arch. Dermatol.*, 98, 445, 1968.
28. Plewig, G., Hofman, C., and Bran-Falko, O., Photoallergic dermatitis from 8-methoxypsoralen, *Arch. Dermatol. Res.*, 261, 201, 1978.
29. Bjellerup, M., Bruze, M., Hansson, A., Krook, G., and Ljunggren, B., Liver injury following administration of 8-methoxypsoralen during PUVA therapy, *Acta Derm. Venereol. Stockholm*, 39, 371, 1979.
30. Pariser, D. M. and Wyks, P. I., Toxic hepatitis from oral methoxalen photochemotherapy (PUVA), *J. Am. Acad. Dermatol.*, 3, 248, 1980.
31. Blechan, S. S., Freckles induced by PUVA treatment, *Br. J. Dermatol.*, 99, 70, 1978.
32. Gschnait, F., Wolff, K., Hönigsmann, H., Slingl, G., Brenner, W., Jaschke, E., and Konrad, K., Long-term photochemotherapy: histopathological and immunofluorescence observations in 243 patients, *Br. J. Dermatol.*, 103, 11, 1980.
33. Forman, A. B., Roenigk, H. H., Jr., Caro, W. A., and Magid, M. L., Long-term follow-up of skin cancer in the PUVA-48 cooperative study, *Arch. Dermatol.*, 125, 513, 1989.
34. Stern, R. S., Lange, R., et al., Non-melanoma skin cancer occurring in patients treated with PUVA, 5 to 10 years after first treatment, *J. Invest. Dermatol.*, 91, 120, 1988.
35. Henseler, T., Christophers, E., Hönigsmann, H., Wolff, K., et al., Skin tumors in the European PUVA study, *J. Am. Acad. Dermatol.*, 16, 108, 1987.

36. Stern, R. S., Laird, N., Muski, J., Parrish, J. A., Fitzpatrick, T. B., and Bleich, H. L., Cutaneous squamous-cell carcinoma in patients treated with PUVA, *N. Engl. J. Med.,* 310, 1156, 1984.

37. Lindelöf, B., Sigurgeirsson, B., Tegner, E., Larkö, O., Johansson, A., Berne, B., Christensen, O. B., Andersson, T., Törngren, M., Molin, L., Nylander-Lundqvist, E., and Emtesatam, L., PUVA and cancer: a large-scale epidemiological study, *Lancet,* 338, 91, 1991.

38. Abdullah, A. N. and Keczkes, R., Cutaneous and ocular side-effects of PUVA photo chemotherapy — a 10-year follow-up study, *Clin. Exp. Dermatol.,* 14, 421, 1989.

39. Ljunggren, B., Bjellerup, M., and Carter, M. D., Dose-response reactions in phototoxicity due to 8-methoxypsoralen and UV-A in man, *J. Invest. Dermatol.,* 76, 73, 1981.

29

X-Ray Treatment of Hand Eczema

Bernt Lindelöf

CONTENTS

0-8493-7355-7/94/$0.00 + $.50

I. HISTORY OF X-RAY THERAPY

Dermatologists have successfully used X-ray therapy for the treatment of benign and malignant skin disorders since 1899.[1] The reason for the early use of X-ray therapy in dermatology was that the effect of ionizing radiation on the skin quickly became apparent. Radiation-induced dermatitis, epilation, and pigmentation led to recognition of the biological effects of the X-rays. Treatment with soft X-rays for benign inflammatory skin diseases became available in 1923, when Gustav Bucky succeeded in devising an apparatus that produced ultrasoft X-rays. Today, dermatologic X-ray therapy can be divided into two main groups: grenz-ray therapy and superficial X-ray therapy (Table 1).

II. PHYSICS

The quality of X-rays is defined by their penetrating ability. The most frequently used definition for various X-ray qualities is the half-value layer (HVL). It is defined as that thickness of a given filter material (in dermatology, usually aluminum [Al]) that reduces the intensity to 50% of the original incident radiation. Grenz-rays are referred to as soft (HVL up to 0.02 mm Al), medium (HVL 0.023 to 0.029 mm Al), and hard (HVL 0.030 to 0.036 mm Al). Superficial X-ray radiation has a HVL of 0.7 to 2 mm of Al. The HVL is influenced by multiple factors, but for practical purposes only two of them are important: kilovoltage and additional filtration. An X-ray beam produced by higher kilovoltage has shorter wavelengths and greater penetrating power. By placing a filter in the X-ray beam the quality is changed in such a way that the higher the atomic number of the filter, the greater the reduction in beam intensity. The intensity or dose rate of radiation is influenced by kilovoltage (kV), milliamperage (mA), filter, exposure time, and target skin distance (TSD). It increases when the kV and mA are increased. It decreases as the distance is increased, approximately in inverse square proportion, and it is also reduced as the thickness and the atomic number of the filter are increased. The radiation dose is directly proportional to the exposure time, if all other factors remain constant. The X-ray dose in roentgen (R) specifies the exposure to a certain quantity of radiation, based on its ability to ionize air. It is not identical with the observed dose in the tissue, which is expressed in rads. The unit of the absorbed dose (tissue dose) used today is Gray (Gy): according to the International System of Units (SI) standards, 1 Gy equals 100 rads.

III. BIOLOGICAL EFFECTS

Low voltage X-rays are absorbed predominantly through the photoelectric effect. Since their energy is small at the outset, the path of the photoelectron is short, so that its entire quantum of energy is absorbed within one cell. However, thousands of collisions occur along that short path. This produces ions and excited atoms and molecules that are able to enter into chemical combinations with free radicals or other molecules to form new molecules of unpredictable effect on the tissue.[2] Recent research has shown that grenz-ray therapy, superficial X-ray therapy, and soft X-ray therapy decrease the number of Langerhans' cells in the epidermis. After a single dose of 4 Gy of 10 kV grenz-rays on human epidermis, it was found that the number of Langerhans' cells (OKT-6 positive) was slightly reduced after 30 min and markedly reduced 1 and 3 weeks after irradiation.[3] By counting the Langerhans' cells at electron microscopic resolution in human epidermis before and after grenz-ray therapy, it was confirmed that the Langerhans' cells disappeared from the epidermis after treatment. No consistent differences in keratinocyte morphology was observed.[4] By pretreating nickel-sensitive patients with grenz-rays and then applying nickel patch tests on the treated area and on untreated control skin, it has been shown that grenz-ray therapy can almost totally suppress allergic contact dermatitis.[5] This suppression lasts for about 3 weeks after treatment and is paralleled by a suppression of the number of Langerhans' cells in the epidermis.[6] Superficial X-ray (90 kV) treatment has also proved to reduce the number of S-100 (+) dendritic cells by an average of 80% 1 week post-irradiation in humans[7] and soft X-ray therapy has been found to reduce the number of ATPase and Ia-positive cells by approximately 70% 1 week post-irradiation in the mouse system.[8]

TABLE 1 Radiation Methods For Benign Skin Disorders

Therapy	Sources and synonyms	kV	Wavelength (nm) (average)	Half-value layer (aluminum)	Half-value depth (tissue)
Superficial X-ray	Low voltage, standard X-ray, pyrex window	60–100	0.05	0.7–2 mm	7–10 mm
Soft X-ray	Beryllium window	20–100	0.015	0.1–2 mm	1–20 mm
Grenz-ray	Ultrasoft, super-soft, Bucky rays	5–20	0.2	0.03 mm	0.2–0.8 mm

IV. GRENZ-RAY THERAPY OF HAND ECZEMA

Most inflammatory dermatoses have their pathology in the first millimeter of the skin and the rest in the first 3 mm of the skin. Grenz-ray therapy may be expected to be beneficial because 50% of grenz-radiation administered is absorbed by the first 0.5 mm of the skin. This form of radiation is extremely suitable if one considers the sparing effect on hair roots, sebaceous and sweat glands, eyes, and gonads. There have been a few papers published in recent years concerning grenz-ray therapy of hand eczema. In one study, the effect of grenz-ray therapy as an adjunct to topical therapy in chronic symmetrical eczema of the hands was assessed in 24 patients by randomly allocating active treatment to one hand while the other, which received simulated therapy, served as a control — 3 Gy of grenz-rays were applied on 6 occasions at intervals of 1 week. There was a significantly better response to active treatment 5 and 10 weeks after the start of treatment compared with the untreated control.[9] In another study of 30 patients with bilateral symmetrical constitutional hand eczema, resistant to previous treatment, there was no difference in efficacy between grenz-rays and placebo treatment.[10] However, the dosage regimens in these two studies were quite different. In the latter study, only 3 doses of 3 Gy with a 3-week interval were given, in contrast to the former study, where 6 doses of 3 Gy were given with a 1-week interval. This points out the need of different treatment schedules for different X-ray qualities. The schedule using 3 doses with a 3-week interval is commonly used for superficial X-ray therapy, but was apparently not sufficient for the grenz-ray therapy.

Allergic contact dermatitis of the hands is a main indication of grenz-ray therapy owing to the suppressive effect on Langerhans' cells.[3-6] After a grenz-ray course, the allergic contact reaction is suppressed to a minimum for approximately 3 weeks.[6] This period is very important in order to heal the eczema.

A. Radiation Technique

The most common radiation quality used for grenz-rays is 10 kV. The interval between treatments recommended by different authors varies from 1 to 3 weeks. In this author's opinion, an interval of 1 week is suitable, and four to six treatments are usually necessary. The areas of skin vary in their radiosensitivity, which must be taken into account. Palms, soles, and scalp are the least sensitive areas and 4 Gy for each treatment can be administered safely. Scales absorb an important quantity of the dose and must be removed before treatment by using a salicylic acid ointment. The maximum cumulative dose for a certain area of skin should not exceed an arbitrary limit of 100 Gy. In situations where it seems advisable to go beyond this limit, the patient should be monitored closely and the treated area should be examined for malignant transformations for every 100 Gy.

B. Side Effects

Possible side effects of grenz-ray therapy are qualitatively identical to those of conventional X-rays. The principal adverse effects are erythema and pigmentation. Grenz-ray erythema is relatively asymptomatic, and its latent period is shorter than that of conventional X-ray erythema. It is normally not followed by sequelae other than pigmentation.[10] The intensity of this cutaneovascular reaction varies greatly, not only among different individuals but also among different body regions of the same individual.[11] Pigmentation may result from grenz-ray therapy and close shielding should be avoided in order not to produce a sharp line at the edge of the treated area. The induced pigmentation varies with race, age, and body region, but is never permanent.[12] Large doses may occasionally give rise to a peculiar pigment displacement — a spotty hyperpigmentation instead of uniform hyperpigmentation.[10]

The only large-scale study of the carcinogenic effect of grenz-ray therapy[13] did not reveal any increased risk of cancer development in 481 patients who had received at least 100 Gy on the same body area.

The incidence of carcinoma after grenz-ray therapy is small indeed, but may follow extremely high doses in persons who are abnormally sensitive to X-rays.[14]

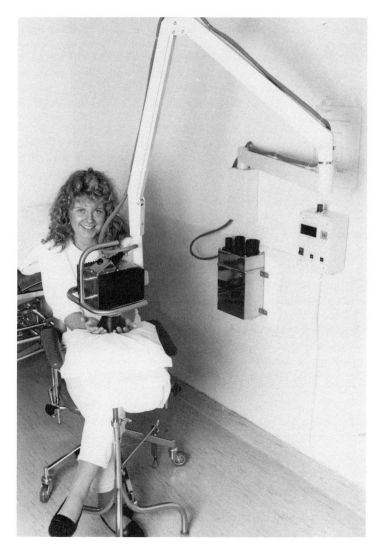

FIGURE 1. A modern grenz-ray unit.

C. Radiation Protection

The exposure to grenz-rays of office personnel handling a grenz-ray unit at 10 kV and a dose rate of 1 Gy/10 s has been investigated for different treatment situations. Scattered and leakage radiation and primary radiation at some distance from the grenz-ray unit were measured. Air absorption was found to be the most important factor. Direct exposure of the operator to the primary grenz-ray beam at a distance of 4 m was practically nil. At a distance of 2 m from the unit, the operator was permitted to be exposed 100 h/year; at a distance of 1 m, the permitted exposure of the direct beam was 3 h/year. Scattered and leakage radiation from the unit was of no importance and certain clothing was demonstrated to promote absorption.[15]

V. SUPERFICIAL X-RAY THERAPY OF HAND ECZEMA

Superficial X-ray therapy is not in common use today as grenz-ray therapy has superseded conventional dermatologic X-ray therapy for benign conditions in most cases, mainly for safety reasons.

However, it is well established that small fractional doses of superficial X-rays have a beneficial effect on the course of eczematous disorders. The efficacy of superficial X-ray therapy has been assessed in the treatment of constitutional eczema of the hands.[16-18] In a double-blind fashion it has been shown that a significantly better therapeutic result was recorded on the hand which received active X-ray therapy (50 kV, 1 mm Al filter, HVL = 0.85 mm Al). The advantage bestowed was optimal 6 to 9 weeks after the start of treatment, but was still present after 18 weeks.

A. Radiation Technique

As in the case of grenz-rays, there are different recommendations by different authors. According to Rowell,[19] 1 Gy of superficial X-rays at 3-week intervals for 3 doses is a suitable treatment schedule; in this way, 3 courses of 3 Gy can be given quite safely in a lifetime. It has been found that a total cumulative dose of 10 Gy per area is quite safe. During the X-ray treatment the patients usually wear a lead apron extending from the knees to the neck.

B. Side Effects

Radiodermatitis may be acute or chronic and results only from overdosage; hence, it can be prevented. The palms and soles are also considered to be the least radio-sensitive areas of the body and, therefore, this side effect should be minimized. In a follow-up study by Rowell[23] it was noted that keratoses and telangiectases on hands were more common in those who had 20 Gy to the hands than in control subjects, but the skin of a particular person may also resist the effect of radiation completely, though high doses have been administered.

X-ray-induced neoplasms have been extensively reported in the literature.[19] Many of them arise as a consequence of the use and misuse of X-rays for a variety of outdated indications, and again, in treating hand eczema, this sequela should be minimized.

REFERENCES

1. Leigh, S., Use of Roentgen rays in inflammatory disease, *Am. J. X-rays,* 4, 559, 1899.
2. Bucky, G., *Grenz Ray Therapy,* Macmillan, New York, 1929.
3. Lindelöf, B., Lidén, S., and Ros, A.-M., Effect of grenz rays on Langerhans' cells in human epidermis, *Acta Derm. Venereol.,* 64, 436, 1984.
4. Lindelöf, B. and Forslind, B., Electron microscopic observation of Langerhans' cells in human epidermis irradiated with grenz rays, *Photodermatology,* 2, 367, 1985.
5. Lindelöf, B., Lidén, S., and Lagerholm, B., The effect of grenz rays on the expression of allergic contact dermatitis in man, *Scand. J. Immunol.,* 21, 463, 1985.
6. Ek, L., Lindelöf, B., and Lidén, S., The duration of grenz ray-induced suppression of allergic contact dermatitis and its correlation to the density of Langerhans' cells in human epidermis, *Clin. Exp. Dermatol.,* 14, 206, 1989.
7. Edwards, E. K., Jr. and Edwards, E. K., Sr., The effect of superficial X-radiation on epidermal Langerhans cells in human skin, *Int. J. Dermatol.,* 29, 731, 1990.
8. Groh, V., Meyer, J., Panizzon, R., and Zortea-Caflisch, C., Soft X-irradiation influences the integrity of Langerhans' cells. A histochemical and immunohistological study, *Dermatologica,* 168, 53, 1984.
9. Lindelöf, B., Wrangsjö, K., and Lidén, S., A double-blind study of Grenz ray therapy in chronic eczema of the hands, *Br. J. Dermatol.,* 117, 77, 1987.
10. Hollander, M. B., Ultrasoft X-rays. An historical and critical review of the world experience with grenz rays and other X-rays of long wave-length, William & Wilkins, Baltimore, MD., 1968.
11. Kalz, F., Observations of grenz ray reactions, *Dermatologica,* 118, 357, 1959.
12. Rowell, N., Adverse effects of superficial X-ray therapy and recommendations for safe use in benign dermatoses, *J. Dermatol. Surg. Oncol.,* 630, 1978.
13. Lindelöf, B. and Eklund, G., Incidence of malignant skin tumors in 14,140 patients after grenz ray treatment for benign skin disorders, *Arch. Dermatol.,* 122, 1391, 1986.

14. Frentz, G., Grenz ray-induced nonmelanoma skin cancer, *J. Am. Acad. Dermatol.*, 21, 475, 1989.

15. Lindelöf, B., Karlberg, J., Lyckefält, S., and Gerhardsson, A., Grenz ray therapy: practical aspects of protecting office personnel from radiation, *Photodermatology*, 5, 248, 1988.

16. Fairris, G. M., Mack, D. P., and Rowell, N. R., Superficial X-ray therapy in the treatment of constitutional eczema of the hands, *Br. J. Dermatol.*, 111, 445, 1984.

17. King, C. M. and Chalmers, R. J. G., A double-blind study of superficial radiotherapy in chronic palmar eczema, *Br. J. Dermatol.*, 111, 451, 1984.

18. Fairris, G. M., Jones, D. H., Mack, D. P., and Rowell, N. R., Conventional superficial X-ray vs. Grenz ray therapy in the treatment of constitutional eczema of the hands, *Br. J. Dermatol.*, 112, 339, 1985.

19. Rowell, N., Adverse effects of superficial X-ray therapy and recommendations for safe use in benign dermatoses, *J. Dermatol. Surg. Oncol.*, 4(8), 630, 1978.

20. Rowell, N., Ionising radiation in benign dermatoses, in *Recent Advances in Dermatology*, Rook, A., Ed., Churchill Livingstone, Edinburgh, 1977, 329.

21. Crossland, P. M., Dermatologic radiation therapy in this nuclear age, *J. Am. Med. Assoc.*, 165, 647, 1957.

22. Sulzberger, M. B., Bear, R. L., and Borota, A., Do roentgen-ray treatments as given by skin specialists produce cancer or other sequelae?, *Arch. Dermatol. Syphilol.*, 65, 639, 1952.

23. Rowell, N. R., A follow-up study of superficial radiotherapy for benign dermatoses: recommendations for the use of X-rays in dermatology, *Br. J. Dermatol.*, 88, 583, 1973.

30

Protective Gloves

Tuula Estlander, Riitta Jolanki, and Lasse Kanerva

CONTENTS

0-8493-7355-7/94/$0.00 + $.50
© 1994 by CRC Press, Inc.

I. INTRODUCTION

The hands are frequently exposed to environmental hazards. Elimination of the numerous hazards would, of course, be the most effective way to prevent their noxious effects, but this is often impracticable. Personal hand protection, the use of gloves in particular, is then necessary in both the work environment and at home or during hobbies.

Protective gloves can be used to protect the hands from chemical, physical, mechanical, and biologic hazards. Especially in work situations where advanced technical solutions are not possible or available, the proper use of gloves is important. It may be the only way to protect the hands against hazards or even modify their effects. For example, many jobs in the manufacturing and service branches often entail the simultaneous exposure of workers' hands to chemical (organic solvents, mineral oils, cutting fluids, synthetic resins and detergents, wet and dirty work) and mechanical (friction, cuts) hazards. Hand protection with gloves may be necessary despite the use of automated processes, because even automation does not protect the hands completely. The hands may come in contact with noxious agents during installation or adjusting, maintenance, repair, or sampling, especially in workplaces where these functions are not well organized.[1,2] Apart from hand protection, the use of gloves may be necessary to protect the product being manufactured from the workers' dirty hands, or to protect patients from the microbes on the hands of the personnel.

II. HAZARDS TO HANDS AND THEIR EFFECTS

A. Chemicals

1. Occupational Dermatoses and Caustic Skin Disorders

Chemical substances constitute most of the hazards to the hands. These substances may have allergenic, irritant, toxic, poisonous, and even carcinogenic effects. Chemicals affect the skin of the hands especially in work environments; accordingly, hand dermatitis is the most common form of occupational dermatosis. Conversely, one-third of all hand eczema patients have occupationally derived eczema.[3,4] Occupational dermatoses constitute a notable proportion (20 to 80% of all occupationally derived diseases.[5-7] About 70 to 80% of the cases are due to primary irritation, one explanation being that at work the exposure to irritants is probably more common than exposure to allergenic chemicals.[8] The rest of the cases are caused by the development of an allergy, mostly delayed or Type IV allergy.[7,9] Some chemical substances, such as strong alkalis and acids, certain organic solvents, metal salts, and gases may accidentally come into contact with the skin and cause chemical burns leading to ulcerations.[10]

2. Percutaneous Absorption of Hazardous Substances

The skin of the hands may also be the route by which poisonous and carcinogenic chemicals enter the body, in amounts sufficient to evoke universal adverse effects. Examples of such chemicals are pesticides, herbicides, aromatic nitro and amino compounds, phenols, hydrocarbons (*m*-xylene, polychlorinated biphenyls), and organic and inorganic cyano compounds.[11-15]

B. Mechanical and Physical Damage

The hands and fingers are injured in a significant number of industrial accidents. Hand injuries caused by mechanical and physical hazards include damage due to friction and pressure, cuts, lacerations, abrasions, burns (either high or low burns), vibration, and radiation. In addition, isomorphic responses and reactions to foreign bodies are injurious.[16,17]

C. Biologic Agents

The skin of the hands is also an important port of entry for many biologic agents, especially if the skin is lacerated or abraded. The list of the biological causes of occupational dermatology is a long one. It includes bacteria, fungi, rickettsiae, chlamydiae, parasites, toxins, and viruses (herpes simplex, hepatitis B virus and the human immunodeficiency virus HIV, orf, milkers' nodules, and cat scratch disease).[18,19]

III. GENERAL ASPECTS OF THE CHOICE AND USE OF GLOVES

A. Analysis of Hazards

All environmental hazards (both work-related and those not related to work)[3,7,20-31] must be identified before appropriate preventive measures can be planned. The choice of protective gloves should be dictated by the actual conditions in each workplace.[32,33] The need for preventive measures should be considered separately for everyone at each worksite. The health risks of maintenance and repair workers and cleaners as well as of workers substituting permanent employees during sick leaves and holidays and of those in rarely repeated tasks should also be taken into account.

B. Chemical, Physical, and Mechanical Resistance of Gloves

The chemical, physical, as well as mechanical protective properties of the gloves must be taken into consideration. These include abrasion resistance, cut and impact resistance, puncture, tear, and tensile strength, cold and heat resistance, resistance to radiant heat and flames, insulation against electricity, resistance to perspiration, and chemicals (water, chemicals, fumes, gases).[34,35]

C. Assessment of the Appropriateness of Gloves

The assessment of the appropriateness of gloves entails consideration of the following factors: whether the material 'breathes' (water penetrability, ability to absorb humidity), whether it is pliable and elastic, whether the size, gripping, and friction qualities (dry and wet) are suitable, and what is the need of tactile sense. In addition, the construction of the gloves, including roughness of seams, reinforcements, supports, and the pattern requires consideration.[34,35] The length of the work shift, temperature during the use of gloves, availability of gloves and their suitability for glove care and the control program are among other important factors affecting the choice of gloves.[32,33] Other aspects include disadvantages connected with the use of gloves: sensitization and irritation caused by gloves, slowing of the work, and hindering the dexterity necessary for the task.[8]

D. Assessment of the User's Individual Characteristics

It is also to be remembered that the technical suitability of gloves alone is not enough, the workers' and patients' individual characteristics should also be kept in mind. The most important factors affecting the choice of gloves are the user's state of sensitization: delayed allergy to rubber or plastic additives and preservatives[36-41] and chromium,[42] and immediate allergy to natural rubber[41,43] or rubber additives,[39,41,44,45] or to glove powder,[41,46,47] the health state of the skin of the hands, and an assessment of perspiration (always dry or sweaty hands). Especially, polymer gloves are primarily designed to protect healthy skin, but they can also be used to protect inflamed skin, though only temporarily. Gloves should not be the only solution to the problem of diseased skin.[8]

IV. TYPES OF GLOVES

A. Classification According to General Construction

Protective handwear can be classified into three main types: five-finger gloves, three-finger gloves, and mittens. Five-finger gloves are used when precise manual dexterity is necessary. Three-finger gloves can be used in jobs where dexterity is less important, e.g., welding and forestry. Mittens are usually used to insulate the skin from heat and cold but they can also be used, e.g., in handling rough materials or sharp-edged metal plates. Gloves may be equipped with short or long gauntlets. In addition, several types of cuffs are available, e.g., spring cuffs, protective cuffs, and long cuffs. Long cuffs may extend up to the upper arm. Cuffs may contain splits to improve donning of the cuff and wrist movement.[8,48]

B. Classification According to Intended Use

Plastic and rubber gloves can be classified according to their intended use:[8,49]

- Disposable gloves (thickness 0.07 to 0.25 mm) — surgical or examination gloves or the like.
- Household gloves (thickness 0.20 to 0.40 mm) — usually unsupported or unlined, or with nappy inside.
- Industrial gloves (thickness 0.36 to 0.85 mm) — usually supported or lined.
- Special industrial gloves — durable surface material, special supports, thick linings.
- Gloves for special purposes (cold, heat) — additional linings or length.

V. GLOVE MATERIALS

A. Rubbers and Plastic (Polymers)

Rubber and plastic gloves are used mostly to protect the hands against water and liquid chemicals.[50-55] Thick household or industrial or special industrial gloves are used in jobs of long duration. They can also be used as disposable gloves in tasks requiring excellent chemical resistance. Disposable gloves made of plastic or rubber materials are generally suitable for short work periods, e.g., in laboratories, in care work (hairdressing, hospitals, dentistry), in the food industry and groceries, and in other branches of industry when sensitizers[31,56] or irritants[30] are handled.

The common materials of rubber gloves are natural rubber (NR), butyl rubber (IIR), nitrile (NBR), chloroprene (Neoprene®, CR), fluororubber (Viton®, FPM) and styrene-butadiene rubber. Plastic gloves are usually made of polyvinylchloride (PVC) and polyethene (PE). Other plastic materials include polyvinylalcohol (PVA), two-layered (ethylene/methacrylate, EMA) and multi-layered materials.[49] Folio-type multilayered materials are especially resistant to organic solvents, epoxy resin compounds, and acrylates, which easily penetrate most of the previously mentioned materials. An example is a Danish laminated glove, in which etene-vinylalcohol-copolymer is laminated by polyethene on both sides (EVOH/EVAL).[55] Protective gloves can also be prepared by mixing plastic and rubber materials, thus creating a combination with the good properties of both types of materials. Glove materials can be manufactured by combining butyl and neoprene rubber (lamination), polyvinylchloride (PVC) and nitrile rubber (mixture) and natural, neoprene, and nitrile rubbers (mixture).[8,49,52]

B. Leather

Leather gloves are suitable for the handling of dry materials. They give protection against irritant solids, dusts, and mechanical damage. They can also be used to insulate the hands from cold and heat. Leather is resistant to wear. Leather gloves are comfortable because the material 'breathes', and is able to absorb humidity. It is soft and pliable even in cold.[8] If better protection is needed, disposable chemical-resistant multilayered plastic gloves can be used as inner gloves.[30]

C. Textiles

Textile gloves can be made of woven fabrics, knits, or terry cloth. Woven fabrics display good friction resistance, whereas knitted fabrics have good cut resistance. The heat-insulating properties of terry cloth gloves can be improved by using various insulating materials, e.g., cotton, fibrous materials, artificial furs, felt cloth, or laminated fabrics. Synthetic materials are more wear resistant than natural fibers. Materials made of natural fibers or viscose are more comfortable to use, however, because they absorb more sweat than synthetic materials. Natural fibers are especially suitable as materials of inner gloves. Textile gloves are also made of natural and synthetic fibers mixed together, thereby combining the good properties of both materials.[8,57] Textile gloves can be partially or totally coated with rubber or plastic materials. Totally coated gloves are suitable for the handling of water and liquid chemicals, depending on the quality of the surface material. Textile gloves impregnated with rubber or plastic materials are water repellent, but not watertight. They can be regarded as the intermediate between leather and textile gloves. They are pliable and cheaper than leather gloves, and they are machine washable.[8] They can be used to protect the product being manufactured (e.g., shiny painted or polished metal objects) from the workers' sweaty hands.

D. Special Materials

Wire cloth made of steel- or nickel-plated brass can be used in the prevention of cuts. Some experiments have also been performed on the suitability of aluminum or titanium mixtures in the manufacture of wire cloth. Asbestos cloth has previously been used as protection against heat. Its use is no longer recommended because of the well-known health risks connected with asbestos.[8,57] Asbestos cloth can be replaced with aramide fibers, e.g., Kevlar® and Nomex®.[58]

VI. CHOICE OF GLOVES FOR PROTECTION AGAINST CHEMICAL HAZARDS

A. General Aspects

Plastic and rubber gloves are generally used to protect the hands from the hazardous effects of chemical substances.[32,33,47,49,50,52] The prevention or minimization of the hazards to the hands requires that the glove material is more or less impermeable to the chemicals to be handled. The following aspects should therefore be taken into account before selecting gloves. No one material is suitable for protection from all possible chemicals. All plastic and rubber materials allow the penetration of chemicals to some extent. There are chemicals against which no gloves give protection for more than an hour.[8,32] Two contradictory statements also need to be weighed in each individual case. It is widely accepted that working with gloves that are permeable to chemicals or impregnated with chemicals may even be more harmful than working without gloves.[31,59,60] In some work tasks, however, the use of any type of gloves is better than no gloves at all.[30,56]

B. Permeability of Gloves

The glove materials distributed by different manufacturers vary greatly in their resistance to chemicals even though the materials have the same-type names, e.g., natural rubber and nitrile rubber.[33,49,61,62] Permeability to chemicals depends on many factors, e.g., on the raw materials and additives used in the manufacture, the type of manufacturing process, and the thickness and uniformity of the structure of the material.[32,49,61] For instance, defective uniformity, including superficial leaks, dimples, and thin spots in the material, facilitates the permeation of chemicals though the glove material. The protective capacity of an individual glove also depends, e.g., on the specific properties and the concentration of the chemicals which have come into contact with the glove materials, as well as the duration of the contact, and the temperature and humidity of the environment.[8,32,33,62] The following special problems should be noted: some chemicals are able to transform the structure or constitution of polymer materials, e.g., to dissolve plasticizers, resulting in hardening, fragility, or swelling of the material.[62-64] Machine washing of the gloves may have a similar effect on the material. Thus, reuse of the gloves may decrease their protection capacity. Additional problems encountered in the handling of chemical mixtures are (1) all the components of a chemical mixture are usually not known when the handling of the mixture begins, (2) the mixture may possibly have more noxious effects than its separate components,[33] (3) some components, e.g., an organic solvent, may penetrate the glove material and thus enhance the penetration of other components,[33,65] and (4) on the other hand some components may even lessen the skin absorption.[54]

The safest way to determine the proper glove type is to perform permeation tests using whole gloves and the chemicals to be handled at work, and then select for use the gloves with the best test results.[33,49,54] In practice, the gloves are selected on the basis of information on materials and their chemical resistance properties found in various guidebooks,[33,48,51,52] data bases,[49,66,67] and manufacturers' chemical resistance charts, and sometimes using only information on the wrappings of the gloves. Guidebooks usually contain lists of the manufacturers and distributors of personal protectors. Detailed advice for selection is obtained from the results of permeability tests contained in these books. The protective capacity of a glove material can be estimated principally by determining the breakthrough times of chemicals, i.e., the time that elapses between initial contact with a certain chemical and the appearance of the chemical on the inside of the material. Less important in the selection is the permeation rate of the chemicals, i.e., the amount of chemical which passes through a certain area of the material in a unit of time.[49,52] Experimental breakthrough times usually express the highest rate at which chemicals permeate through materials. Thus the results are usually reliable for the selection of gloves. Some information is available on the practical application of the results of testing materials for degradation and penetration. Such guides help in deciding whether the materials can be used.[68] Examples of recommendations for use are shown in Tables 1 and 2.

VII. CHOICE OF GLOVES FOR PROTECTION AGAINST MECHANICAL AND PHYSICAL HAZARDS

Gloves are less important in the prevention of serious industrial or other accidents to the hands, but they give good protection against minor hand injuries. Leather and textile gloves offer protection

TABLE 1 Selection of Gloves For Protection against Organic Solvents and Certain Other Chemicals[8,51,53]

Group of chemicals	Recommended glove materials[a]
Aliphatic hydrocarbons	Nitrile rubber (NBR)
	Viton (FPM)
	Polyvinyl alcohol (PVA) cyclohexane excluded
Aromatic hydrocarbons	Polyvinyl alcohol (PVA) ethyl benzene excluded
	Viton (FPM)
	(Nitrile rubber, NBR)
Halogenated hydrocarbons	Polyvinyl alcohol (PVA)
	Viton (FPM) methyl chloride and halothane excluded
Aldehydes, amines, and amides	Butyl rubber (IIR) butylamine and triethylamine excluded
Esters	Butyl rubber (IIR) butyl acrylate excluded
	Polyvinyl alcohol di-*n*-octyl phthalate excluded
Alkalies	Neoprene rubber (CR)
	Nitrile rubber (NBR)
	Polyvinyl alcohol (PVA)
Organic acids	Neoprene rubber (CR) acrylic acid and methacrylic acid excluded
	Butyl rubber (IIR)
	Nitrile rubber (NBR) acrylic acid, metacrylic acid, and acetic acid excluded
Inorganic acids	Neoprene rubber (CR) chromic acid excluded
	Polyvinyl chloride (PVC) hydrofluoric acid, 30–70%, excluded
	Natural rubber (NR) chromic acid, nitric acid 30–70%, sulfuric acid over 70% excluded
	Nitrile rubber (NBR) hydrofluoric acid 30–70%, nitric acid 30–70%, sulfuric acid 30–70% excluded

[a] Laminated plastic materials of folio type or Teflon are suitable for protection against most chemicals.[53]

TABLE 2 Glove Recommendations for Some Branches of Industry/ Occupations[8]

Industry/occupation	Glove recommendation
Services/cleaning work	PVC household gloves
Metal industry, car repair/machine and engine mechanics, maintenance crew	According to the solvents used (Table 1), usually nitrile rubber, PVA or Viton
Manufacture of plastic products (reinforced plastics)	According to the solvents used (Table 1), usually PVA or Viton
Manufacturing/painters, lacquerers	According to the solvents used (Table 1), usually nitrile rubber, PVA or Viton
Graphics industry/printers	According to the solvents used (Table 1), usually butyl rubber, PVA, or nitrile rubber
Manufacturing/plywood and fiberboard workers	Thick industrial PVC gloves
Chemical industry/other occupations	According to the chemicals used (Table 1)
Biologic science, technical work/ laboratory workers	Usually PVC examination gloves, EM laboratory/embedding resins rubber disposable gloves and PE disposable gloves (inner) together, for special tasks according to the chemicals used (Table 1)
Manufacturing/dyeing, manufacture of leather	According to the chemicals used (Table 1), usually neoprene rubber, nitrile rubber, or PVC
Services/hairdressers, barbers	Disposable gloves of PVC or PE (two pairs together)
Manufacturing/concrete mixer operators, concrete product workers	Thick industrial PVC gloves
Social science/handlers of acrylic monomers (dental technicians, orthopedic surgeons, nurses)	Disposable gloves (a minimum of two pairs together
Agriculture, forestry/handling of pesticides	Neoprene® rubber gloves

against abrasions, lacerations, and cuts. They protect from brief exposure to heat and minimize the effect of impacts. Leather gloves also protect the hands from flying hot slugs in welding.

Leather gloves can be reinforced by steel staples or studs to improve their cut resistance. The cut resistance of textile gloves can be improved by plastic or rubber coatings, which also ensure a slip-resistant grip. Special gloves, e.g., metal mesh gloves, have been developed for butchers. Metal mesh gloves are made of welded nickel-plated brass or stainless steel. They are sometimes used in the textile industry.[8]

VIII. PROBLEMS IN GLOVE USAGE AND THEIR PREVENTION

A. Problems Encountered in the Use of Gloves

Each material has its advantages and disadvantages. Although gloves are chosen to give the best possible protection against hazards, their use entails many problems. The most important of these include dirt, development of allergy to glove material and donning powder, irritant dermatitis and maceration of the skin, and getting caught in moving or revolving parts of machinery.[8]

B.   Prevention

If protective gloves are chosen and used without careful forethought, there is a great risk that their effect will be merely a sensation of false security. The following points should be taken into account in the prevention or minimization of the disadvantages encountered in the use of protective gloves:[8]

- A detailed job analysis should be done, and all materials to be handled should be specified before the gloves are selected.
- The use of protective gloves should be started at the same time as the handling of hazardous materials.
- Every worker with long-lasting hand dermatitis should be referred for a dermatological examination including skin testings.
- Only high-quality gloves clearly marked as to the type of material should be worn. The cheapest gloves are not the safest ones.
- The gloves should fit the contours of the hands well and they must not be too small.
- The gloves should be inspected for any imperfections and any disruption of the seams before they are used.
- The seams of gloves must be smooth enough not to irritate the skin by friction or by rubbing chemicals into the skin.
- The cuffs or gauntlets should be long enough to prevent irritant dusts, solids, spillages, or splashes from getting inside the gloves. Otherwise separate sleevelets should be used.
- There should be a specific place at every worksite where gloves can be left without risk of becoming soiled or mechanically damaged.
- Plastic gloves are always preferable to rubber gloves if both materials are otherwise equally suitable.[37,38]
- Persons allergic to rubber should use gloves made of plastic materials or sometimes gloves made of synthetic rubber with separate textile inner gloves. Rubber gloves free of thiram accelerators are available.[41]
- Separate textile gloves should be worn under unlined polymer gloves, especially when there are symptoms of skin irritation or dermatitis of the hands, or the hands sweat profusely. Alternatively, the use of gloves should be restricted to the most irritating jobs and for relatively short periods (up to 30 to 40 min) whenever possible.
- Inner gloves should be made of soft cotton or viscose, or wool.
- Better protection is ensured if at least two pairs of gloves are available for every work shift.
- The thicker the glove material, the better protection it gives. However, the thickness reduces both flexibility and dexterity. One alternative would be simultaneous use of two pairs of thinner, more flexible gloves. Another even better alternative would be the simultaneous use of thin gloves made of different materials (e.g., a disposable pair of polyethene gloves, and another pair of natural rubber to be worn uppermost).
- Gloves, the material of which is hardened or cracked, should be discarded, as should gloves entirely impregnated with chemical substances known to be hazardous to the skin.
- Discarded gloves should be collected into disposable plastic bags so that other workers or family members do not come into contact with hazardous chemicals.

IX.   SUMMARY

The use of protective gloves entails many problems. On the one hand, there is a wide variety of individual differences in skin types among various groups of human beings. The chemicals to be handled and the working methods used in various work places are even more varied. On the other hand, there are great differences in the degree of experience and education between different groups of workers and, consequently, their ability to understand the importance of instructions on safe working methods and the use of personal protective equipment. Therefore preemployment selection is an important and demanding task for the occupational health care personnel and for dermatologists. Appropriate hand protection, however, is essential in the prevention and also in the care of many skin disorders and minor injuries of the hands.

REFERENCES

1. Fregert, S., Possibilities of skin contact in automatic process, *Contact Dermatitis,* 6, 23, 1980.
2. Estlander, T., Jolanki, R., and Kanerva, L., Occupational dermatitis from 2,3-epoxypropyl trimethyl ammonium chloride, *Contact Dermatitis,* 14, 49, 1986.
3. Agrup, G., Hand Eczema and Other Dermatoses in South Sweden, thesis, *Acta Derm. Venereol.,* Suppl. 61, 1969.
4. Goh, G. L. and Soh, S. D., Occupational dermatoses in Singapore, *Contact Dermatitis,* 11, 288, 1984.
5. Fisher, A. A. and Adams, R. M., Occupational dermatitis, in *Contact Dermatitis,* 3rd ed., Fisher, A. A., Ed., Lea & Febiger, Philadelphia, 1986, 486.
6. Mathias, C. G. T. and Morrison, J. H., Occupational skin diseases, United States. Results from the Bureau of Labor Statistics annual survey of occupational injuries and illnesses, 1973 through 1984, *Arch. Dermatol.,* 120, 1202, 1988.
7. Estlander, T., Occupational skin disease in Finland. Observations made during 1974–1988 at the Institute of Occupational Health, Helsinki, thesis, *Acta Derm. Venereol.,* Suppl. 155, 1990.
8. Estlander, T. and Jolanki, R., How to protect the hands, *Dermatol. Clin.,* 6, 105, 1988.
9. Adams, R. M., Allergic contact dermatitis, in *Occupational Skin Disease,* 2nd ed., Adams, R. M., Ed., W. B. Saunders, Philadelphia, 1990, 26.
10. Lammintausta, K. and Maibach, H. I., Contact dermatitis due to irritation, in *Occupational Skin Disease,* 2nd ed., Adams, R. M., Ed., W. B. Saunders, Philadelphia, 1990, 1.
11. Feldman, R. J. and Maibach, H. I., Absorption of some organic compounds through the skin in man, *J. Invest. Dermatol.,* 54, 399, 1970.
12. Feldman, R. J. and Maibach, H. I., Percutaneous penetration of some pesticides and herbicides in man, *Toxicol. Appl. Pharmacol.,* 28, 126, 1974.
13. Lange, M., Nitzshe, K., and Zesch, A., Percutaneous absorption of lindane in healthy volunteers and scabies patients, *Arch. Dermatol. Res.,* 271, 387, 1981.
14. Riihimäki, V., Studies on the Pharmacokinetics of *m*-Xylene in Man, thesis, Helsinki, 1979.
15. Andersen, K. E., Systemic toxicity from percutaneous absorption of industrial chemicals, in *Occupational Skin Disease,* 2nd ed., Adams, R. M., Ed., W. B. Saunders, Philadelphia, 1990, 73.
16. Gellin, G. A., Physical and mechanical causes of occupational dermatoses, in *Occupational and Industrial Dermatology,* Maibach, H. I. and Gellin, G. A., Year Book Medical Publishers, Chicago, 1982, 109.
17. Kanerva, L., Physical causes of occupational skin disease, in *Occupational Skin Disease,* 2nd ed., Adams, R. M., Ed., W. B. Saunders, Philadelphia, 1990, 41.
18. Harwood, R. F. and James, M. T., *Entomology in Human and Animal Health,* 7th ed., Macmillan, New York, 1987, 342.
19. Ancona, A. A., Biologic causes, in *Occupational Skin Disease,* 2nd ed., Adams, R. M., Ed., W. B. Saunders, Philadelphia, 1990, 89.
20. Cronin, E., *Contact Dermatitis,* Churchill Livingstone, New York, 1980.
21. Lammintausta, K., Risk Factors For Hand Dermatitis In Wet Work. Atopy and Contact Sensitivity in Hospital Workers, thesis, Turku, 1982.
22. Björkner, B., Sensitizing Capacity of Ultraviolet Curable Acrylic Compounds, thesis, Lund, Sweden, 1984.
23. Bruze, M., Contact Sensitizers in Resins Based on Phenol and Formaldehyde, thesis, Lund, Sweden, 1985.
24. Fisher, A. A., *Contact Dermatitis,* 3rd ed., Lea & Febiger, Philadelphia, 1986.
25. Hausen, B. M., Allergiepflanzen - Pflanzenallergene: Handbuch und Atlas der allergie-induzierenden Wild- und Kulturpflanzen, ecomed Verlagsgesellschaft mbH, München, 1988.
26. Adams, R. M., *Occupational Skin Disease,* 2nd ed., W. B. Saunders, Philadelphia, 1990.
27. Jolanki, R., Occupational Skin Diseases From Epoxy Compounds. Epoxy Resin Compounds, Epoxy Acrylates and 2,3-Epoxypropyl trimethyl ammonium chloride, thesis, *Acta Derm. Venereol.,* Suppl. 159, 1991.

28. Tarvainen, K., Salonen, J.-P., Kanerva, L., Estlander, T., Keskinen, H., and Rantanen, T., Allergy and toxicodermia from shiitake mushrooms, *J. Am. Acad. Dermatol.*, 24, 64, 1991.

29. Tarvainen, K., Kanerva, L., Tupasela, O., Grenquist-Norden, B., Jolanki, R., and Estlander, T., Allergy from cellulase and xylanase enzymes, *Clin. Exp. All.*, 21, 609, 1991.

30. Tarvainen, K., Jolanki, R., and Forsman-Grönhom, L., Reinforced plastics industry: exposure, skin disease and skin protection, in *Proc. 4th Scand. Symp. Protective Clothing Against Chemicals and Other Hazards* Mäkinen, H., Ed., (NOKOBETEF IV), Finland, 1992, 147.

31. Estlander, T., Jolanki, R., and Kanerva, L., Occupational dermatitis from exposure to polyurethane chemicals, *Contact Dermatitis*, 27, 161, 1992.

32. Mansdorf, Z. S., Risk assessment of chemical exposure hazards in the use of chemical protective clothing — an overview, in Performance of Protective Clothing, ASTM STP 900, Barker, R. L. and Coletta, G. C., Eds., American Society for Testing and Materials, Ann Arbor, MI, 1986.

33. Roder, M. M., A guide for evaluation the performance of chemical protective clothing (CPC). U.S. Department of Health and Human Services, National Institute for Safety and Health, Division of Safety Research, Morgantown, WV, June 1990.

34. Dionne, E. D., How to select proper hand protection, *Natl. Saf. News*, 19, 44, 1979.

35. Berardinelli, S. P., Prevention of occupational skin disease through use of chemical protective gloves, *Dermatol. Clin.*, 6, 115, 1988.

36. Lammintausta, K. and Kalimo, K., Sensitivity to rubber. A study with rubber mixes and individual rubber chemicals, *Dermatosen*, 33, 204, 1985.

37. Estlander, T., Jolanki, R., and Kanerva, L., Dermatitis and urticaria from rubber and plastic gloves, *Contact Dermatitis*, 14, 20, 1986.

38. Frosch, P. J., Born, C. M., and Schutz, R., Kontaktallergien auf Gummi-, Operations- und Vinylhandschuhe, *Hautarzt*, 38, 210, 1987.

39. Turjanmaa, K. and Reunala, T., Latex-contact urticaria associated with delayed allergy to rubber chemicals, in *Current Topics in Contact Dermatitis*, Frosch, P. J., Dooms-Goossens, A., Lachapelle, J.-M., Rycroft, R. J. G., and Scheper, R. J., Eds., Springer-Verlag, Berlin, 1989, 460.

40. Maso, M. J. and Goldberg, D. J., Contact dermatoses from disposable glove use: a review, *J. Am. Acad. Dermatol.*, 23, 733, 1990.

41. Heese, A., von Hintzenstern, J., Peters, K.-P., Koch, H. U., and Hornstein, O. P., Allergic and irritant reactions to rubber gloves in medical health services, *J. Am. Acad. Dermatol.*, 25, 831, 1991.

42. Fregert, S. and Gruvberger, B., Chromium in industrial leather gloves, *Contact Dermatitis*, 5, 189, 1979.

43. Turjanmaa, K., Latex Glove Contact Urticaria, thesis, University of Tampere, 1988.

44. Helander, I. and Mäkilä, A., Contact urticaria to zinc diethyldithiocarbamate (ZDC), *Contact Dermatitis*, 9, 326, 1983.

45. Geier, J. and Fuchs, Th., Kontakturtikaria durch Gummihandschuhe, *Z. Hautkr.*, 335, 912, 1990.

46. van der Meeren, H. L. M. and van Erp, P. E. J., Life-threatening urticaria from glove powder, *Contact Dermatitis*, 14, 190, 1986.

47. Fisher, A. A., Contact urticaria due to cornstarch surgical glove powder, *Cutis*, 38, 307, 1986.

48. Mellström, G., Protective gloves and barrier creams. 1983: 28. Part I: a survey of documentation concerning protective effects and side-effects of plastic and rubber protective gloves and barrier creams (in Swedish: 15.1983.29). Part II: market survey — plastic and rubber gloves — barrier creams (in Swedish; 16.1983:30). Part III: compilation of test results to be used as guidance when choosing plastic and rubber protective gloves. National Board of Occupational Safety and Health, Occupational Dermatology Unit, Research Department, Solna, Sweden, Investigation reports, 1983, (in Swedish).

49. Mellström, G., Protective Gloves of Polymeric Materials. Experimental Permeation Testing and Clinical Study of Side Effects, thesis, Arbetsmiljöinstitutet, Arbete och Hälsa, 1991, 10.

50. Figard, W. H., Intensifying the efforts of proper glove selection, *Occup. Health Saf.*, 7, 30, 1980.

51. Forsberg, K. and Olsson, K., Guidelines for the Selection of Chemical Protective Gloves (in Swedish), Föreningen Teknisk Företagshälsovård, FTF, Stockholm, 1985.

52. Schwope, A. D., Costas, P. P., Jackson, J. O., Stull, J. O., and Weitzman, D. J., Guidelines for the Selection of Chemical Protective Clothing, 3rd ed., Vol. II and III, Am. Conf. Gov. Ind. Hyg. Inc., Cincinnati, Ohio.

53. Anon., Arbetsmiljöfonden, Informations Producenterna Gbg, Select proper chemical protective gloves, 2nd rev. ed., Stockholm, 1987 (in Swedish).

54. Boman, A., Factors Influencing the Percutaneous Absorption of Organic Solvents. An Experimental Study in the Guinea Pig, thesis, Arbetsmiljöinsitutet, Arbete och Hälsa, 1989, 11.

55. Anon., Chemical Protection List, 4 H, Safety 4 A/S Lyngby, Denmark, 1992, 1.

56. Jolanki, R., Kanerva, L., Estlander, T., Tarvainen, K., Keskinen, H., and Henriks-Eckerman, M.-L., Occupational dermatoses from epoxy resin compounds, *Contact Dermatitis*, 23, 172, 1990.

57. Hobbs, N. E., Oakland, B. G., and Hurwiz, M. D., Effects of barrier finishes on aerosol spray penetration and comfort of woven and disposable nonwoven fabrics for protective clothing, in Performance of Protective Clothing, ASTM STP 900, Barker, R. L. and Coletta, G. C., Eds., American Society for Testing Materials, Ann Arbor, MI, 1986.

58. Dixit, B., Development and testing of asbestos substitutes, in Performance of Protective Clothing, ASTM STP 900, Barker, R. L. and Coletta, G. C., Eds., American Society for Testing and Materials, Ann Arbor, MI, 1986.

59. Wester, R. C. and Maibach, H. I., Percutaneous absorption relative to occupational dermatology, in *Occupational and Industrial Dermatology*, Maibach, H. I. and Gellin, G. A., Eds., Year Book Medical Publishers, Chicago, 1982, 201.

60. Jolanki, R., Estlander, T., and Kanerva, L., Contact allergy to an epoxy reactive diluent: 1,4-butanediol diglycidyl ether, *Contact Dermatitis*, 16, 87, 1987.

61. Sansone, E. B. and Tewari, Y. B., Differences in the extent of solvent penetration through natural rubber and nitrile gloves from various manufacturers, *Am. Ind. Assoc. J.*, 41, 527, 1980.

62. Mellström, G., Lindberg, M., and Boman, A., Permeation and destructive effect of disinfectants on protective gloves, *Contact Dermatitis*, 26, 163, 1992.

63. Williams, J. R., Permeation of glove materials by physiologically harmful chemicals, *Am. Ind. Hyg. Assoc. J.*, 40, 877, 1979.

64. Williams, J. R., Evaluation of intact gloves and boots for chemical permeation, *Am. Ind. Hyg. Assoc. J.*, 42, 468, 1981.

65. Linnarson, A., Permeation of solvents through plastic materials studied by mass spectrometry, *Adv. Mass Spectrom. Biochem. Med.*, 8, 1959, 1980.

66. Goydan, R., Schwope, A. D., Loyd, S. H., and Huhn, L. M., CPCbase, a chemical protective-clothing data base for personal computer, in Performance of Protective Clothing: 2nd Symp., ASTM STP 989, Mansdorf, S. Z., Sager, R., and Nielsen, A. P., Eds., American Society for Testing and Materials, Philadelphia, 1988, 403.

67. Mellström, G., Lindahl, G., and Wahlberg, J., DAISY: reference database on protective gloves, *Semin. Dermatol.*, 8, 75, 1989.

68. Leinster, P., Bonsall, J. L., Evans, M. J., and Lewis, S. J., The application of test data in the selection and use of gloves against chemicals, *Ann. Occup. Hyg.*, 34, 85, 1990.

31

The Role of Corticosteroid Allergy in Hand Eczema

Antti I. Lauerma and Howard I. Maibach

CONTENTS

0-8493-7355-7/94/$0.00 + $.50
© 1994 by CRC Press, Inc.

I. INTRODUCTION

Awareness of contact sensitization to topical corticosteroids has improved markedly during recent years[1] and there is also evidence that the true prevalence of this condition has increased.[2,3] Eczema patients are prone to develop contact allergy to topical medicaments, including corticosteroids, used in treatment of the disease. Hand eczema patients are not an exception, because hand eczema patients use corticosteroids as a major form of treatment, raising the susceptibility of sensitization to them. There is also a considerable number of hand eczema patients reported as having contact allergy to corticosteroids.

II. CONTACT ALLERGY TO CORTICOSTEROIDS

A. Prevalence

Corticosteroid allergy is not rare. As testing methods become more accurate and sensitive, remarkable prevalences have been found. In a recent study 10.7% of the patients undergoing the standard series had corticosteroid allergy.[4] From Belgium a recent figure was 2.9%[5] and from Finland 4.1%[2]. Note, however, that these figures are from patients undergoing a standard patch series, and the true prevalence in dermatologic patients and population in general should be much smaller.

B. Cross-Reactions

Cross-reactions between corticosteroids in corticoid allergy have been reported. Such reactions are important, because they may enable use of only some corticosteroids as screening markers for detection of allergy to a larger number of different corticosteroids. An attempt to determine the cross-reaction pattern was performed by Coopman and colleagues, who in a literature review suggested that corticosteroids may be classified into four groups according to differences in the D-ring of the corticosteroid skeleton or the side chains in carbons 17 and/or 21 (see Figure 1 for corticosteroid structure).[6] The classes were hydrocortisone type, triamcinolone acetonide type, dexamethasone type, and hydrocortisone-17-butyrate type. However, cross-reactions have been reported frequently between corticosteroids of the hydrocortisone and hydrocortisone-17-butyrate classes.[2,7,8] Moreover, a study by Wilkinson and English revealed that in intradermal tests in hydrocortisone allergy the antigenic determinant seemed to be in rings A to C, rather than in ring D of the steroid skeleton.[9] A further study by Dooms-Goossens et al. suggested that the hydroxyl group in carbon 11 could also be important.[10] Classification of cross-reaction patterns in corticosteroid contact allergy needs more prospective research before it can be conclusively determined.

One cross-reaction pattern between two corticosteroids has been well documented: hydrocortisone and tixocortol pivalate. Intradermal testing with hydrocortisone sodium phosphate showed that allergic patch test reactions to tixocortol pivalate in most patients are caused by contact allergy to hydrocortisone.[11] Patch testing with hydrocortisone is problematic, presumably because of inadequate penetration, and therefore tixocortol pivalate may be used as a patch test preparation to detect hydrocortisone contact allergy.

C. Diagnostic Procedures

Testing for corticosteroid contact allergy is usually done with patch testing. Some screening markers for detection of corticoid allergy in the standard series have been suggested: hydrocortisone-17-

TABLE 1 Proportions of Hand Eczema Patients among Corticosteroid-Allergic Patients from Different Countries

Patients with corticosteroid allergy	Patients with hand eczema	Country	Ref.
80	17	Finland	2,7,8
80	23	Belgium	5,12
11	4	England	4

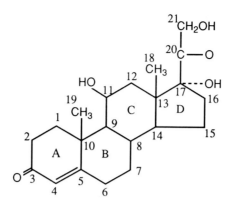

FIGURE 1. The chemical structure of hydrocortisone.
(From Lauerma, A. I. and Reitamo, S.,
J. Am. Acad. Dermatol., 28, 618, 1993.
With permission.)

butyrate,[8] budesonide,[5] and tixocortol pivalate.[12] The latter detects hydrocortisone contact allergy because of a cross-reaction.[11] Hydrocortisone-17-valerate has, in our experience, also been a useful marker. Of these compounds, tixocortol pivalate (as Pivalone Nasal Spray, Jouveinail Laboratoires, France) diluted 1/10 in ethanol is superior to 1% hydrocortisone-17-butyrate (Gist-Brocades, The Netherlands) in ethanol as a screening marker.[2]

For further detection of specific contact allergies to different corticosteroids, a corticosteroid patch test series is recommended. In such series the corticosteroids most commonly used in a particular country should be incorporated. To avoid false-negative reactions due to insufficient penetration, an ethanol vehicle is recommended instead of petrolatum,[7] although some problems due to degradation during storage may be involved.[13] We have successfully utilized therapeutic concentrations, i.e., those in commercial preparations, and tenfold concentrations of them.[2,7,8] However, saturation in ethanol limits the concentration of hydrocortisone to 2.5%. Controls with ethanol and petrolatum vehicles should be performed.

If pure compounds are not available, commercial preparations have to be used. These have the theoretic advantage of optimized penetration of the active compound (corticoid), which increases the sensitivity of the patch test. However, after a positive result the other ingredients in the preparation have to be separately tested, with negative results, to have conclusive evidence of corticosteroid allergy.

Intradermal testing has been introduced to corticosteroid contact allergy diagnostics.[9,11] It seems to be a more sensitive method than patch testing.[4] In intradermal testing, 1 mg of the corticosteroid allergen is introduced in a parenteral preparation to the skin. Reading is done at 48 h and an indurated erythema of at least 0.5 cm in diameter should be considered positive.[4] To avoid anaphylactoid reactions, prick tests with the same preparations may precede the intradermal tests.

III. CORTICOSTEROID ALLERGY IN HAND ECZEMA

It seems that many hand eczema patients are sensitized to corticosteroids, because in recent studies which included screening in standard patch test series, up to 40% of corticosteroid allergy patients were reported as having hand eczema.[2,4,5,7,8,12] A summary of the results is in Table 1.

Few studies reveal information about the frequency of corticosteroid allergy in hand eczema patients (Table 2). In a study by Dooms-Goossens and Morren, 2.2% of hand eczema patients had corticosteroid allergy when tested with a large battery of corticosteroid patch tests; in this study the overall prevalence of corticosteroid allergy was 2.9%.[5] In another study by Wilkinson et al., where intradermal tests also were employed, 9% of hand eczema patients had allergic reactions to corticosteroids while the overall prevalence was 10.7%.[4]

While the studies by Dooms-Goossens and Morren[5] and Wilkinson et al.[4] are the only ones providing some information on the frequency of corticosteroid allergy in hand eczema patients,

TABLE 2   Prevalence of Corticosteroid
Contact Allergy among Hand
Eczema Patients

Hand eczema patients	Corticosteroid-allergic patients	Ref.
871	19	5
44	4	4

their figures are probably high because these patients were already suspected of having contact allergy. Unfortunately, there are no truly prospective studies available about the prevalence of corticosteroid allergy in hand eczema patients.

IV. CONCLUSIONS

Because hand eczema is a chronic and disabling disease, any factors that may worsen it must be considered. As the main therapeutic agents used in hand eczema are topical corticosteroids, contact allergy to them is a factor which may remarkably contribute in keeping the hand eczema chronic. As more corticosteroids are usually applied when the eczema worsens, a vicious cycle may result.

To avoid problems due to corticosteroid allergy, it is strongly recommended that screening patch tests with tixocortol pivalate, budesonide, hydrocortisone-17-butyrate, and/or hydrocortisone-17-valerate be performed. Considering the chronic character of hand eczema, it is also wise to routinely test the topical preparations, including corticosteroids, that the patient is using to be certain of the beneficial effect of the therapy.

REFERENCES

1. Dooms-Goossens, A., Contact dermatitis to topical corticosteroids: diagnostic problems, in *Exogenous Dermatoses: Environmental Dermatitis,* Menne, T. and Maibach, H. I., Eds., CRC Press, Boca Raton, FL, 1991, 299.
2. Lauerma, A. I., Screening for corticosteroid contact hypersensitivity. Comparison of tixocortol pivalate, hydrocortisone-17-butyrate and hydrocortisone, *Contact Dermatitis,* 24, 123, 1991.
3. Lauerma, A. I., Förström, L., and Reitamo, S., Incidence of allergic reactions to hydrocortisone-17-butyrate in standard patch test series, *Arch. Dermatol.,* 128, 275, 1992.
4. Wilkinson, S. M., Heagerty, A. H. M., and English, J. S. C., A prospective study into the value of patch and intradermal tests in identifying topical corticosteroid allergy, *Br. J. Dermatol.,* 127, 22, 1992.
5. Dooms-Goossens, A. and Morren, M., Results of routine patch testing with corticosteroid series in 2073 patients, *Contact Dermatitis,* 26, 182, 1992.
6. Coopman, S., Degreef, H., and Dooms-Goossens, A., Identification of cross-reaction patterns in allergic contact dermatitis from topical corticosteroids, *Br. J. Dermatol.,* 121, 27, 1989.
7. Reitamo, S., Lauerma, A. I., Stubb, S., Käyhkö, K., Visa, K., and Förström, L., Delayed hypersensitivity to topical corticosteroids, *J. Am. Acad. Dermatol.,* 14, 582, 1986.
8. Reitamo, S., Lauerma, A. I., and Förström, L., Detection of contact hypersensitivity to topical corticosteroids with hydrocortisone-17-butyrate, *Contact Dermatitis,* 21, 159, 1989.
9. Wilkinson, S. M. and English, J. S. C., Hydrocortisone sensitivity: an investigation into the nature of the allergen, *Contact Dermatitis,* 25, 178, 1991.
10. Schoenmakers, A., Vermorken, A., Degreef, H., and Dooms-Goossens, A., Corticosteroid or steroid allergy?, *Contact Dermatitis,* 26, 159, 1992.
11. Wilkinson, S. M., Cartwright, P. H., and English, J. S. C., Hydrocortisone: an important cutaneous allergen, *Lancet,* 337, 761, 1991.

12. Dooms-Goossens, A. E., Degreef, H. J., Marien, K. J. C., and Coopman, S. A., Contact allergy to corticosteroids: a frequently missed diagnosis?, *J. Am. Acad. Dermatol.*, 21, 538, 1989.
13. Förström, L., Lassus, A., Salde, L., and Niemi, K. M., Allergic contact eczema from topical corticosteroids, *Contact Dermatitis*, 8, 128, 1982.

INDEX